JAN   2009

"A serious handbook for healthy aging."

—Cheryl Melton, MS, RD
Editor, *Relish* magazine

Prevention

Positively Ageless

A 28-Day Plan for a Younger, Slimmer, Sexier You

Cheryl Forberg, RD
Nutritionist for NBC's *The Biggest Loser*

Foreword by **Bradley J. Willcox, MD, MSc**
Coauthor, *The Okinawa Program* and
The Okinawa Diet Plan

RODALE

Direct edition published as *Prevention's You Only Younger* in 2007.

Rodale books may be purchased for business or promotional use or for special sales. For information, please write to:

Special Markets Department, Rodale, Inc., 733 Third Avenue, New York, NY 10017

Prevention is a registered trademark of Rodale Inc.

Printed in the United States of America

Rodale Inc. makes every effort to use acid-free ∞, recycled paper ♻.

Book design by Carol Angstadt

Library of Congress Cataloging-in-Publication Data

Forberg, Cheryl.
    Prevention positively ageless : a 28-day plan for a younger, slimmer, sexier you / Cheryl Forberg ; foreword by Bradley J. Wilcox.
      p.   cm.
    Includes bibliographical references and index.
    ISBN-13 978–1–59486–616–6 paperback
    ISBN-10 1–59486–616–3 paperback
    1. Longevity. I. Title.
RA776.75.F6715 2008
613.2—dc22
                                           2008006799

2 4 6 8 10 9 7 5 3 1 paperback

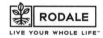

RODALE
LIVE YOUR WHOLE LIFE™

We inspire and enable people to improve their lives and the world around them

For more of our products visit **rodalestore.com** or call 800-848-4735

*For my stepfather, Bill Treible, who believed
that I could do anything I tried. Bill was deeply interested
in everything I said and did. He championed my every
undertaking as though I were his own daughter.
He encouraged my fascination with and interest
in antiaging nutrition. He cheered when I subsequently
launched my career as an author. And he celebrated
when I began to write this book,
which I now dedicate to him.*

CONTENTS

Acknowledgments..vii

Foreword..xi

Preface...xiii

Introduction 1

WEEK ONE: KEEP YOUR VITAL FUNCTIONS STRONG

    chapter 1: **A Healthy Heart for Life** **37**

    chapter 2: **Preventing Common Cancers with Dietary Changes**. **54**

    chapter 3: **Digestion: Keep Things Moving Properly**...............................**72**

    chapter 4: **The Immune System: Stay Safe from Invaders (and Yourself!)** **84**

    chapter 5: **Fight Fatigue for a High-Energy Life**...................................**97**

    chapter 6: **The *Positively Ageless* Program for Age-Proofing Your
                  Vital Functions** **106**

    chapter 7: **Eat Smart, Live Long Menus** **116**

WEEK TWO: AGE-PROOF YOUR HORMONES AND YOUR MIND

    chapter 8: **Diabetes: A Condition with Many Age-Robbing Consequences** **127**

    chapter 9: **Menopause: Navigating "The Change" with Health
                  and Happiness** **142**

    chapter 10: **Stress: Let Off Steam to Protect Your Health** **151**

    chapter 11: **Stay Safe from Stroke Damage**...**157**

    chapter 12: **Alzheimer's: Enjoy a Fit Mind and Body in Your Boomer Years
                  and Beyond**..**164**

    chapter 13: **Eat Smart, Live Long Menus**..**174**

WEEK THREE: MUSCLES AND BONES: STRONG IS SEXY

    chapter 14: **Strong Bones Support a Healthy Body**................................**185**

    chapter 15: **Maintaining Muscle: Much More Than an Exercise in Vanity** **195**

    chapter 16: **Eat Smart, Live Long Menus** **208**

WEEK FOUR: YOUR OUTSIDE PARTS

chapter 17: **Protect the Skin You're In** 219

chapter 18: **Hair: There's Plenty You Can Do to Protect Your Mane** 231

chapter 19: **Bite into Good Health** 234

chapter 20: **Keep Your Eyes on the Prize** 238

chapter 21: **Eat Smart, Live Long Menus** 246

POSITIVELY AGELESS RECIPES

Breakfast 258

Beverages 268

Condiments 279

Snacks 290

Soups and Stews 296

Grains 304

Salads 310

Entrées 318

Vegetables and Legumes 330

Desserts 336

On the Web 349

Shopping Resources 351

Sources 355

Index 368

ACKNOWLEDGMENTS

This book would not have been possible without the generous support of a lengthy list of academics, clinicians, and researchers, many of whom I have the honor of calling my friends.

The outstanding scientists I met through the American Aging Association (founded by Dr. Denham Harman) facilitated my initial research. What the libraries could not offer was readily provided by experts such as Donald Ingram of the National Institute on Aging at the National Institutes of Health; Dr. Eric Ravussin, chief, division of health and performance enhancement at the Pennington Biomedical Research Center in Baton Rouge, Louisiana; Dr. Bill Evans of the Nutrition, Metabolism, and Exercise Laboratory at the University of Arkansas; Dr. Ronald Prior of the USDA at the Arkansas Children's Nutrition Center; and many others. Special thanks to Donna Cini, who made it possible to meet most of the experts.

Many thanks to Dr. Nicholas Perricone for his inspiration and guidance and to Anne Sellaro for her ongoing support and encouragement.

I am so appreciative of my friend and colleague Susan Bowerman, MS, RD, of the UCLA Center for Human Nutrition, who continually opened doors and exchanged ideas with me. She enlightened me to studies I would not have known about otherwise and patiently read sections of the manuscript, discussed many ideas in great detail, and added much value to the final product. Susan, I am indebted for your support and treasure your friendship.

Marie Chrabaszewski, RD, of the Encino Medical Group, provided considerable assistance and support as she generously reviewed the final sections and provided valuable feedback. Thanks for your wisdom, for your humor, and for being so incredibly reliable—you are truly a cherished friend.

Robin Kline, MS, RD, keeps me tethered across the miles with culinary wisdom, scientific curiosity, spiritual guidance, over-the-top generosity, and heartwarming good cheer. I am so blessed to know you!

I am forever indebted to my friends and family who patiently (and diplomatically) tested and tasted my recipes, especially Patricia Treible; Paul Skittone; John and Bette Forberg; Claudia and Rob Hampton; Paul Franson; Karen and Steve Price; David and Erica Ettinger; Paula, John, Jack, and Beau Beritzhoff; Betty Teller; Pam Elder; Leigh Corshen; Julie Logue-Riordan; Carolyn Harber and Bob Fiorella; John Pugh; Gloria Marth; Jill Hunting; Annie Baker; and Brooke Austin. And a special thanks to my friend Bill Frazier, of Frazier Winery in Napa, for the delicious infusions of antioxidant-rich red wine, which made our tastings even more enjoyable.

Diana Erney, senior research librarian of the impressive Rodale Library, provided me with rare published material I did not think was still available. She also shared additional studies that I may never have found nor read. Thank you, Diana, for your valuable input.

Eric Metcalf translated volumes of technical research into entertaining prose. He patiently kept me on the right track and helped me to condense and substantially rethink my ideas concerning this book and this incredibly fascinating topic. Thank you, my friend!

I am thankful to the members of the Food & Culinary Professionals Dietary Practice Group of the American Dietetic Association, the International Association of Culinary Professionals, Les Dames d'Escoffier, and the Association of Food Journalists for their knowledge, support, and camaraderie that continually inspire and motivate me.

I am grateful to Chad Bennett and Mark Koops of Reveille LLC, first for selecting me as the nutritionist for NBC's *The Biggest Loser* fitness reality show. Once I had begun to write this book, they subsequently derailed me with another exciting book project (*The Biggest Loser Complete Calorie Counter*), which ultimately gave me the research expertise I needed to understand one of the many facets of this project. I am indebted for your support and for your belief in me and in my work.

Thank you to Dr. Alexa Altman, Dr. Michael Dansinger, Dr. Rob Huizenga, Lisa, Tiare, Jennifer, Terry, Juliana, Elayne, Allison, and Kat, as well as all of the contestants on *The Biggest Loser 3*. I wish I could list each of you by name. You were with me in spirit as I wrote this—especially the recipes. I cannot thank you enough for letting me be a part of your transformation and life's journey. You have each inspired me personally and for that, you have inspired this book.

Amy Super of Rodale, you have been a joy to work with and a wellspring of encouragement. My unending thanks to you for the invitation to meet at Grand Central Station that fateful afternoon. Who knew that a cup of tea and a fruit plate could lead to this?

I must acknowledge those people whose influence extends well beyond this project. Barbara Sutherland, PhD, of the University of California, Davis, has been my mentor and friend since I first attended one of her classes at UC Berkeley. Since then, she has been a perpetual source of support, encouragement, advice, and laughter, which aided my studies, my career, and my life. Thank you, Barbara!

Dr. Bradley Willcox has inspired me (and many others) over the years with his unprecedented research in the Okinawa Centenarian Study. I am indebted for your insights, for your wisdom, and for illuminating this path for me.

My most profound thanks to scientists around the world who devote their work and their lives to the study of diet and disease to afford better health for us all.

Aging is inevitable. We cannot stop or reverse it, but numerous studies have suggested that *we do have enormous control over the rate at which we age.* My research work, funded by the US National Institute on Aging and the Japan Ministry of Health and Welfare, has focused on healthy aging. In other words, my research attempts to understand why some of us end up living to exceptional ages in good health, like many centenarians who live into the mid to late nineties in vibrant health, and why others don't make it much past their sixties. My work has mainly been with the centenarian population of Okinawa, as co-principal investigator of the Okinawa Centenarian Study, and more recently with long-lived people in Hawaii, as principal investigator of the Hawaii Lifespan Study, a 40-year study of healthy aging in men. Both studies show that lifestyle plays a key role in healthy aging. There is no disputing that genetics is important for healthy aging, but after several decades of research by our team, it is clear that how we live our lives accounts for the greater part of the human life span.

It is easy when one is younger not to be concerned with aging because many of us have feelings of immortality, and most of us do not wish to live to an age where we feel "old and decrepit." But we should be concerned. Our research has shown that centenarians achieve such long and healthy lives precisely because they aged more slowly *from a young age.* In other words, aging is a lifelong process. The early start in healthy aging for centenarians appears to have decreased their risk for many age-associated diseases and has resulted in the delay or, in some cases, complete absence of age-associated diseases, such as coronary heart disease, stroke, cancer, and Alzheimer's disease. On the other hand, our 40-year Hawaii Lifespan Study, among the largest and longest studies of aging men ever conducted, shows that midlife risk factors, including diet and physical activity, are extremely important for late-life health. So it really is never too late.

It is remarkable that, as a percentage of the population, more people in Okinawa achieve centenarian status than anywhere else. But more remarkable is the quality of their lives. This continues to inspire me and our research team's work. Okinawans not only survive longer and delay or avoid many chronic diseases but have fun doing so. They have survived and thrived despite hardships of war, deprivation, and other stressors in younger years. Their diets and indeed their lives are akin to "Japanese with salsa." Their food and, indeed, the Okinawans themselves tend to be livelier, spicier, and more vibrant than other Japanese. And really, that's what it's all about, isn't it? Life is meant to be enjoyed, and good food is among our greatest pleasures.

This is why dietitian extraordinaire Cheryl Forberg's new book—*Positively Ageless*—is so timely and important. Cheryl has always striven to bring her readers and clients wonderful food with strong health benefits, but she has outdone herself here. In her new book, Cheryl brings us a highly readable and engaging eating and exercise program that teaches the reader, over 4 weeks, important lessons in healthy aging. This delightful and engaging book will introduce you to some remarkably healthy foods that just happen to have the added benefit of great taste and satisfaction for your palate. Indeed, if you follow her advice closely enough, perhaps you will be joining the ranks of healthy centenarians yourself one day! In any event, *Positively Ageless* should put you firmly on the path to a healthier and more vibrant life—and let you enjoy the journey. *Bon appétit!*

Bradley J. Willcox, MD, MSc
Co-principal investigator, Okinawa Centenarian Study
Coauthor, *The Okinawa Program* and *The Okinawa Diet Plan*

By the early 1990s, I knew a lot about food . . . or at least I *thought* I did.

I was a graduate of the California Culinary Academy and had continued my studies in several of the top restaurants in France. Upon returning to America, I earned a slot among the first team of chefs in Wolfgang Puck's first restaurant in San Francisco.

I knew how to whip up creamy sauces and rich, tantalizing desserts. I could prepare an exquisite entrée and arrange it on the plate like a tiny, edible work of art. I could perfect one creation after another for the most demanding customers during the most fast-paced dinner-hour rush.

However, I realized that talent in an award-winning kitchen didn't necessarily translate into a comfortable savings account, so I started moonlighting as a chef for private clients.

And I quickly learned that though I could make food that was pleasing to the palate, I didn't know so much about making food that was good for the *body*. Many of my clients had particular dietary needs—they were following the low-fat Pritikin diet, or they had heart conditions that necessitated low-sodium or low-cholesterol eating. My training hadn't prepared me for these challenges.

During all that time I spent learning how to prepare cuisine in some of the finest establishments on two continents, we never focused on how to make *healthy* food. So I started buying books on different diet plans and teaching myself the basic principles of nutrition. Then I'd tweak these healthy recipes to add color and flavor without compromising nutritional value.

The more I learned, the more I discovered that I didn't know *any* chefs who were well versed in healthy cooking. Nor did I see many dietitians who knew much about cooking! Here were two professions that knew so much about different aspects of food, but at the time, there were very few people who could serve as a bridge between these two fields.

Eventually, I stopped working at restaurants and began working full-time as a personal chef for well-heeled clients who wanted their meals to taste great yet support their health. And I decided that studying on my own was merely scratching the surface of the fascinating world of nutrition. So I went back to college, taking nutrition classes during the day and cooking dinner for my celebrity clients in the evenings.

My last job as a private chef was to cook for a famous movie director and his family in northern California for 3 years. After he put the finishing touches on the screenplay for his latest lasers-and-spaceships blockbuster, he flew off to an exotic locale to begin filming it. I headed off to my remaining chemistry classes at Berkeley and finally earned my nutrition degree and RD certification at the age of . . . let's say 40-something!

I moved to Los Angeles and took a job as a clinical researcher at Cedars-Sinai Medical Center, where I worked with menopausal women who had breast cancer. I taught them how they could alter recipes to make them more nutritious, and in exchange I learned more about how food choices affect the aging process.

Through a series of happy developments, I wound up writing the first antiaging cookbook—*Stop the Clock! Cooking*. Although it focused primarily on recipes, I learned a lot while I was developing it about how the unseen nutrients in our foods play a crucial role in the invisible processes that cause our bodies to either break down or keep working properly as we get older.

I've since had the good fortune to work for several seasons as the nutritionist for the popular reality show *The Biggest Loser*. The show has allowed me to work with dozens of inspiring people who have made the decision to break their old eating habits and gain control of their weight and their health.

These are folks who are determined to change the way they eat so they can finally lose weight—sometimes *hundreds* of pounds—and keep it off for the rest of their lives. That requires lots of permanent change . . . so the foods I direct them toward had better be appealing!

Many of the contestants initially subscribe to the common view that improving one's eating habits means trading in favorite foods for bland, yucky, "good for you" stuff. They think that "healthy eating" will be a three-times-daily schedule that alternates between boredom and torture.

That's because they probably haven't met many dietitians with chef's training! After I've worked with clients for a while, opening the door to a world of new, delicious flavors and wonderful textures, they realize that the foods they'd indulged in for years don't taste so good after all. The foods filled with white sugar and flour; the heavily processed and overpackaged junk; and the heavy, fatty fast foods are not prizes to be treasured. Not when you can have fruits and vegetables in a palette of colors so rich and varied that you can go days—weeks, even—before you touch the same one.

When your meals carry the lusciousness of extra-virgin olive oil and the flavors of sweet, pungent or complex, mouthwatering herbs and spices, you'll never feel deprived of those pale imitations of food that used to crowd your plate. When you can eat huge portions of vegetables, whole grains, and fruits, your stomach will stay full and happy. When a diet allows you to have red wine or cocoa or Brazil nuts, are you really missing anything?

Most important, when you have more energy; a strong, fit body; and good prospects for a long, healthy life, would you ever want to let go of the new lifestyle that bestowed all of these improvements?

There are so many seductive choices in flavors and textures that are good for your health that you really can eat these foods for the rest of your life! Better yet, you'll savor every bite.

This book will offer you hundreds of food choices and lifestyle improvements that will slow down or even prevent the conditions that we often associate with aging: diabetes, cancer, heart disease, weakened bones and muscles, wrinkling, and many more.

It's not enough for me to tell you that nutritious food and exercise are somehow "good for you"—you'll learn in this book exactly *why* particular changes improve your health and prevent illness. When you can actually picture the improvements going on inside (and outside) your body, making these changes becomes downright easy.

And it's certainly not enough for the dietitian in me to tell you to "eat these foods because they're healthy." That's why the chef in me has written dozens and dozens of delicious recipes so this book can be a welcome companion for years to come.

You can't keep yourself from getting older, but you can keep yourself from getting *old*. Are you ready? Let's stop the clock on your aging!

A LOT OF PEOPLE ARE JOURNEYING TOWARD A LONG, HEALTHY LIFE SPAN . . . HOW ABOUT YOU?

We baby boomers have packed a lot of living into our lifetimes already: We watched a man walk on the moon and saw a woman—then *two* women—join the Supreme Court. We woke up to Jimi Hendrix's guitar at Woodstock and, decades later, could download songs over the Internet. Some of us became hippies, many became yuppies, and lots of us became parents. Now some of us are grandparents, and some are getting our first taste of retirement.

That's a lot of good times. But people in their fifties and sixties have many more experiences to enjoy. Some of us are going to see a *lot* more in our lifetimes, in fact.

According to the US Census Bureau, when the year 2050 rolls around, about 834,000 Americans will be at least 100 years old. That's a group larger than the population of San Francisco! This rise in the number of *centenarians*—the term for people who are at least 100 years old—will be absolutely enormous. In the year 2000, there were only about 72,000 centenarians in America.[1]

What wonderful things will these people see in coming years? What landmark events will they witness? What new technological breakthroughs will they get to use? How many new family members will they welcome into the world?

And will you be one of them?

But here's an even more important consideration than what age you will reach: Will the remaining years of your life—however many are awaiting you—be free from disease and disability?

It's tempting to measure your health by how long you live. And 100 years is certainly a sizable, impressive number to reach. Indeed, blowing out this many candles is certainly a sign that your body has held up well. However, even though we're learning more and more about how to lengthen our lives, *living to be 100 doesn't have to be your goal.* Let's make that point clear: Aging successfully doesn't mean you have to reach a magic number, whether it's 90, 100, or beyond. After all, even though the ranks of centenarians may swell to over 800,000 in the coming decades, only a small percentage of the population will actually make it to this age.

A 2005 poll by *USA Today* and ABC News found that, on average, people would be happy just to live to the age of 87. But along the way, they really want to keep their health and maintain functions such as taking care of themselves, being able to drive, and living on their own. Their top two concerns about aging were losing their health and becoming unable to take care of themselves.[6]

Instead of trying to hit 100, a more reasonable goal is to aim for a long life but, more important, push back—or avoid entirely—the diseases and functional impairments that crop up in older age. The experts call this "compression of morbidity"—we call it antiaging. It simply means that instead of slowly and steadily declining and growing weaker in your forties, fifties, sixties, and beyond, you can stay healthy, active, and youthful deep into your senior years. You may wind down toward the very end of your life, but you'll have had decades of life without cancer or the disabilities of diabetes or heart disease. You'll enjoy more years of being active, running your own errands, and playing with your grandkids—with strong muscles and unflagging energy levels.

If you make the right choices day after day, you can certainly improve your chances of enjoying a long, fit, healthy life. The right choices are explained in full throughout this book, presented as strategies to prevent, reverse, or in some cases cure the diseases that age the body.

Doctors and researchers are tackling the issue of aging at an unprecedented rate, and they're discovering more than they ever knew about what helps some people enjoy long, healthy lives.

In laboratories around the world, these experts are peeking into our very cells to observe what kind of changes occur as we age. They're learning to tell the difference between the signs that accompany normal aging and those ailments that shouldn't be happening at all. And they're making breakthroughs in extending the longevity of many creatures, from a simple yeast cell or a fly to more complex animals like mice and monkeys. Although they're only now figuring out how to apply this knowledge to humans, many researchers can't keep the excitement out of their words when they describe the potential benefits these discoveries may hold in improving our quality of life and extending our life span.

You have keen advantages in your favor as you strive to enjoy a healthy long life. For starters, women on average live a lot longer than men. Throughout the 1900s, everyone's life expectancies were greatly extended with the advent of antibiotics and improved sanitation . . . but women made the bigger gains. Baby boys born in 1900 could only expect to live to 46, on average. But girls born alongside them would live to 48, on average. Fast-forward to 1950, and boys born in the era could expect to see the age of 66, but girls could expect to live more than *5 years* longer.[2]

Jump forward again to the present day and you'll find that roughly 83 percent of American centenarians are female. They're expected to hold this big lead over men all the way to 2050, when centenarians in this country will be more than 10 times more common than they are today.[1]

Part of this increased longevity is due to the fact that women tend to negotiate the turbulent teen years and their young adulthood in a safer and healthier manner than men do. Think accidents, homicides, and suicides, which kill off more young males than females. But new research shows that on the microscopic level, a natural process in the body that's harmful to cells may not be as damaging to women as it is to men. We'll talk more about that later.[3]

You also benefit from a great deal of recent knowledge on how to live a lifestyle that's conducive to a long life. It's true that your genes play a significant role in how long you'll live . . . but it may not be as large a role as you think. A Swedish study on twins who were raised in the same household versus different ones (thus being influenced by the same genes but perhaps different environments) estimated that longevity differences are about 35 percent genetic and 65 percent environmental. Other studies on twins have found that inherited factors account for only 25 to 30 percent of longevity.[4]

You can't go back and pick different parents, but you *can* choose the foods you eat, how much exercise you'll do, and whether or not you'll smoke. These environmental factors go a long way toward determining how successfully you'll prevent and avoid diseases that are associated with unhealthy aging.

Another study divided up more than 400 centenarians by whether they'd had common age-related diseases such as cancer, diabetes, heart disease, hypertension, or stroke before the age of 80 (they were called survivors), after the age of 80 (delayers), or never (escapers). A majority of the people who made it to 100 were either delayers or escapers. They avoided many common serious diseases until they were already living beyond their normal life expectancy. In this book, you'll learn to reduce the chances of developing these conditions. In short, you'll learn to make the choices that could lead you to become a "delayer" or "escaper."[4]

Researchers are also looking at several populations around the world in which a high percentage of individuals live to old age. These include Okinawans, who enjoy the longest life expectancy on Earth, have lower rates of heart disease and cancer than Americans, and tend to stay surprisingly active even at extremely old ages; and Seventh Day Adventists, a religious group whose members' life expectancy is 10 years longer than average Americans'. This may be due to their vigilant attitude toward not smoking, choosing a vegetarian diet, exercising regularly, and staying leaner.[5,4]

There are no promises or guarantees that good nutrition, exercise, and other lifestyle improvements will allow you to avoid serious ailments. But growing evidence says that a few simple steps can greatly improve your chances of enjoying a long, healthy life that would have been unattainable to most people just a few generations ago.

Since I've focused my career on antiaging nutrition, I've given countless seminars and presentations to groups of people who were curious about slowing down the telltale signs of aging and sidestepping the conditions that often plague the later years. I've been surprised to see more than my fellow boomers—a group that has *always* been eager to squeeze as much enjoyment out of life as we can—in the audience. College students and 30-somethings are already concerned about how they're going to look and feel decades in the future. Senior groups want to know if they can still make changes to improve their health and longevity. The answer is yes—it's never too late or too early to slow the aging clock with changes in your lifestyle choices.

And my audiences have been surprised at many of the things they've learned, too: chiefly, that they can do a lot to influence their health and appearance. Their destiny is not solely at the mercy of their internal pre-programmed genes and an external environment they can't control.

There's no doubt we're very concerned about aging on the *outside* of our bodies. We're spending millions in an effort to postpone it. In the last decade, the number of cosmetic surgeries soared, and it promises to continue rising. According to the American Society for Aesthetic Plastic Surgery, 11.4 million cosmetic surgical and nonsurgical procedures were performed in 2005. We're lining up for face-lifts, tummy tucks, and injections to fill furrows and freeze creases so our faces won't wrinkle.

If our quest to preserve our youthful vitality is so strong that these options seem reasonable, then eating the right foods and getting a little exercise shouldn't be difficult changes to make. After all, we have to eat every day. Why not choose foods that will protect us, rather than harm us?

Are you ready to start? Over the course of this book, you're going to see a lot of recommendations for foods and beverages you should consume and those you should avoid. Some of these suggestions may look familiar. I'm sure someone has already told you to eat your vegetables. You know that gorging on pie and cookies won't improve your health. But you may be surprised to learn *why* eating certain foods is so important to preserving your youth and your health, even down to the cellular level. Many of my clients have told me that after they learned to envision the microscopic damage that accumulates with age, they found it downright seductive to make the healthy changes I'm about to suggest.

Let's zoom in and take a close look at what can happen to the human body to make it lose health and functionality over the long term.

What Exactly *Is* Aging?

The human body has an incredibly complicated array of processes that keep it ticking properly, and scientists have found all kinds of problems that tinker with this delicate machinery as time progresses. Let's take a look at some of the key changes occurring in your cells that influence aging.

Many longevity researchers agree that *free radicals* are the main culprit involved in damaging our bodies as we age. Free radicals are oxygen molecules with one or more unpaired electrons. Some of them have an extra electron—or even more than one electron without a partner—and some are missing one or more electrons. That may not seem like a big problem to you, but it certainly does to the oxygen molecule. It zips around in your body, trying to steal an electron from or donate an electron to another molecule to satisfy or neutralize its charge. Once it accomplishes its mission, the other molecule becomes a free radical in turn, and the problem cascades. Free radicals are highly reactive, meaning they easily affect the healthy cells in your body. The damage resulting from this process is referred to as oxidation or oxidative stress.[16]

Free radicals inflict a variety of types of injury within your body. They damage your DNA, which can cause mutations that transform normal cells into cancerous ones. They oxidize cholesterol, making it more likely to develop deposits of plaque on the walls of your arteries, leading to heart disease. And they damage proteins, which are the building blocks of your body. The older you get, the more you accumulate free radical damage in your DNA, lipids (fats in your body), and proteins. Damaged proteins can affect the structure and function of your tissues, resulting in problems from wrinkles to heart disease.[7]

Some sources of free radicals are avoidable. Smoking introduces a huge number of them into your body, as does pollution. Radiation from sunlight can create them in your skin, causing signs of aging such as wrinkles and pigment changes.[7]

Unfortunately, your body also naturally creates a steady flow of these troublemakers during everyday metabolism. For that you can blame your mitochondria, the powerhouses inside your cells that produce energy. They do this by using oxygen to convert fuel within the cell into usable energy. This process is wonderful in that it gives your cells the spark to keep you moving and functioning properly. On the other hand, all this energy production generates a lot of free radicals.[7]

We're not talking just a few troublemakers here and there—scientists believe that at least 2 percent of the oxygen you breathe goes into making free radicals.[15] It's important to understand that this is a steady, significant onslaught against your body that intensifies with age. Fortunately, your body has a built-in system for neutralizing free radicals so they cause less damage. This process primarily utilizes powerful enzymes produced by your body, as well as protective chemicals derived from your diet.[7,16]

USEFUL KNOWLEDGE

Need more evidence that free radicals should stay at the front of your mind when you're planning your food choices each day? Experts think that the DNA in each cell in your body could take a damaging hit from free radicals 104 times a day! Will the next food you eat protect or damage your genetic material? The choice is yours.[17]

When you're young, your internal antioxidant system is very effective at preventing free radical damage. However, as you get older, your mitochondria churn out free radicals in greater quantities, and your protective system is less proficient and becomes overwhelmed. The damage accumulates faster as you age.[7]

Here's a good way to envision this damage. Picture your healthy body as a sturdy and freshly painted new home and an attack of free radicals as a hailstorm. As the storm reaches your home, the first few pieces of hail bounce off with no problem. After all, what's a pellet or two of ice against a sturdy roof? But the hail gradually pummels the place faster and harder. Fortunately, you happen to have a repair crew already working in your home, and they agree to go up on the roof, fix the damage, and replace broken shingles to fortify your defenses. The storm shows no sign of weakening, but for a while, this efficient crew keeps your roof solid and unblemished. But as the hail falls harder, the workers get tired, and they can't keep up with repairing the damage.

The storm lasts for years without stopping. Eventually the hail burrows holes in your roof and ravages your attic. It keeps pounding away until it has punched holes in your ceiling, damaging the walls, floor, wiring, and furniture. The outside of your home looks pretty worn, too.

Even though each piece was no bigger than a pea, over time the hail turned your sturdy new home into a dwelling that's faded, ragged around the edges, and shaky. The hailstorm of free radicals, growing stronger as your natural defenses wane, can have the same effect on your body: It can ravage you inside and out. Sometimes it even shows.

So that's the bad news. But that's only part of the story.

EVEN APPLES NEED ANTIOXIDANTS

When I'm teaching a class and we reach the discussion on antioxidants, I like to use the following example. I slice an apple the day before class and divide the slices between two plates, then dip one batch in lemon juice.

By the time class rolls around, the untreated apple is brown and oxidized. This is because the sugars in the untreated apple have oxidized. The treated apple, however, remains fresh, crisp, and white because it is drenched in natural antioxidants (vitamin C) found in the lemon juice.

Think of the cells in the tissues throughout your body as apple slices. They're under constant attack by free radicals—do you want them to remain fresh and intact, or do you mind if they become disfigured and damaged? This is the difference an antioxidant-rich diet can make.

Researchers have recently discovered that women's mitochondria produce fewer free radicals than men's mitochondria do. Women also have higher levels of naturally protective chemicals to fight free radicals, and the DNA within our mitochondria have only a fraction of oxidative damage, compared with men. Estrogen hormones in women may be to thank for these beneficial results, since they may help encourage production of the protective chemicals.[8,9]

Plus, you don't have to let your body try to defend itself against free radicals on its own. What if you put a strong, trusty shield over your home that would deflect more hail so it doesn't cause harm? Even better, what if you could somehow *make the hailstones slow down and become fewer in number?*

When it comes to free radicals, you can strengthen your protection by eating foods containing antioxidants. You've probably heard of antioxidants before, perhaps without really considering what they are and why they're helpful. But if you consider that free-radical damage is called oxidation, it becomes obvious that antioxidants help by working against oxidation. They circulate in your body and break the chain reactions that occur when free radicals rob or donate electrons from or to other molecules, thereby turning them into free radicals, too. Antioxidants offer up their own electrons so the roving bands of free radicals don't have to vandalize your cells to get what they want. And when dietary antioxidants give up electrons, they don't become free radicals themselves—they remain harmless.[16]

Since free radicals may only "live" for the tiniest fraction of a second, it's important to always have plenty of antioxidants available to quickly handle them before they damage something vital . . . like before they cause a mutation in a cell's DNA or make a little bit of cholesterol in an artery wall especially dangerous.

Remember that your body creates powerful antioxidant enzymes and also bolsters its defenses with nutrients from your food choices. The antioxidants from your diet include vitamins A, C, and E; minerals that support your body's antioxidant enzymes; and certain plant chemicals called phytochemicals. As we get older, our internal antioxidant enzyme system runs less efficiently. It becomes more and more important to include fruits, vegetables, and whole grains in meals so you're armed with an ample supply of antioxidants to support your waning defenses.[16]

In essence, these antiaging foods are like adding a protective barrier on your roof to make more of those hailstones bounce off harmlessly.

It's important to stress that these vital external antioxidants should come from *food*. Antioxidant supplements are selling like hotcakes, now that boomers are realizing the power of the free-radical fighters. But supplements are *supplemental* to what you get in your food. Research has found that antioxidants from a bottle can actually have *pro*aging or *pro*oxidant effects when we take too many. A classic example is a large Finnish study in which male smokers who took beta-carotene supplements actually increased their risks for lung cancer. There is an inexplicable synergy of Mother Nature's antioxidants that are naturally found in food. Somehow their sum is larger than their individual parts. This is the protection we're looking for—not high doses of supplemental antioxidant pills.

In addition, scientists are starting to think that simply cutting back on calories may reduce the number of free radicals that your mitochondria churn out and help you live longer. That's like making the hailstorm decrease in intensity! They don't know for sure that this happens in humans, but countless studies have found that cutting back on calories is associated with a longer life span in numerous animals, insects, and other creatures. You'll see some fascinating details on this process in a few pages.[18]

The take-home message is this: Your genes do play a role in how healthy you'll be and how long you'll live. But genetics is only one factor, and perhaps a relatively minor one, in determining the rate at which we age. Since you can't choose your genes (not yet, anyway), why not focus on things you can do something about, like free radicals, which appear to be responsible for much of the aging process? And the best part is that you can find most of the tools you need at your grocery store.

Glycation and Blood Sugar

Although free radicals play a crucial role in aging, they're certainly not the only problem wreaking havoc in your body and influencing how healthy you remain as you age. Another factor is called advanced glycation end products, or AGEs.

AGEs are created when blood sugar—in the form of glucose—becomes attached to proteins. Proteins are strings of amino acids that act as building blocks in your body, with many different functions, depending on the type of tissue in which they're found. When glucose attaches to a protein, it becomes *glycated*. This changes the structure and function of the protein, says Jaime Uribarri, MD, a kidney specialist at Mount Sinai School of Medicine in New York who studies AGEs. For example, AGEs cause proteins to cross-link, or make connections to each other. If you put a sample of collagen—a component of skin—into a test tube containing glucose, it gradually stiffens due to the AGEs. When this occurs in your own skin, it contributes to the wrinkling process, he says.

AGEs are linked to many diseases associated with aging. They can cause proteins in the lenses of your eyes to become cross-linked, leading to the cloudiness of cataracts. They can damage cartilage in your joints, leading to osteoarthritis. They can make your arteries stiff and can contribute to heart disease. They're also linked to Alzheimer's disease.

But cross-linking is only one way they damage your body. AGEs can also activate cells in your immune system, causing them to release chemicals that initiate inflammation (you'll see in a few pages why unwanted inflammation is bad). AGEs also cause cells to form more free radicals.

AGEs get into your body in two ways. First, they can form inside your body. Elevated blood sugar, which is a problem in people with diabetes and a condition leading to it, called prediabetes, can lead to a significant buildup of AGEs in your system.[19]

AGE BETTER BY AVOIDING AGE

The following chart reflects approximate AGE amounts for some common foods. The research is still emerging on the recommended limit of AGEs in your daily diet, so it is too early to recommend an acceptable amount. However, in a small screening, it was found that median dietary AGE intake was about 16,000 kilounits per day. Thus, low and high AGE intake may be defined as lower or greater than 16,000 kilounits per day, respectively. As with nutrients, the combination of food types and amounts over the day would be more important than the specific AGE content of any food item.

FOOD	SERVING SIZE	AGE CONTENT
Frankfurter, broiled 5 min	1 large (90 g)	10,143
Pizza, thin crust	1 slice (100)	6,825
Frankfurter, boiled 7 min	1 large (90)	6,736
Chicken breast, fried 8 min	1 small (90 g)	6,651
Philadelphia cream cheese	2 Tbsp (30 g)	3,265
Chicken breast, microwaved 5 min	1 small (90 g)	1,372
Potato chips	1-oz package (30 g)	865
Puffed rice cereal	2 cups (30 g)	600
Pepper and mushrooms, grilled	½ cup (100 g)	261
Canned red kidney beans	½ cup (100 g)	191
Pasta, cooked 8 min	1 cup (100 g)	112
Popcorn, microwaved, low-fat butter	1 cup (192 g)	64
Bagel, toasted	½ small (3 inch) (30 g)	50
Tomato, raw	½ large (100 g)	23
Apple	½ large (100 g)	13
Bran flakes	½ cup (30 g)	10
Vegetable soup, homemade	1 cup (250 ml)	3
Honey	2 tsp (15 g)	1
Milk, fat-free	1 cup (250 ml)	1

Adapted from "Advanced Glycoxidation End Products in Commonly Consumed Foods," Goldberg, et al, *Journal of the American Dietetic Association* (August 2004).

Note: 100 grams of solid foods equals 3.53 ounces; 250 milliliters of liquid foods equals 8.45 fluid ounces.

In addition, outside sources—namely, food and smoking—can usher AGEs into your body. Foods that are high in fat and protein and cooked with high heat are especially likely to contain AGEs. High-carbohydrate foods are less likely to have them, although some processed carbs contain an ample amount. In general, saturated fats have 30 times more AGE contents than carbs, and meats have 12 times more.[19,21]

In 2004, Dr. Uribarri and other researchers from Mount Sinai School of Medicine measured the AGE content in hundreds of foods and found particularly high levels in butter, roasted nuts, cream cheese and many other forms of cheese, and broiled and fried meats. High-temperature methods of cooking such as frying and broiling were also associated with higher AGE levels. Fat-free milk, fruits, vegetables, and whole grain bread were low in AGEs.[20]

Dried and cured tobacco leaves also contain AGEs, which enter your body through your lungs when you smoke. For many reasons, smoking is not going to help you preserve your health as you go through life. In addition to dramatically raising the risk of lung cancer, smoking tobacco also results in AGE damage—yet another reason to avoid the nasty habit.[19]

When you fill your antiaging pantry, avoid fatty, heavily processed foods and focus instead on foods low in AGEs: fruits, vegetables, and whole grain foods. When you occasionally choose to eat lean meat, be sure it hasn't been cooked with a high-temperature method, such as broiling or frying. Meats containing more moisture tend to be lower in AGEs, so a good way to prepare them is with a moist-heat cooking method such as boiling, stewing, or poaching, Dr. Uribarri says.

Inflammation

A third factor that accelerates the aging process has benevolent effects, too. Inflammation is a process that attacks germs and helps your body heal itself from injury. When it needs to deal with a wound or an onslaught of germs, your body sends special cells in your immune system to confront the matter via your bloodstream. A sprained wrist, for example, or a cut on your foot probably feels hot and swollen because so many blood and inflammatory cells are called to the area.

On the other hand, when inflammation gets stuck in the on position for too long, it can cause major damage to your body. Immune cells can unleash chemicals that are harmful to your tissues—and can also release free radicals. For example, some of the damage in Alzheimer's disease and Parkinson's disease is caused by free radicals from immune-system cells that oxidize substances in your body and cause glycation of proteins. (All these sources of aging—free radicals, AGEs, and inflammation—can become interconnected.)[28] Inflammation also contributes to many other conditions associated with aging, including arthritis, heart disease, and cancer. Skin damage that contributes to outward signs of aging can be inflammatory in nature, too.

The foods you eat can increase or decrease inflammation in your body. Based on what you've already learned about how both nutritious and unwholesome foods interact with your system on the cellular level, which foods do you think will encourage inflammation and which will protect you from it? Antioxidants and healthy oils (such as the omega-3s found in fish and flaxseed oils) help protect you from inflammation. Conversely, heavily processed foods and items containing sugar can encourage inflammation.

So now we've identified some of the most important issues causing aging in your body on the microscopic level: oxidation, damage from AGEs, and inflammation. Let's move on to the bigger picture. Certain problems and diseases are more likely to strike as you get older. Some of these can prematurely end your life, while others prematurely create wrinkles or cause disability, decreased functioning, and difficulty interacting with your surroundings. Avoiding these—or at least postponing them—can help you look and feel younger longer.

Bypass the Big Obstacles to a Life Brimming with Good Health

Hopefully, the glimpse you've had deep inside your body has given you an understanding of why good nutrition is mandatory for healthy aging and disease avoidance and prevention. It's not always easy to eat something nutritious just because you heard that "healthy foods are good for me." Making nutritious choices—say, eating almonds for vitamin E and red peppers for vitamin A—is easier when you know that you're giving your body a much-needed burst of antioxidants to neutralize a cloud of free radicals.

You've peered through the microscope to see the damage happening on

(continued on page 16)

ADD UP YOUR ANTIOXIDANTS TO GET AMPLE PROTECTION

Most of us are unaware that the antioxidants we eat actually swoop in to halt free radicals before they can hurt us. But for Ronald Prior, PhD, watching these helpful food components do their job is all in a day's work. Dr. Prior, a senior investigator with the USDA, is at the forefront of developing ways to quantify the antioxidant ability of food by measuring how it interacts with sources of free radicals in the laboratory.

The ORAC (oxygen radical absorbency capacity) score indicates a food's antioxidant brawn, or its ability to neutralize cell-damaging free radicals in a test tube or lab measurement. We're still not sure how this translates to the role of antioxidant-rich foods in our diet, but preliminary studies indicate they may also neutralize harmful free radicals in our bodies, potentially slowing the aging process.

Dr. Prior knows exactly how well the antioxidants in hundreds of foods, from berries to cocoa, are capable of protecting us. But to enjoy their protection, we have to eat these foods first. And many Americans just aren't doing it.

Based on calculations of eating habits surveyed by the federal government, Americans consume about 4,500 to 5,500 ORAC units per day. This is equal to about 2½ servings of fruit and vegetables daily, and "clearly that's not enough," Dr. Prior says. Though his work in estimating just how many ORAC units people need per day is still preliminary, a better target would be 12,000 to 13,000 daily ORAC units, he says. Since the amount of free radicals your body produces is related to how much food you eat, this number applies to someone who eats 2,500 calories daily. If you eat more calories, you need more antioxidant foods. Following are some of the findings, to date, of studies tracking the consumption of antioxidant-rich foods.

- Men and women had up to a 15 percent increase in the antioxidant power of their blood after increasing their daily fruit and vegetable intake, compared with what they consumed before the study.

- A small study of elderly women showed the antioxidant power of their blood was raised as much as 25 percent after consuming approximately 1½ cups sliced strawberries, 1¾ cups cooked spinach, *or* two 5-ounce glasses of red wine per day.

- An Italian study demonstrated that subjects who drank two 4-ounce glasses of red wine per day experienced a 30 percent increase in total plasma antioxidant capacity.

- In a cardiac study, patients who consumed 6 ounces of pomegranate juice each day for 1 year realized a 130 percent increase in total antioxidant status as well as a decrease in blood pressure.

- Healthy men who consumed 4 tablespoons of dark buckwheat honey had a 7 percent increase in serum antioxidant levels.

- A study of cardiac patients revealed that a daily intake of about 4 cups of black tea for 4 weeks raised beneficial antioxidant catechin levels by 33 percent.

You'll find the ORAC content of many foods starting on page 19. It would be unwise, however, to look at the list and think that eating three plums would satisfy your antioxidant needs for the day.

About 85 percent of the antioxidants in fruits and vegetables are water soluble. This means that 5 hours after you eat a piece of produce, the water-soluble antioxidants have left your system, Dr. Prior says. We do store up fat-soluble antioxidants for a few weeks, however.

"You've got to have antioxidant compounds in the vicinity of where free radicals are," Dr. Prior says. "The hydroxyl radical [a very destructive type of free radical] can do a lot of damage. But it doesn't travel far, either. It does this damage in the locale of where it's produced. If there aren't antioxidants there to neutralize them, [hydroxyl radicals] will interact with cellular components—like DNA or lipids—and start the process that might lead toward cancer or cardiovascular disease."

That's why you should make sure you have a good source of antioxidants every few hours throughout the day in meals, snacks, and beverages. While cooking can reduce the amount of water-soluble antioxidants (such as vitamin C), it increases the bioavailability of fat-soluble antioxidants, like lycopene, which is found in tomatoes. That said, raw or cooked, one source is not necessarily better. Besides, some people don't tolerate raw foods well. Just as a variety of antioxidant-rich foods provide an inexplicable synergy of health benefits, a mix of antioxidant-rich foods, both raw and cooked, will provide a great balance of these clock-stopping nutrients.

an invisible level. Now let's take a look at the big screen and see what happens to American women as they age. It plays out in numbers you can't ignore.

Here are some of the major problems that strike millions of women as they age. Throughout the book, you'll learn more about why these are more likely to occur as you get older and, specifically, how you can reduce your risk of them—and slow the aging clock—through food choices and other lifestyle changes.

Heart disease. One out of every three women will die of heart disease. In 2003, nearly 500,000 women died of cardiovascular disease. However, women often forget that they're at risk for heart problems. One survey found that only 13 percent of women felt that heart disease was the most serious threat to their health. This may be because men start having heart disease about 10 years younger than women do.[10,11,12,13,14]

But as we get older, our risk catches up to men's. According to the American Heart Association, rates of coronary heart disease—in which the heart doesn't get enough bloodflow through the arteries feeding it—are two to three times higher in women *after* menopause than in women the same age who haven't entered menopause. According to the Centers for Disease Control and Prevention (CDC), if all forms of major cardiovascular disease could be eliminated, people could expect to live *nearly 7 years longer.*[22] Now that's really stopping the clock!

Cancer. In 2006, nearly 700,000 women developed new cases of cancer, and about 275,000 died from the disease, according to the American Cancer Society (ACS).[23] The most common sites where new cancer developed were the breast, the lung and bronchus, and the colon and rectum. These accounted for more than half of all the cases. The most common types of *fatal* cancer were the same three, but in a different order. Women were most likely to die of lung cancer, followed by breast and colorectal cancer.[23]

Your risk of all these diseases rises sharply with age. According to the ACS, until you turn 39, you have only a 1 in 209 chance of developing breast cancer. From ages 40 to 60, your odds climb to about 1 in 24, and they jump even higher later in life.[23]

Your risk of colorectal cancer takes an even more worrisome climb. Until the age of 39, your odds of the disease are only about 1 in 1,567. Over the next 2 decades, they rise to 1 in 143. Then, during your sixties, the odds climb to 1 in 86.[23]

Finally, your odds of lung cancer increase, too. Up to age 39, only 1 in 3,100 women get it. During the next 2 decades, 1 in 125 will be struck. And among women in their sixties, 1 in 60 will develop the disease. Remember: More women die of lung cancer than breast cancer![23]

The foods you eat and other choices you make can help protect you from these and other cancers, and you'll learn plenty about how to make the right choices in this book. As far as lung cancer goes, one very straightforward step will protect you from the most important risk factor: Avoid smoke, whether by not lighting up or avoiding other people's smoke.[23]

Stroke. More women than men have strokes, and more women die from them, too. In 2003, American women had 373,000 strokes, which killed nearly 100,000 women. Men, in comparison, had 327,000 strokes, and 62,000 of them were fatal.[22]

As you get older, your risk of stroke rises; the vast majority of people who die of a stroke are 65 or older. Keep in mind that these events aren't only worrisome because they can be fatal—they're also one of the leading causes of major disability. The damage from a stroke can rob you of the quality of life you've always enjoyed, including communicating with others, walking, and taking care of yourself.[22] Successful aging includes maintaining a high quality of life—and preventing a stroke goes a long way toward that goal.

Diabetes. Your risk of diabetes goes up with age. Fewer than 5 percent of adults up to the age of 39 have it. That number climbs to 10 percent in people between 40 and 59 and 20 percent in those age 60 and over.[24]

Diabetes is a major cause of many forms of disability. It causes around 24,000 people to go blind from retinal damage each year. It makes people up to four times more likely to die of stroke or heart attack. And most people with diabetes develop nerve damage, commonly leading to problems such as numbness in the feet. Any of these problems can hinder your ability to enjoy your life on your own terms.[24]

Osteoporosis. Although men do get osteoporosis, a condition marked by fragile bones, women bear most of the burden of the disease. Your risk goes up with age, particularly after menopause. After the age of 50, women who are white or Asian have about a 20 percent chance of developing osteoporosis and about a 50–50 chance of having low bone mass, which puts them at risk for the disease.[25] In black women over age 50, about 5 percent have osteoporosis, and another 35 percent have low bone mass. In Hispanic women over 50, 10 percent have osteoporosis, and 49 percent have low bone mass.[25]

As you're making changes to your lifestyle that will allow you to live a long, active life, preventing osteoporosis should be a priority. If your bones become fragile and break easily, your ability to move around and take care of yourself can become seriously impaired. And that's not what healthy aging is all about.[25]

Loss of muscle mass. As you progress past young adulthood, your muscles steadily dwindle in size and strength. Many women don't put as high a priority on gaining and keeping muscle as men do, but staying strong should be a goal as you move through life. Your muscles burn a lot of calories each day, and as they shrink with age, you naturally start burning fewer calories. This means that as muscle decreases, body fat increases. In addition, when you reach your later years, the amount of muscle you've maintained will help determine how easily you can get up and down from a chair, climb in and out of your car, and carry groceries and other items. It will also dictate your ability to retain bone mass. But those worries can be decades away if you make the right choices now.

Skin damage. As you get older, your skin naturally goes through changes, including thinning, developing wrinkles and age spots, and losing its youthful elasticity. However, a number of controllable factors can speed up (or slow down!) the aging process on your skin. Sunlight and smoking are two important factors in causing your skin to become deeply wrinkled, leathery, and blotchy at an accelerated pace. By protecting yourself from the sun and avoiding smoking, you can slow these visible signs of aging. In addition, as experts in skin health are learning, eating particular nutrients will keep you looking younger longer.

Vision problems. Your risk of cataracts—which bring clouding of the clear lens at the front of your eye—climbs steeply from your fifties to your seventies and beyond. After the age of 40, about one in six Americans has the condition.[26] Another common eye condition, called age-related macular degeneration (AMD), typically strikes only after age 50. It involves damage to the retina, which is the lining within the eye.[26] Experts think that a healthy diet rich in antioxidants may help reduce the risk of each of these conditions. So will avoiding smoking.[26]

ANTIOXIDANTS—HOW MANY WILL *YOU* GET TODAY?

The following chart will help you get a sense of which foods are good sources of antioxidants and what you need to eat each day to get an adequate supply. The top foods in 15 different categories are listed below. Comprehensive lists for each category will be found throughout the book in appropriate sections.

POSITIVELY AGELESS FOOD	SERVING SIZE	ORAC
Sorghum flour	¼ c	9,378
Beans, mature small red, dry	¼ c	6,864
Blueberry, lowbush (wild)	½ c	6,314
Blackstrap molasses	1 Tbsp	5,366
Red wine	6 oz	4,585
Natural cocoa powder	1 Tbsp	4,100
Artichoke hearts, cooked	½ c	3,952
Dried plums	¼ c	3,646
Cloves, ground	½ tsp	3,144
Green tea, brewed	1 c	2,951
Coffee, brewed	1 c	2,860
Pecans	2 Tbsp	2,548
Ginger, fresh, chopped	2 Tbsp	1,781
Tarragon, fresh	1 Tbsp	933
Extra-virgin olive oil	2 Tbsp	303

Dental health. In the not-so-distant past, getting fitted for dentures was a common rite of passage for older people. However, plenty of people nowadays maintain healthy teeth very late in life. A 2004 survey found that only 21 percent of people age 65 and older had lost or replaced all their teeth.[27]

Teeth and gums require a steady supply of nutrients and regular maintenance to stay healthy. If you don't maintain good oral health, your body can pay a price in more ways than you might realize. Losing teeth leaves you less able to chew nutritious raw fruits and vegetables and nuts. Gum disease is a major risk factor for heart disease, too!

The American Diet: A Fast, Cheap Ticket to a Short, Unhealthy Life

Okinawa is a chain of tiny islands south of Japan with a big population of centenarians. The elderly residents there who have captured the world's attention for their remarkable health and spryness tend to eat:[5]

- Seven servings of fruits and vegetables each day

- Seven servings of grains a day, such as rice and wheat noodles

- Two servings of soy per day

- Fish several times a week

- Minimal meat and dairy foods

They also eat a variety of plant foods, rather than the same few over and over, according to Bradley Willcox, MD; Craig Willcox, PhD; and Makoto Suzuki, MD, in their book *The Okinawa Program*. In addition, Okinawans place careful attention on their food and make eating sort of a ceremony. Plus, they have a practice of deliberately eating until they're 80 percent full.[5]

In short, they don't eat a huge amount of food; when they are eating, they pay attention to what's going into their mouths; and most of their calories come from a variety of vegetables, grain foods, and fish.

However, you don't have to convert to an authentic Okinawan diet in order to adopt eating habits that support a long, healthy life. You don't have to give up all of your favorite things or fill your plate with unfamiliar foods. American supermarkets and health-food stores are filled with familiar choices suitable for a diet that will slow the aging clock. You just have to start incorporating them into your daily life and adjusting your approach to food. Making several small changes can make a big difference.

Compared with the Okinawans, we eat and drink too much of the wrong types of food and beverages, eat too little of the right kinds of foods, and don't pay attention to what or how much goes into our mouths.

Most of the excess calories are empty—few if any are antioxidant-rich and nutrient-dense.

Take a look at the American approach to eating. Everything is backward when compared with how the Okinawans do it. See if you can find factors that can be improved.

- Red meat, fast foods, and processed foods take precedence.

- Loads of cholesterol, salt, and sugar are added to the mix.

- Fruits and vegetables are sorely lacking.

- Fiber and antioxidants are at a bare minimum.

- Feeling overstuffed is the cue to end a meal, rather than stopping when satisfied and comfortable.

According to the federal government, in 2002 only 22.7 percent of adults said they ate five or more servings of fruits and vegetables a day. An alarming number barely have one serving per day. We've learned a lot in recent years about why plant foods are so important for maintaining health, but it doesn't seem like the message is getting through. Way back in 1994, a similar number—20 percent—ate at least five servings per day . . . so people still aren't racing toward the produce section.[29]

In the 1990s, government surveys found that whole grains accounted for only about 15 percent of people's grain foods. Most of the grain products you choose should be whole grain—like brown rice, whole grain bread, and whole wheat pasta—and little to none should come from foods containing processed grains, such as white bread and pasta and baked desserts.[30]

Americans get 33 percent of their calories from fat, including 11 percent from saturated fat and 2.6 percent from trans fats in particular. Ideally, no more than 25 percent of your daily calories should come from fat. Only 10 percent, at most, should come from saturated fat, since it contributes to higher levels of "bad" cholesterol and raises your risk of heart disease. And you should omit or limit trans fats—a harmful, processed kind of fat often found in baked goods, margarine, chips, and the fryer in fast-food restaurants—to a bare minimum.[30]

Results of a survey of Americans' eating habits, presented at a conference of supermarket executives in 2006, found that even the idea of eating microwaveable TV dinners at home is becoming a dated concept. Not only are people eating fewer meals at home or in restaurants, more of us are eating take-out food, most often in the car. In fact, one out of every four times that people order a meal from a restaurant, *they never get out of the car!* When we do eat at home, only 47 percent of meals contain a fresh item. The fastest-growing breakfast item is soda.

It's clear that when it comes to following a diet that helps us negotiate the slippery slope between sickness and health, many Americans are taking a radically different path than the long-lived Okinawans have chosen.

Over the course of this book, you'll learn how to change your diet to combat the microscopic sources of aging you learned about earlier—free radicals, AGEs, and inflammation—and you'll see the specific eating habits you can adopt to reduce your risk of cancer, heart disease, osteoporosis, and the other diseases that can interfere with your journey toward your healthy later years. Now, though, let's take a quick overview of the basic *Positively Ageless* principles that will form the foundation for the antiaging action steps throughout this book.

Make Every Calorie Count

In the early 1990s, an odd science experiment captured headlines—and late-night talk-show monologues. It was called Biosphere 2, a mostly self-contained steel-and-glass structure rising into the Arizona sky, in which eight people lived for 2 years. One of them was Roy Walford, MD, a pioneer in calorie restriction studies conducted on mice.[15]

The residents of Biosphere 2 weren't able to grow as much food as they'd expected, and they all lost a lot of weight. Interestingly enough, Dr. Walford observed a number of changes in their blood tests indicating that their bodies were rewarded with some of the same improvements noted in rodents when their calories were restricted in his earlier studies.[15]

When lab mice don't get enough to eat, they live longer. This process, called calorie restriction, or CR, also extends the longevity of yeast, worms, and flies. It seems to help monkeys live longer, too, which is bringing our knowledge about CR closer and closer to human applications.[15,31]

Experiments have shown that calorie restriction, over time, lowers insulin levels in rodents and primates. It lowers their body temperature and the amount of energy they expend. As you've just learned, this means fewer free radicals are generated. Thus, they have lower oxidative stress and improved sensitivity to their insulin.[15]

There are now some observational studies of people indicating that a lower calorie intake may lengthen our lives, too. Research on Okinawan adults has found that they eat 20 percent fewer calories than Japanese on average . . . and they have 31 percent fewer cancer deaths and 41 percent fewer heart disease deaths than the rest of Japan.[15]

Experimental studies—in which researchers control people's food intake rather than simply observing what they eat—are starting to show some interesting results, too. A 2006 NIH study looked at CR at three study sites in the United States. At one site, Louisiana State University (LSU), researchers followed 48 overweight men and women for 6 months, dividing them into four groups. A control group merely maintained their weight; one group cut their calorie intake by 25 percent; another cut their intake by 12.5 percent and burned off 12.5 percent more calories through exercise (12.5 + 12.5 = 25 percent energy decrease); and a fourth group followed a very low-calorie diet of 890 calories a day until they'd lost 15 percent of their weight, then maintained that weight loss.

The authors concluded that CR decreased people's fasting insulin level and body temperature, which are two biomarkers that have been associated with an increased life span in humans. A "biomarker" is a factor that allows you to measure an internal bodily process. The people in the experimental groups also showed signs of less DNA damage.[32]

"I think that there's no reason to think that calorie restriction would not work in humans as it does in animals," says Eric Ravussin, PhD, the study's senior author and an obesity and diabetes researcher at LSU. Some scientists, including him, feel that CR could work by reducing the body's oxidative stress. By reducing your calorie intake, you reduce the rate at which mitochondria convert fuel into energy, which in turn reduces the number of free radicals they produce. "To me, this is the most appealing of theories. We know that species with lower metabolic rates live longer," says Dr. Ravussin. "There's no question that reactive oxygen species [another term for free radicals] are damaging lipids [fats], proteins, and the genetic code [DNA]. They are also triggering some forms of cancer." Simply losing weight causes your body's metabolism to lower, but his study found that subjects' metabolic rate was dropping even more than what the researchers would have expected from weight loss alone. Coupled with the reduction in DNA damage, these preliminary results "are quite appealing in relationship to the theory of aging emphasizing the rate of living," he says.

Relax—it's too early yet for you to develop a strict calorie-reduced diet in the expectation that it will help you live longer. It's a theory that's just beginning to be studied in humans, and scientists are still grappling to find good ways to measure just how the benefits that CR confers will translate to human longevity.

However, it's worth keeping in mind that being overweight puts you at a higher risk of diabetes, arthritis, high blood pressure, heart disease, and certain cancers, which can cause disability, lower your quality of life, and shorten your life span. In short, being overweight contributes to faster and unhealthier aging. Restricting calories to where you're only getting what you need will help you avoid all these complications. That's assuming that you're optimizing the quality of those calories, too.

Ensuring that your diet is generous with nutrients and frugal with calories may reduce the amount of free radical damage you incur over your lifetime. Let this serve as an extra reason to skip the second portions and avoid empty calories. And if you happen to overindulge on one day, make up for it the next by eating less or exercising a little more. When science one day shows how CR can help humans live longer, you'll be glad you've avoided overeating in the meantime.

Eat Right, Live Long

Throughout this book, you'll see specific suggestions on how to gradually improve your eating habits over the course of 4 weeks to protect your heart, brain, skin, bones, muscles, and the rest of your body from the ravages of aging. Here are the primary guidelines to get you in the right mind-set.

Vegetables: Eat at least 4 cups of vegetables and fruits each day. Most of your choices should be vegetables, with a few fruits tossed in—not vice versa. Vegetables should cover half your plate at lunch and dinner so that you get enough. Aim for a wide variety of deeply colored vegetables. Having lots of dark greens, reds, and purples in different kinds of produce will ensure you're getting a variety of the thousands of phytochemicals that fight disease and keep your body working properly. Keep starchy vegetables—like potatoes, peas, and sweet potatoes—to a minimum.

Fruit: Eat a variety of fresh whole fruits. Most fruit juice doesn't contain the fiber found in whole fruits. This means it's more concentrated in sugar and calories. In addition, choose fruits with a low glycemic index, like apples, grapefruit, oranges, berries, pears, and melons. We'll be talking more about GI (glycemic index) later, but in essence, high-GI foods raise your blood sugar quickly, and your body responds with a surge of insulin to handle the sugar. The goal of *Positively Ageless* eating is to keep your blood sugar and insulin on a steady level.

A final note on fruits and vegetables: Most are low in caloric density. This means they occupy a lot of space in your stomach because they're high in water and fiber, but they're lower in calories. Not only are they packed with antiaging nutrients, but they make you feel full on fewer calories! That's a good reason to start lunch and dinner with a salad: It'll help you fill up before you move on to more calorie-dense items.

Carbohydrates: Most of your carbohydrates each day should come from vegetables, fruits, and whole grains such as kasha, oats, bulgur, brown rice, wild rice, whole grain couscous, and tortillas. Spread them out throughout the day rather than having a gargantuan bowl of cereal for breakfast or several slices of bread with dinner.

Cut out the "white stuff." That means white flour, sugar, pasta, bread, and processed baked goods. They affect your blood sugar and insulin too quickly, and—as you'll see many times throughout this book—you don't want an excess of either in your bloodstream. And unlike their whole grain counterparts, these foods lack antioxidants and fiber, which is good for your digestion and can help prevent colorectal cancer. In fact, they don't offer much of anything, other than calories. The *quality* of your calories is as important as the *quantity*—so choose wisely.

Protein: They may not contain the antioxidants and vitamins found in fruits and vegetables, but a variety of lean protein sources contain valuable nutrients that are integral to slowing the aging process. Calcium, iron, selenium, and zinc are essential for bone formation, nerve transmission, fighting cancer, and maintaining a strong immune system. Protein is also required for building and preserving muscle, tissue repair, and making important enzymes and hormones. In addition to fish, excellent sources of lean protein include skinless white meat of chicken and turkey, pork tenderloin, lean cuts of beef such as top round (limit red meat to twice a week at most), and fat-free and low-fat dairy products. Beans and legumes are also a healthy source of protein.

Include some form of protein with every meal and snack. It slows the rise in blood sugar that carbohydrates will trigger, and it helps fill you up so you don't become as hungry as quickly as you would with carbs alone.

Fish: Eat fish rich in omega-3 fatty acids, such as tuna and salmon, at least four times per week. These healthy fats are good for your heart and help counteract inflammation—a major contributor to unhealthy and fast aging. More omega-3 benefits are detailed on page 64.

Dairy: Eat organic, unsweetened, lean dairy products in moderation, including fat-free or low-fat ricotta and cottage cheese and low-fat or fat-free yogurt and kefir. Aim for two servings per day. An alternative to drinking fat-free or low-fat cow's milk is calcium-fortified soy milk.

Fats: Fats should make up no more than 25 percent of your total calories. Most of your fat calories will come from lean protein, dairy, nuts and seeds, and "healthy" oils. When you use oil for cooking, choose olive oil. It contains vitamin E and components called polyphenols, which are antioxidants. Olive oil use helps increase your "good" HDL cholesterol, which helps protect your heart. If you need oil spray to coat your cooking surfaces, buy a pump bottle and fill it with your own fresh olive oil, so you can avoid the chemicals and hydrocarbons that are loaded into spray cans.

Fiber: Many professional health organizations recommend that you consume 25 to 35 grams of fiber a day. However, the typical American eats only half this amount or less. That's unfortunate, since fiber helps protect you from colorectal cancer, which is one of the most common types of cancer that women develop, and reduces your risk of heart disease. Additionally, fiber gives a feeling of satiety, which means it makes you feel full. The best way to get more fiber is to serve yourself more whole grains, fruits, vegetables, and other complex carbohydrates.

If you follow the *Positively Ageless* plan, you'll have no problem reaching the daily recommendations for fiber. If you're unaccustomed to the foods in the *Positively Ageless* pantry, you may want to add fiber to your diet gradually over the 4-week period. This will allow you to avoid abdominal consequences such as bloating, diarrhea, and gas that can occur if you introduce too much fiber too fast.

Meal timing: Eat small, frequent meals throughout the day; aim for three small meals and two or three snacks. This will help keep your energy steady and your blood sugar and insulin levels stable. Also, since many clock-stopping antioxidants from foods linger in your bloodstream for only a few hours, this ensures that you continually keep your internal supply replenished.

Fluids: You should take in plenty of fluid throughout your waking hours, primarily water and tea. Aim for 8 to 10 glasses of water each day. If you don't drink water, focus on antioxidant-rich green tea or black tea, calcium-rich organic fat-free or low-fat milk, and the occasional cup of coffee. Don't waste an opportunity to take in vital nutrients by choosing empty calories in soft drinks or artificially sweetened beverages.

Why is fluid so important for health and vitality? When you're young, your cells are plumped up with water (including the cells in your skin, which imparts a youthful look). Over the years, as cells become damaged, their water content dwindles. Keeping yourself hydrated will help keep your skin—and the rest of your body—looking and feeling good. In addition, you need lots of water to keep all the fiber you'll be eating moving through your system.

Seasonings: Limit your salt intake. Sodium in the diet is often associated with high blood pressure (a key aging biomarker), though its effect varies among individuals. African Americans are more sensitive to salt's ability to raise blood pressure. And as we age, salt generally has more of an effect.

One way to lower sodium intake is to simply eat fewer processed foods, which contain higher amounts of the stuff. Loading up on fresh fruits, vegetables, and whole grains will naturally decrease the amount of sodium you consume.

Another way is to leave the saltshaker in the cabinet. Instead, flavor your foods with the antioxidant-rich herbs and spices listed on page 108. Not only will they add some zing to your foods, they're another way to infuse your body with clock-stopping antioxidants.

Sweeteners: If you must use sweeteners, add them sparingly, and go

SATISFY YOUR SUGAR CRAVING
WITH WHOLESOME SWEETENERS

When you sprinkle sugar onto foods, you're getting a burst of sweetness . . . and that's it. You've put some calories into your body and you have no antioxidants or nutrients to show for it. Plus, sugar rapidly affects your blood sugar and insulin, so you're losing the longevity game; the goal is to keep these on an even keel.

Instead of sugar—or artificial replacements—consider these alternative sweeteners, which contain antioxidants, affect your blood sugar more slowly, and bring other potential health benefits. For more information on where to find these, consult the Shopping Resources section at the back of the book.

Agave nectar. This tasty topping, which is extracted from the pineapple-shaped wild agave plant, is similar to honey, though a bit thinner in texture and with a lighter taste. Due to its proportion of fructose to glucose, it has a relatively low glycemic index (see page 138 for an explanation of glycemic index and how certain foods can affect your blood sugar). Even better, it also contains some antioxidants! You can substitute agave nectar for an equal amount of sugar in terms of sweetness. But in recipe substitutions, tweaking is required because this sweetener is liquid (and darker than white sugar).

Brown rice syrup. This sweetener is similar in appearance to honey, but it's less sweet. It's made from sprouted brown rice and provides a

with natural choices such as agave nectar, brown rice syrup, sorghum syrup, or dark honey.

A lot of controversy surrounds artificial sweeteners, even though many think they're perfectly safe. It's becoming increasingly clear that natural foods are better for our bodies than man-made foods. In my opinion, sweeteners are no exception. My view is to steer clear of anything artificial. Period.

In addition, when you need a condiment to dress up a food, stick with a mustard, salsa, balsamic vinegar, or barbecue sauce that isn't loaded with sugar. Avoid high-fat toppings such as mayonnaise, salad dressing, or mar-

decent supply of antioxidants. You can substitute brown rice syrup for an equal amount of honey or use 1½ cups of rice syrup for each cup of sugar.

Honey. Don't forget about this gift from our friends the bees. Honey contains antioxidants, and if you seek out a dark-colored one, such as the kind that bees produce from buckwheat nectar, you'll find even more of these free-radical-fighting components.

Blackstrap molasses. This product is made during sugarcane processing; it's the syrup that remains after the sugar has crystallized from the cane's juices. As a result, it has a relatively low sugar content—and a low glycemic index. Its color is dark and its flavor is intense. Blackstrap molasses provides calcium, iron, magnesium, and potassium, as well as a rich supply of antioxidants.

Sorghum syrup. Like sugarcane, stalks of the sorghum cane plant are crushed to extract clear juices. Impurities are removed before the liquid is simmered and reduced to a viscous amber syrup, which is similar to molasses but milder in flavor and less sweet than honey. Unlike molasses, sorghum syrup is not a by-product, as sugar crystals are not extracted from its juices. Therefore, sorghum tastes sweeter and probably has a higher glycemic index. Currently, there are no GI values available for sorghum syrup. Nutritionally, it is rich in antioxidants and minerals. When substituting sorghum for sugar, the general rule is to increase the amount of sorghum by one-third over the amount of sugar, and decrease the liquids by the same amount.

garine, including their low-fat versions. Why? Because if you're in the habit of using low-fat products, you're much more likely to use full-fat versions if they're the only thing available away from home. Plus, using fake/substitution products regularly may keep your tastebuds accustomed to added fat. Try to adjust to the alternative choices suggested here and use *Positively Ageless* condiment recipes, too.

Label reading: Even if you aren't trying to lose weight, read labels and nutrition information in restaurants until you develop a sense of how many calories your body needs and how many calories are in the portions of food you choose.

KNOW YOUR CALORIE NEEDS

An important step in maintaining long-lasting health is to make sure you don't eat too much. Not only may restricting your calories help you live a longer life (see page 23), but being overweight is linked to cancer, diabetes, heart disease, and a host of other maladies that are more likely to strike as you get older.

A great way to get a sense of how many calories you need each day is called the Harris Benedict Equation. For most people, it offers a good estimate of daily caloric needs, though it may underestimate your needs if you're very muscular or overestimate them if you're overweight.

The On the Web section (page 349) will direct you to a Web site that performs this calculation for you. If you'd like to do it on your own, here's how. (It involves some math, so you'll find it much easier to do with a calculator.)

1. Multiply your weight in pounds by 4.35.
   Write it here: _____

2. Multiply your height in inches by 4.7.
   Write it here: _____

3. Multiply your age in years by 4.7.
   Write it here: _____

4. Add the numbers you wrote down in Steps 1 and 2, then add another 655. Next, subtract the number you found in Step 3. Write your final answer here: _____

5. The amount of exercise and other movement you do each day plays a role in how many calories you need. Multiply your number from Step 4 by:

1.2 if you get little to no exercise

1.375 if you get light exercise 1 to 3 days a week

1.55 if you get moderate exercise 3 to 5 days a week

1.725 if you exercise vigorously 6 or 7 days a week

1.9 if you exercise vigorously more than once a day, or you exercise vigorously daily plus have a physical job

Write your final number down here. This is how many calories you should take in each day: _____

And if you're trying to lose weight, subtract 20 percent from that number. However, as noted earlier, this book is not a replacement for personal medical advice. Consult your doctor before beginning any weight-loss program.

Alcohol in moderation: If you're going to drink alcohol, stick mostly with red wine, a rich source of antioxidants. Beer and white wine also contain antioxidants (just not as many), so they're decent alternatives. Whichever you choose, limit yourself to one or two drinks daily.

How to Use This Book

Positively Ageless builds on a core eating-and-exercise program divided into 4 weeks: The first week teaches you about vital antiaging issues such as heart health and cancer prevention; the second covers hormone-related issues and your mind; the third discusses your musculoskeletal system; and the fourth covers your "outside parts," including your skin, teeth, and eyes.

You'll learn about biomarkers, which are measurements of conditions or processes that can help us analyze how well our body is moving through the aging process. Biomarkers for skin health, body weight, and muscle mass are visible. Other biomarkers of processes such as immune function, blood sugar control, and blood pressure are more subtle. Collectively, these powerful aging biomarkers dictate our longevity and the quality of life we'll enjoy during the years we have.

Positively Ageless will help you evaluate your age-related biomarkers and determine where you stand on the ruler called the aging process. In each section, you'll learn about the physiological processes that determine these biomarkers and, more important, how to change them with your diet and other lifestyle factors. Four weeks from today, you will have an exhilarating running start down the path toward healthier longevity!

Since food is such an integral part of our lives, and it can take time to change our eating habits, *Positively Ageless* is designed so that you make small changes to your meals at first, gradually building up until you're following all the dietary steps you need to improve your health and longevity. At the end of each weekly section, you'll find specific recommendations on foods to eat and avoid, broken down into the following four stages.

"Make One Change": This section spotlights the most important self-care strategies to adopt if you want to achieve your optimum biological age for these biomarkers. If you're not ready to commit to a completely new lifestyle, these tips and strategies will give you a good introduction to an antiaging lifestyle.

FIBER'S EASY TO FIND WHEN YOU STICK WITH PLANT FOODS

Health experts recommend that we include 25 to 35 grams of fiber in our diets each day, though most Americans eat less than half that amount. It's no wonder, with the emphasis we place on processed, pre-packaged, and fast foods. It's nearly impossible to get adequate fiber eating that way. However, when you switch to the *Positively Ageless* eating program, you'll find that it's heavy on grains, vegetables, and other plant foods. The fiber quota pretty much takes care of itself.

When you read labels, keep in mind that:

- A food with 2.5 to 4.9 grams of fiber per serving is a *good* source of fiber.

- A food with 5 grams or more per serving is an *excellent* source of fiber.

Here are some sources, measured by grams of fiber.

FOOD	SERVING SIZE	FIBER (G)
All-Bran cereal	½ c	9
Kidney beans, cooked	½ c	8.2
Lentils, cooked	½ c	7.8
Spinach, cooked	1 c	7
Whole barley, cooked	½ c	6.8
Garbanzo beans	½ c	6.2
Apple	1 large	5
Plums, dried	3 medium	4.7
Orange	1 large	4.4
Popcorn, air popped	3½ c	4.2
Pear	1 medium	4.1
Raspberries	½ c	4
Edamame, shelled	½ c	3.8
Banana	1 medium	3.8
Strawberries	1 c sliced	3.3
Rice, brown, long-grain, cooked	½ c	2
Blueberries	½ c	2

"Quick Start": To ensure that you soon reap the rewards from your antiaging efforts, this section presents tips and techniques that produce measurable results in a short period of time.

"Young for Life": This section identifies essential lifestyle changes that may require more time and effort, but their dramatic and lasting impact on your biological age can reward you for the rest of your life.

Finally, each week of the program includes menu plans for 7 days of meals and snacks. The ingredients are chosen to slow the aging process and help you improve the biomarkers covered during that week. Everything you need to embrace the ultimate antiaging diet is here—except the food! Once you know where to look for the ingredients in the supermarket, you'll be set for life.

KEEP YOUR VITAL FUNCTIONS STRONG

Smooth, glowing skin and a gorgeous body are probably the first things that come to mind when you think of living youthfully. However, your vital functions—including heart and digestive health, the strength of your immune system, and your day-to-day energy levels—are the most important things to age-proof. Why? Because avoiding major diseases that are associated with age is the single best strategy for living younger with a higher quality of life. In the following sections, I'll show you the most important aging biomarkers for your vital functions—and introduce you to easy-to-follow strategies for turning back your internal clock.

chapter 1

A HEALTHY HEART FOR LIFE

As time marches forward, the changes that may or may not develop in your cardiovascular system (the term for your heart and the blood vessels connected to it) are crucial in determining whether you'll stay young and healthy longer or grow old and sick faster. That's because all the cells in your body require a constant blood supply of food and oxygen. If your heart can't do its job, the result can be disability or even an early death. The foods you eat and many other lifestyle habits that you maintain will play a major role in your heart's health.[1,2]

The Heart: A Hard Worker That Needs Nourishment

Your heart is a pump that sends blood on a complicated journey. It draws blood *in* from your body, where your cells have taken out the oxygen they need, then sends the blood to your lungs, where it's recharged with oxygen. Your heart then pumps the blood *back* from your lungs and out through a major blood vessel called the aorta, sending it out to your body again. Your heart beats about 100,000 times each day.[1,2]

The walls of the organ contain muscle, which also needs a steady supply of oxygen to keep working properly. As blood exits your heart, some of it is immediately diverted into several arteries—called your coronary arteries—that branch off your aorta and cling to the surface of your heart. These arteries feed oxygen-rich blood to the constantly working muscle in the walls of your heart.[1,2]

Your arteries aren't just simple pipes: Their walls are actually made of layers of different tissues. A thin lining helps protect the artery from harmful substances in the blood. A deeper layer contains muscle cells, allowing the artery to expand and contract as blood passes through it.

(continued on page 40)

MEASURE YOUR RISK
OF APPROACHING HEART DISEASE

The National Institutes of Health recommends the following test to measure your risk of developing coronary artery disease in the next 10 years. This provides a handy tool to discuss your risk with your doctor and weigh the necessity of diet and other lifestyle changes or whether you should also consider medications.

The test assigns points to the following factors: your age, total and HDL cholesterol, smoking status, and systolic blood pressure. Get a calculator and a notebook and check your own score. If you don't know your blood pressure or cholesterol, now may be a good time to schedule a checkup to get yours tested.

Let's run through the formula with a hypothetical woman: She's 45, has a total cholesterol of 205, doesn't smoke, and has an HDL of 53 and systolic blood pressure of 124, for which she's getting treatment. Thus, her final score is 12 points, which puts her at a low risk of developing coronary artery disease in the next 10 years.

ESTIMATE OF 10-YEAR RISK FOR WOMEN (FRAMINGHAM POINT SCORES)

AGE	POINTS
20–34	−7
35–39	−3
40–44	0
45–49	3
50–54	6
55–59	8
60–64	10
65–69	12
70–74	14
75–79	16

TOTAL CHOLESTEROL	POINTS				
	AGE 20–39	AGE 40–49	AGE 50–59	AGE 60–69	AGE 70–79
< 160	0	0	0	0	0
160–199	4	3	2	1	1
200–239	8	6	4	2	1
240–279	11	8	5	3	2
> 280	13	10	7	4	2

	POINTS				
	AGE 20–39	AGE 40–49	AGE 50–59	AGE 60–69	AGE 70–79
Nonsmoker	0	0	0	0	0
Smoker	9	7	4	2	1

HDL (MG/DL)	POINTS
> 60	−1
50–59	0
40–49	1
< 40	2

	POINTS	
SYSTOLIC BP (MMHG)	IF UNTREATED	IF TREATED
< 120	0	0
120–129	1	3
130–139	2	4
140–159	3	5
> 160	4	6

POINT TOTAL	10-YEAR RISK %
< 9	< 1
9	1
10	1
11	1
12	1
13	2
14	2
15	3
16	4
17	5
18	6
19	8
20	11
21	14
22	17
23	22
24	27
> 25	> 30

When you press your fingertip to the inside of your wrist to check your pulse, you're actually feeling an artery expand with each heartbeat![3]

When they're healthy, your arteries are flexible and allow blood to pass smoothly through them. However, a very common process called atherosclerosis, which stiffens and narrows the arteries, can make it difficult or impossible for arteries to do their job. This can put your heart in serious danger.[3]

The first changes leading toward atherosclerosis often begin during the teen years. By the time we are in our forties (and sometimes younger), some of us already have a hefty buildup in our arteries, resulting in a significant narrowing.[3]

Age-Related Heart Problems

Atherosclerosis tends to become more of a problem as you get older because cells in the lining and the wall of the artery may not be as resistant to injury as they were when you were younger. However, you may also be more likely to develop the condition simply because the risk factors that contribute to it have silently been wreaking havoc for many years. Either way, many researchers believe it is "the most important disease in old age" because it is responsible for so many deaths and so much disability in the later years.[3]

Atherosclerosis seems to begin when the artery sustains some sort of injury. Arterial damage may come from LDL (or "bad") cholesterol that is too excessive or has become oxidized; cigarette smoking; high blood pressure; diabetes; or infections.[3] Once the lining of the artery becomes injured, cells from the bloodstream are able to sneak through it and enter the wall of the artery, and a variety of substances begin to accumulate. These include immune system cells, cholesterol, and calcium. This causes the whole artery to grow stiff, so it can't expand and contract like it should when the heart pumps blood through it. The inner passage narrows, too, interfering with the flow of blood.[4]

If the stiff, narrowed artery is a coronary artery, which feeds the heart muscle with oxygen-rich blood, the process can cause angina—or chest pain—when the blood supply to the heart muscle dwindles. Plus, an accumulation of material in the artery wall can rupture, causing blood to stick and form a clot on the site, which totally blocks the flow. The sudden loss of blood to the heart muscle can result in a heart attack.[5,6]

Since the heart muscle needs steady oxygen, the disruption of the blood supply in a heart attack can cause permanent damage to the organ. Heart attacks and angina can also result in heart failure, a condition in which the heart is unable to pump blood strongly enough.[7,6]

Underlying Causes of Atherosclerosis

The following factors play a role in atherosclerosis—thus putting you at higher risk for heart disease. As you'll learn later in this section, you can help reduce all these factors with lifestyle changes.

Cholesterol. This is a fatty substance that actually has many useful functions in the body: It helps insulate nerves, create hormones, and maintain the integrity of each of our cell walls. However, when you have too much of it in your blood, it puts you at greater risk of coronary artery disease.[8,9]

To travel through the body, cholesterol must be attached to a carrier called a lipoprotein. There are several different types of lipoproteins, which are classified by density.[8]

- HDL: High-density lipoprotein is a good cholesterol. Remember HDL as "highly desirable lipoprotein." It transports cholesterol to the liver, which disposes of it.[8]

- LDL: Low-density lipoprotein builds up in the walls of your arteries, contributing to plaque. A higher concentration of this stuff in your bloodstream means that more can get into your artery walls. Think of it as "least desirable lipoprotein."[8] Researchers have been learning more lately about the role that oxidation—damage caused by free radicals—plays in making LDL cholesterol more harmful. LDL particles wedged into the walls of arteries are prone to developing free-radical damage. The oxidized LDL prompts the lining of your artery to attract cells from the immune system, which move into the arterial wall and "eat" these oxidized particles of LDL. The immune cells then release inflammatory chemicals, attracting even more immune cells. This creates a vicious cycle of inflammation and more accumulation of debris in the artery.[10,3,11]

- Triglycerides: "Triglyceride" is the chemical name for both dietary fat and body fat. Triglycerides in our plasma are made from either carbohydrates or fat that we eat. Any calories that are not immediately used for energy are converted to triglycerides and then stored in our fat cells. If we need energy in between meals, hormones regulate the release of triglycerides from fat tissue for that purpose. Like elevated cholesterol, too many triglycerides in plasma can cause heart disease. Elevated triglycerides can also be caused by untreated diabetes.

High blood pressure. This condition deserves its moniker as "the silent killer": There are often no symptoms whatsoever. Your blood pressure is a measure of the force of blood exerted on the inside walls of your blood vessels. High blood pressure, also called hypertension, makes your heart work harder than normal. It also makes your arteries more likely to develop atherosclerosis. Years of untreated high blood pressure can in itself lead to heart failure.

Several risk factors for high blood pressure are unique to women. Research has found that menopause is linked to higher systolic blood pressure that's even more pronounced than the elevated effect associated with weight gain (which often occurs around menopause). The use of birth control pills has also been linked with higher blood pressure.

Since blood pressure directly impacts how hard the heart must work, it's no surprise that some scientists consider healthy blood pressure levels to be a key biomarker for longevity. Although aging itself may not directly cause hypertension, many of the changes associated with aging, such as weight gain and decreased exercise levels, can.

Diabetes and metabolic syndrome. Your pancreas produces insulin, a hormone that helps blood sugar enter your cells, where it's used as fuel. Type 2 diabetes—the most common kind—occurs often with boomers who gain weight. Their bodies either can no longer produce enough insulin or they don't use it properly. As a result, their blood sugar can't enter their cells efficiently and it rises in their blood.[12]

Insulin resistance means the pancreas can still produce insulin, but the body doesn't use it efficiently. High blood glucose appears to play a role in the development of atherosclerosis and blood vessel disease; people with diabetes are much more likely to develop heart disease than people without it.[9,12]

In addition, a problem called metabolic syndrome puts people at higher risk of both coronary artery disease and diabetes. People with metabolic syndrome are typically obese, with most of their extra weight around the belly. They have low HDL cholesterol and high LDL cholesterol and triglycerides. They usually have high blood pressure and insulin resistance. Their blood has a greater tendency to form clots, and they have evidence of more inflammation in their bodies. With this combination of problems, it's no surprise that the stage is now set for heart disease.[13]

Smoking. This is the most avoidable of all the risk factors for heart disease. Experts haven't nailed down exactly how smoking contributes to heart disease, but the toxins it releases into your system cause damage to cells in your artery walls, making them less resistant to atherosclerosis.[3]

Biomarkers for Heart Disease

Your doctor can measure many factors that may be increasing your risk of heart disease. By establishing your baseline and learning whether these factors are elevated, you can get a sense of what steps you need to take to lessen your chance of developing heart disease. By having these biomarkers measured again later, you can track your progress in terms of how much the *Positively Ageless* dietary and other lifestyle changes are helping.

Blood Pressure

Your blood pressure rises and falls throughout the day, so your doctor will want to measure it several times on different days before diagnosing you with hypertension, or high blood pressure. Systolic blood pressure is the pressure that's measured when the heart beats and pumps blood out; diastolic is the pressure between heartbeats. These make up the two numbers you see when your blood pressure is measured, such as "120 over 80."[14,15] The National Institutes of Health (NIH) has issued the following criteria for determining whether your blood pressure is okay or too high.[14]

- Normal: Your systolic is less than 120, and your diastolic is less than 80.

- Prehypertension: Your systolic is between 120 and 139, and your diastolic is between 80 and 89.

- High blood pressure: Your systolic is 140 or higher, and your diastolic is 90 or higher.

(continued on page 46)

GET A CONCENTRATED BURST OF ANTIOXIDANTS WITH FRUIT

Although whole fruits are, in general, excellent sources of antiaging nutrients, pomegranates, blueberries, grapefruit, plums, and purple grapes stand out from the pack. Pomegranates are the most concentrated source of antioxidants from fruit. When fresh pomegranates aren't in season, try the refrigerated juice, available year-round.

Plums contain boron, a mineral thought to play a key role in the prevention of osteoporosis. Along with purple grapes, plums also contain phenolic compounds. These rich reserves of antioxidants are believed to reduce the incidence of heart disease by slowing the oxidation process and lowering LDL (bad) cholesterol.

Blueberries contain compounds that not only prevent loss of age-related impairments of memory and motor coordination but may actually help reverse the process. Berries contain anthocyanins, antioxidants with triple the power of vitamin C. These phytochemicals are known to block cancer-causing cell damage and the effects of many age-related diseases. Fresh or dried, plums, grapes, and berries are available year-round and offer a delicious way to protect the body against free radicals, heart disease, and cancer.

Citrus fruits are loaded with antioxidants, including vitamin C, beta-carotene, lutein, zeaxanthin, and beta-cryptoxanthin. Pink and ruby red grapefruit also contain lycopene. Collectively, this army of disease-fighting antioxidants provides protection against chronic conditions that develop over a lifetime, such as heart disease, diabetes, and high blood pressure.

Below you'll find a list of common fruits and their antioxidant power, as measured in ORAC units.

FRUIT	SERVING SIZE	ORAC
Blueberries, lowbush (wild)	$\frac{1}{2}$ c	6,314
Strawberries	$\frac{1}{2}$ c	5,938
Apple, Red Delicious	1	5,900
Apple, Granny Smith	1	5,381

FRUIT	SERVING SIZE	ORAC
Pomegranate	$\frac{1}{2}$ med	5,250
Cherries, sweet	1 c	4,873
Plum, black	1	4,844
Blueberries, cultivated	$\frac{1}{2}$ c	4,509
Cranberries, whole	$\frac{1}{2}$ c	4,492
Plum	1	4,118
Apple, Gala	1	3,903
Blackberries	$\frac{1}{2}$ c	3,850
Apple, Red Delicious, peeled	1	3,758
Apple, Golden Delicious	1	3,685
Apple, Fuji	1	3,578
Avocado, Haas	1	3,344
Pear, green	1	3,172
Raspberries	$\frac{1}{2}$ c	3,029
Pear, Red Anjou	1	2,943
Apple, Golden Delicious, peeled	1	2,829
Orange, navel	1	2,540
Grapes, red	1 c	2,016
Grapefruit	$\frac{1}{2}$ medium	1,904
Peach	1	1,826
Grapes, green	1 c	1,789
Mango, sliced	1 c	1,653
Apricots	3	1,408
Tangerine	1	1,361
Pineapple, diced	1 c	1,229
Banana	1 medium	1,037
Nectarine	1	1,019
Kiwifruit	1	698
Cantaloupe, cubed	1 c	499
Honeydew melon, diced	1 c	410
Watermelon, diced	1 c	216

These numbers are valid only if you aren't already taking medications to lower your blood pressure and you don't have diabetes. If you do have diabetes, anything over 130/80 means you have high blood pressure. Though optimal blood pressure is less than 120 systolic and less than 80 diastolic, you should also be evaluated if your blood pressure is too low. Low blood pressure, also known as hypotension, usually refers to a systolic/diastolic ratio of less than 100/60. Low blood pressure with accompanying symptoms such as lightheadedness or fainting could indicate an underlying condition.[15]

LOWERING YOUR BLOOD PRESSURE

Keeping a normal blood pressure is an important component in protecting your heart's health. Add these steps to your heart-healthy diet, too.

Reduce sodium. Aim to consume no more than 2,400 milligrams of sodium each day. Getting fewer than 1,500 milligrams daily is even better. That's the equivalent of about ⅔ teaspoon of table salt. However, most of the sodium in the American diet comes from processed foods—not a salt-shaker. Be sure to read the labels on all the foods you eat to ensure that your sodium intake stays low. Flavor your foods with fresh herbs and spices, not salt. When you purchase combination flavorings, check the label—these are often high in sodium.[16,17]

Load up on fruits and vegetables. The NIH devised an eating plan called the DASH (Dietary Approaches to Stop Hypertension) diet, designed to help people lower their blood pressure. The plan calls for four to five daily servings each of fruits and vegetables. An example of one serving would be one medium fruit, ½ cup of frozen fruit, ½ cup of cut-up vegetables, or ½ cup of fruit or vegetable juice.[16]

Fruits and vegetables are a rich source of potassium, a mineral that causes you to excrete more sodium. If you have too little potassium in your system, you'll retain sodium. Societies that get a lot of potassium in their diet tend to have fewer people with hypertension. Potassium also plays an important role in muscle contraction. Remember, your heart is one big muscle, so this nutrient is needed for optimal heart health.[18]

Go for low-fat dairy foods. Also aim for two or three servings of low-fat or fat-free dairy products each day. Studies that have looked at large groups of people have found that those who eat lots of calcium have lower blood pressure than those who get less of this nutrient.[16,18] Eating fat-free or low-fat dairy as well as plenty of fruits and vegetables, along with cutting back on saturated and total fat, may reduce your systolic blood pressure (the top number) by 8 to 14 points.[17]

Drink green tea regularly. A cup of antioxidant-rich green tea every day offers many health benefits—including possibly lowered blood pressure. A 2004 study involving 1,507 Taiwanese found that those who drank about 4 to 20 ounces of green or oolong tea daily were 46 percent less likely to have hypertension.[19]

Lose weight. The epidemic of obesity in the United States may be responsible for up to 30 percent of the hypertension in the nation's residents. Strive to maintain or achieve a healthy weight. Losing just 10 pounds if you're overweight can help reduce your blood pressure. Plus, weight loss can help you prevent or reduce the effects of metabolic syndrome.[18]

Drink very little—alcohol, that is. If you drink alcohol, limiting your intake to one drink a day will help prevent high blood pressure. Research has shown a small but significant rise in blood pressure in people who have three or more drinks a day. If you do imbibe daily, make it red wine. It's a rich source of antioxidants.[16,17,18]

Make helpful nondiet lifestyle changes. If you smoke, stopping the habit will help lower your blood pressure. Exercising 30 minutes on most days of the week will lower it, too.[16,17]

Cholesterol and Triglycerides

According to the American Heart Association (AHA), these are the categories of total cholesterol levels (measurements are in milligrams per deciliter of blood, or mg/dL).[20]

CHOLESTEROL LEVEL	CLASSIFICATION
Less than 200 mg/dL	Desirable
200–239 mg/dL	Borderline high risk
240 mg/dL and over	High risk

But those aren't your only important cholesterol numbers. You should also know your LDL and HDL numbers individually. Here's how LDL breaks down.[20]

LDL LEVEL	CLASSIFICATION
Less than 100 mg/dL	Optimal
100–129 mg/dL	Above optimal
130–159 mg/dL	Borderline high
160–189 mg/dL	High
190 mg/dL and above	Very high

The HDL criterion is simple: You want it above 40 mg/dL, since it protects your health by carrying cholesterol out of your system so it can't cause damage.[20]

Another way doctors sometimes weigh the risk from your cholesterol is through the cholesterol ratio. You divide your total cholesterol by your HDL. So if your total cholesterol is 180 and your HDL is 35, the ratio is 5.1 to 1. The ideal ratio is 3.5 to 1, so if your total cholesterol is 180, your HDL would be 51.

Triglycerides are usually measured at the same time as cholesterol testing. According to the AHA, your triglyceride results will fall into one of these categories.

TRIGLYCERIDE LEVEL	CLASSIFICATION
Less than 150 mg/dL	Normal
150–199 mg/dL	Borderline high
200–499 mg/dL	High
500 mg/dL or higher	Very high

LOWERING YOUR CHOLESTEROL AND TRIGLYCERIDES

If your cholesterol is too high (or you want to remain at a healthy level), these dietary changes will help guide your cholesterol biomarkers to where they need to be. The menu plans at the end of this section will also steer you in the right direction.

Eat less saturated fat. This unhealthy fat has the most significant effect on your cholesterol—and reducing it is the most important thing you can do to help your cholesterol. Saturated fat is solid at room temperature. Think butter, cheese, chicken skin, and the visible fat on a lamb chop. It is found in meats, chicken, and turkey fat (the skin is saturated fat, and the meat, especially dark meat, contains less visible saturated fat), whole dairy foods, and coconut and palm oils. That's why it's a good idea to stick with low-fat cuts of meat, remove skin from poultry, and always choose low-fat or fat-free dairy products. Saturated animal fat is also the source of dietary cholesterol.[21]

If you're concerned about your cholesterol, you should keep your daily intake of saturated fat to less than 7 percent of your daily calories. This is even lower than the limit that the average healthy person should maintain, which is 10 percent.[21]

Decrease your intake of total fat. Fat should account for only 25 percent of your daily calories. The table on page 50 will show you how many grams of total fat you can have each day if you're aiming for 25 percent of your calories from fat.

Avoid trans fat as much as possible. Like saturated fat, trans fat also raises cholesterol. If you're eating all whole and unprocessed foods, you don't even have to worry about it. Trans fat is a man-made (artificial) fat created in a process called hydrogenation, which solidifies liquid fat to make food products last longer on the shelves. You'll find this stuff in hard margarines and shortenings (made from liquid vegetable oils), cookies, doughnuts and other baked goods, and foods fried in hydrogenated fat. It's also found in lower levels in some dairy foods and processed meats.[21] Look on labels for the words *hydrogenated* or *partially hydrogenated*. If you see them, put the package back on the shelf.[21]

Cut back on dietary cholesterol. Some foods contain cholesterol, though it doesn't raise your blood cholesterol level as much as saturated fat does. You'll find dietary cholesterol only in animal foods, such as meat, poultry, whole dairy products, and egg yolks. It's not in plant foods.[21] Limit your intake of dietary cholesterol to less than 200 milligrams daily. Our liver produces all the cholesterol our bodies really need, so any amount in the diet is surplus.[21]

Stick with unsaturated fats. Though some unsaturated fats aren't as good as others (e.g., corn oil), many unsaturated fats, known as monounsaturated and polyunsaturated, can actually lower your LDL cholesterol and raise your good HDL cholesterol. Let healthy sources of unsaturated fats make up most of your fat calories.[21,22] Healthy monounsaturated fats include olive and canola oils. Fish contains a polyunsaturated fat known as omega-3 fatty acid, which the AHA says can slow down the growth of atherosclerosis and lower triglyceride levels. (More on omega-3s on page 64.)[23]

FIND YOUR FAT GRAMS
THE QUICK AND EASY WAY

You'll see recommendations in this chapter and the rest of the book on how much fat you can have each day, both total fat and saturated fat in particular. For example, health experts recommend that you get no more than 25 percent of your calories from total fat and 10 percent or less from saturated fat.

Figuring out just how many grams of fat you can have takes a little math. Here's how to do it: If you're taking in 1,400 calories a day and up to 25 percent can come from fat, that means 1,400 × 0.25, or 350 calories can be from fat. A gram of fat contains 9 calories. So simply divide 350 by 9 to get 39 grams.

Here's a table to show you the values for a range of daily calorie intakes. If your daily calorie amount isn't included, get out the calculator to figure your needs.

DAILY CALORIE INTAKE	MAXIMUM TOTAL FAT GRAMS*	MAXIMUM SATURATED FAT GRAMS (10% OF DAILY CALORIES*)	MAXIMUM SATURATED FAT GRAMS (7% OF DAILY CALORIES*)
1,200	33	13	9
1,300	36	14	10
1,400	39	16	11
1,500	42	17	12
1,600	44	18	12
1,700	47	19	14
1,800	50	20	14
1,900	53	21	15
2,000	56	22	16
2,100	58	23	16
2,200	61	24	17
2,300	64	26	18
2,400	67	27	19
2,500	69	28	19
2,600	72	29	20

*Rounded to nearest whole number.

MEDICATION ALERT!

Talk to your doctor about whether lifestyle changes are enough to bring your cholesterol or blood pressure under control. Your doctor can prescribe many different medications to lower your LDL cholesterol, raise your HDL cholesterol, and lower your blood pressure.

Don't overeat. Being overweight or obese (see how to find out if you're at a healthy weight in the muscles section on page 134) raises your risk of high LDL cholesterol and triglycerides and low HDL cholesterol. A small 2004 study from the Washington University School of Medicine shows yet another good reason to limit your calorie intake. The study compared 18 people who practiced calorie restriction (CR) with 18 people of similar age who ate a standard American diet. The people in the CR group were 50 years old, on average, and ate between 1,112 and 1,958 high-quality, nutrient-dense calories daily. The other group ate nearly twice as many calories.[24]

The people practicing CR had extremely low LDL cholesterol and total cholesterol but high HDL cholesterol. In addition, their blood pressure was "remarkably" low. Their insulin and blood sugar levels were lower, too. And their average level of CRP—a marker of inflammation—was only 16 percent of the level found in the standard eaters.[24]

That doesn't mean you need to follow a CR diet. Cutting down your calorie consumption too much can be dangerous if you're not under a doctor's supervision. However, this small study illustrates that the quality of your calories is just as important as the quantity.

Eat more soluble fiber. Fiber is a carbohydrate found in plant foods that your body can't absorb. Hence, you don't get calories from it. Fiber comes in two types, which are distinguished by how they behave in your body. Soluble fiber dissolves in water and becomes a gel-like substance in your digestive tract. Insoluble fiber doesn't dissolve in water, and it helps "bulk up" your stool and improve your digestion.[21]

Though they're both beneficial, soluble fiber is especially important for heart health. As the stuff passes through your intestines, it helps trap fat and cholesterol from the food you've eaten, so they can't pass through the wall of your intestine and into your bloodstream. The NIH recommends that you get at least 5 grams of soluble fiber a day in addition to insoluble fiber. Ten to 25 grams is even better.[21] Look for soluble fiber in apples, bananas, grapefruit, oranges, pears, peaches, prunes, grapes, beans, black-eyed peas, lentils, carrots, barley, rye, oatmeal, and oat bran.

Make nondietary lifestyle fixes. Among the many, many barriers that smoking puts up between you and a long, healthy life, it raises your triglycerides, lowers your HDL, and damages your arteries. If you're still smoking, stop.[21] Also, get at least 30 minutes of moderate physical activity every day. Exercise helps raise your HDL cholesterol, lower your LDL, and prevent excess body weight.[21]

C-Reactive Protein

Inflammation is a process in which your immune system responds to something it regards as a threat. Many stages in the development of atherosclerosis, from when plaque forms to when it ruptures, involve inflammatory cells and chemicals. A substance called C-reactive protein, or CRP, is produced mostly by your liver and shows up when you have inflammation in your system. This test doesn't specifically measure inflammation in your arteries, but it may indicate that you're at a higher risk of heart disease.[26] Experts are still figuring out how your doctor should use the CRP test to help assess your risk of heart disease.

In 2003, the AHA and the Centers for Disease Control and Prevention (CDC) recommended a test called the highly sensitive C-reactive protein test, or hs-CRP, for people who may be at intermediate risk of a heart attack. It's intended to offer more sensitive information when used in addition to better-known biomarkers such as blood pressure and cholesterol.[27] The test itself is based on a blood sample, and results are measured in milligrams per liter (mg/L). A measurement below 1.0 mg/L is considered low risk, 1.0 to 3.0 mg/L is average risk, and above 3.0 mg/L indicates high risk. People in the high-risk category are about twice as likely to develop cardiovascular disease as people in the low-risk category.[27]

LOWERING CRP

As with cholesterol and tryglycerides, C-reactive protein levels can be influenced by our lifestyle choices. Studies [28] have shown that a diet rich in *Positively Ageless* foods (such as omega-3-rich fish as well as whole grains, fruits, and vegetables) [29] coupled with a physically active lifestyle [30] helps to promote optimal levels of CRP for a healthy heart.

Homocysteine

This is an amino acid in the blood that has been related to a higher risk of heart disease. Research suggests that homocysteine may promote plaque deposits in the blood vessels by damaging the lining of arteries. It may also promote blood clots. High blood levels of homocysteine have an inverse relationship to B vitamin levels, such as B_6 (pyridoxine), B_9 (folic acid), and B_{12} (cobalamin). These vitamins help break down homocysteine so that there is less opportunity for it to damage the arteries.

LOWERING HOMOCYSTEINE LEVELS

According to the AHA, high homocysteine levels aren't yet considered a major risk factor for cardiovascular disease, but everyone should include plenty of B vitamins in their diets, especially people at risk for heart disease. The *Positively Ageless* pantry provides ample B vitamins. Citrus fruits, tomatoes, green leafy vegetables, and grain products are excellent sources.

chapter 2

PREVENTING COMMON CANCERS WITH DIETARY CHANGES

As adults, most of us know how to play well with others, follow rules, and do our jobs. The same is true for the trillions of cells in our bodies.[31,32] All cells contain "instructions" in their genes that tell them how to behave properly. Cells work in concert to form tissues and organs. They divide and form new cells to replace those that have become worn-out or injured. Cells are even programmed to know when it's time to die after they've become too damaged to function. Normally they're happy to do so.[31,32] But sometimes a rebel cell disobeys the rules. This renegade cell can cause cancer.[31,32]

According to the American Cancer Society (ACS), the second-leading cause of death in the United States is cancer. Although young people can get it, about 77 percent of cancers are diagnosed in people over the age of 55.[33]

Many kinds of problems can damage the genetic instructions that keep your cells operating properly. Certain chemicals, like those found in toxins in the air, cigarette smoke, and processed foods such as cured meats, can cause this damage. Ultraviolet rays from the sun can harm the DNA in your skin cells. You can inherit defective DNA from your parents. Free radicals can damage it, too.[34]

Though your body can usually repair the problems that develop in DNA, sometimes the damaged cells just willingly die. Your immune system can also detect cells when they've gone bad and wipe them out. But sometimes a wayward cell escapes all these processes. It develops alterations in its DNA that defy natural cell death, and then it divides, reproduces, and creates more abnormal cells at a too-fast rate.[32]

This causes trouble near and far in the body. The growing collection of cancer cells—a tumor—may damage surrounding tissue. In response, the damaged tissue causes blood vessels to grow and supply it with food, depriving other tissues and organs of nutrition. Eventually, the cancer cells may enter a blood vessel or the lymph system and spread to other parts of the body, creating more abnormal growths (a process called metastasis).[35]

Experts aren't sure why cancer is more likely to strike as we get older. Perhaps our bodies become less able to repair faulty DNA. Perhaps our immune systems become less efficient at responding to the threat early in the process. Maybe our cells are more sensitive to carcinogens—the term for cancer-causing substances. Or maybe we're more likely to develop cancer when we're older because we've simply had more years of exposure to factors that increase the risk of the disease.[35] Whatever the cause, there's plenty you can do to reduce the likelihood that it will happen to you.

- About 30 percent of cancers are caused by exposure to cigarette smoke and other forms of tobacco. By not using tobacco—and avoiding other people's smoke—you improve your odds a lot.[2]

- Another 15 percent of cancers are linked to dietary factors: problems like too many calories, too much fat, too many harmful chemicals in certain foods, too few vegetables, and too little fiber. We'll explore all these factors and more later in this chapter.[32]

- Another 30 percent or so, including breast and endometrial cancers, are linked to the influence of hormones. Your food choices may help lower your risk for these cancers, too.[32]

Eating right and not smoking won't guarantee that you won't get cancer, but it will greatly reduce your risk. This chapter will focus on some of the main types of cancer that cause death and major life changes in women: breast, endometrial, and colorectal.

Biomarkers for Cancer

In the section on heart disease, you learned about biomarkers that tell you whether you're at risk of developing heart problems, such as elevated blood pressure and cholesterol. Unfortunately, when it comes to cancer, you don't have as many well-established biomarkers to assess your risk of developing the disease *before* it happens so you can improve your odds. Instead, most cancer screenings try to catch cancers in their earliest stages, before they get worse. Methods for detecting cancers, as well as more specific information on the most common types of cancer found in women, are listed below.

Reducing Risk for Cancer

Go natural. Hundreds of studies have found that as intake of fruits and vegetables increases, the risk of developing many kinds of cancer decreases. In 1992, researchers sifted through roughly 200 studies examining the relationship between fruits and vegetables and cancer risk. They found that people who eat few fruits and vegetables—those whose produce consumption puts them in the bottom one-quarter of the population—have about twice the risk of cancer, compared with people who eat lots of fruits and vegetables. Other research has found that eating fruit more than once daily is associated with a 75 percent lower risk of lung cancer. People who eat beans more than twice a week have been found to have a 42 percent lower risk of developing colon cancer than those who only eat them less than once a week.[36,37] The average American, however, probably doesn't eat enough of these foods to derive optimal cancer protection. [36]

Cancer cells progress through a number of stages in order to manifest a problem, and their progress can be arrested along the way. Many different plant chemicals—or *phytochemicals*—in fruits and vegetables can fight cancer in many different ways, including but not limited to their antioxidant power. Lycopene, for example, is a phytochemical found in tomatoes (and fruit such as watermelon and pink grapefruit) that has potent antioxidant properties. Though many studies have revealed evidence that lycopene may help decrease the risk of prostate cancer while working in concert with other nutrients, they don't support [38] the idea that lycopene works on its own. That's why it's important that you work a variety of foods into your diet each and every day. You want as many protective food chemicals as possible constantly interacting with your cells to prevent cancer.

See the sidebar on page 58 for an overview of just some of the protective chemicals found in fruits and vegetables. Remember: Look for fruits and vegetables with deep, rich hues. Paint your plate with reds, yellows, oranges, greens, and purples. These powerful nutrients and plant chemicals should come from real foods, where they number in the hundreds or thousands. Don't rely on antioxidants in pill form, whose only strength lies in the high price on the bottle. Most are made from individual constituents—they don't have the rich synergy that Mother Nature's vitamins supply naturally.

And remember that whole grains are anticancer plant foods, too. Whole grains contain phytochemicals, vitamins, and minerals with anticancer properties. These foods also tend to be good sources of fiber, which may help reduce your risk of some cancers.[39,40]

Steer clear of animal fats. Fat in the diet has been linked with a higher risk of cancer, but experts are still trying to figure out why. One reason might be that dietary fat packs a lot of calories, raising the risk of obesity, a risk factor for many types of cancer. Saturated fat, which is found in animal foods, seems to be particularly dangerous. A 1998 study of more than 32,000 people found that those who ate meat at least once a week had an 85 percent higher risk of colon cancer than people who didn't eat meat. That's another good reason to stick with lean proteins, fish, and fat-free or low-fat dairy products and keep red meat in your diet to a minimum.[36]

Be sure that fat calories don't provide more than about 25 percent of your daily calories, and stick with monounsaturated olive and canola oils and omega-3 fatty acids from sources such as fish and flax. The healthy omega-3 fats seem to help inhibit breast and colon cancer development.

Maintain a healthy weight. Being overweight and leading a sedentary lifestyle is linked to many kinds of cancers, including breast, colon, kidney, and uterine. Research has shown that obesity may account for 20 percent of all cancer deaths in women![40]

There are many reasons why being overweight could increase your risk. Calorie restriction, as discussed in the first section, might help prevent cancer by reducing inflammation, promoting DNA repair, and encouraging cells to die as programmed (a process called *apoptosis*).[41]

Make sure you keep your calorie intake at a level that will allow you to maintain a healthy weight or shed unnecessary pounds. Getting at least 30 minutes of exercise daily will help, too: A physically active lifestyle has been linked to a lower risk of many cancers. For example, a 2005 study that compiled the results of 19 earlier studies found that physical activity was associated with a 29 percent lower risk of colon cancer in women.[42]

PICK A PECK OF DIFFERENT PLANTS
FOR ALL THEIR BENEFICIAL CHEMICALS

Fruits, vegetables, and grains offer many different phytochemicals that can keep cancer from starting or inhibit its development. Here are just a few of the beneficial components you'll get from a variety of plant foods.

Allium compounds: These substances found in garlic, onions, and chives may make carcinogens less harmful. Allium compounds become primarily available to your system when the foods are cut, crushed, and heated.

Beta-carotene: This carotenoid pigment, when digested, produces more vitamin A than any other carotenoid does. It's also a powerful antioxidant. You'll find it in dark green leafy vegetables like kale and spinach and orange fruits and vegetables like carrots, pumpkins, and sweet potatoes.

Carotenoids: The vivid pigments that give foods their yellow, orange, and red colors act as protective antioxidants in your body. More than 600 carotenoids have been discovered; the more well-known ones include beta-carotene, alpha-carotene, and lycopene. Though high levels of preformed vitamin A from animal sources can be toxic, provitamin A from carotenoids can be very beneficial in fighting aging and decreasing risk of breast, cervical, colon, lung, and skin cancer.

Catechins: These fall into a larger family called phenols and show significant antioxidant power. You'll find them in rich supply in green and black tea and wine.

Ellagic acid: Pop a few strawberries, cranberries, blackberries, or walnuts and you'll get a burst of this cancer-fighting phytochemical.

Epigallocatechin-3-gallate (EGCG): This catechin found in tea possesses powerful antioxidant properties that play an important role in preventing cancer and cardiovascular diseases.

Drink in moderation. Drinking alcohol to excess is a well-known risk factor for a number of types of cancer, including cancer of the mouth and esophagus. One study found that people who drank at least 21 alcoholic drinks weekly had more than nine times the risk of one type of esophageal cancer. Even a drink or two a day can increase your risk of cancer of the breast and colon/rectum. The direct contact of the alcohol against the lining

Flavonoids: These are some of the most potent types of antioxidants found in plants. They've been the subject of lots of research and have been shown to help protect cells from carcinogens. They're found in a wide variety of fruits, vegetables, nuts, legumes, and tea.

Genistein: You'll find this in rich supply in soybeans, soy milk, tofu, and other soy foods. Genistein falls within a group of flavonoids called isoflavones, which are also referred to as phytoestrogens, or plant-based estrogens. Isoflavones may occupy estrogen receptors on cells, keeping your own estrogen from interacting with the cells. The verdict is still out on whether this can reduce your risk of breast cancer.

Indoles: You get these cancer-fighting compounds from cruciferous vegetables such as Brussels sprouts and mustard greens.

Isothiocyanates: These are also found in cruciferous vegetables and have been shown to have significant cancer-fighting ability.

Lignans: The richest source of these phytoestrogens is flaxseed, though you'll also find them in whole grains and soybeans. They may help protect you from cancers such as breast cancer by blocking the effects of your body's estrogen, although again, the evidence is still shaky. They're also antioxidants.

Limonene: This is found in citrus peel and herbs including dill, coriander, and fennel. Research has shown that it can help prevent cancer.

Quercetin: This flavonoid compound, abundant in onions, apples, grapes, and broccoli, works as an antioxidant, decreases inflammation, and helps inhibit cancer formation.

Resveratrol: Another flavonoid found in grape skins, grape juice, and wine, it helps fight cancer by inhibiting cell growth.

Salvestrols: These powerful anticancer phytochemicals, found in bitter flavors in fruits, exist in higher levels in organic produce than in produce treated with fungicide chemicals. Processed fruit products, such as juices, are lower in salvestrols because the bitterness is removed. Good sources of these chemicals are whole organic strawberries, cranberries, red wine (resveratrol is a form of salvestrol), blueberries, broccoli, and cabbage.

of the mouth and esophagus may help explain why it contributes to cancer there; as far as the breasts and colorectal area, experts aren't sure about the connection.[36] Again, if you choose to imbibe, aim for one drink daily.

Skip the cured foods. The rate of stomach cancer in America has dropped considerably since we started using refrigerators. In 1930, more than 30 out of every 100,000 American women died of stomach cancer.

Now fewer than 5 out of every 100,000 women do. Why? Because now that foods can be chilled and stored, Americans eat fewer pickled and cured foods, including vegetables and meats such as bacon and hot dogs, that tend to be high in preservatives called nitrites and nitrates. These are also added to foods to preserve color, enhance flavor, and limit growth of bacteria. They can become converted in your stomach to substances called nitrosamines, which are linked to an increased risk of cancer of the stomach and some other organs.[43,40]

When you're going to eat meat or fish, stick with fresh, nonprocessed choices rather than pickled, salted, or cured selections. Steer toward fresh fruits and vegetables, too. If you do have an occasional hankering for bacon, choose nitrate-free turkey bacon, available in most health food stores. According to some early research, drinking tea or adding garlic or a cruciferous vegetable such as broccoli to your meal may help cut down on the formation of any nitrosamines that are produced.[43,40]

Don't overcook your meats. In the first section of this book, you learned that cooking meats at high temperatures encourages the formation of harmful substances called AGEs. Those aren't the only problems that can arise in heavily cooked meats. Two other types of chemicals can develop: heterocyclic amines (HCAs) and polycyclic aromatic hydrocarbons (PAHs). HCAs are formed in muscle meats at high temperatures. PAHs result from fat dripping onto hot coals during grilling or barbecuing, which creates smoke that then collects on the meat. Both of these chemicals are suspected to be carcinogenic in humans.[40,44]

To reduce the amount of these chemicals in your food, stick with cooking methods that don't char your food. When you do use a grill, drain and blot away any excess oil if marinating the meat. Place your food on foil to prevent fat from dripping on the coals, and cut off any portion of food that gets blackened.[44]

Breast Cancer: What Raises Your Risk?

The breasts contain many lobules (milk-producing glands) and ducts (little channels that link the lobules to the nipples). According to the ACS, most breast cancers start in these structures. Factors that make you more likely to develop breast cancer include:

Your age. Breast cancer seldom strikes women in young adulthood. In

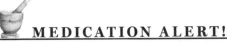

MEDICATION ALERT!

A drug called tamoxifen, which blocks the effects of estrogen in your body, may reduce your risk of breast cancer. If you're at high risk of developing the disease, taking the drug may be a worthwhile step to consider. Talk to your doctor if you're concerned that you need to do more than make lifestyle changes to reduce your risk of breast cancer.

most cases—about 80 percent—women are over the age of 50 when they develop the disease. By the time you reach 85, your chance of getting breast cancer is 1 in 8. One reason the disease becomes more likely with age is that your cells have more time to develop enough DNA damage to become cancerous.[45,46]

Exposure to estrogen. This is a hormone produced by your ovaries and, to an extent, your body fat. The cells in your breasts contain molecules called estrogen receptors. In your breasts, a surge of estrogen during the menstrual cycle causes cells to multiply (in case you were to become pregnant). At the end of the cycle, when your estrogen drops, those extra cells die off. If you have mutated cells in your breasts, the estrogen helps them multiply, too. They may later pick up more mutations that eventually allow them to become cancerous, and the estrogen gives them sort of a helping hand. Women who begin menstruating at an early age (before age 12) or enter menopause late (after 55) have more exposure to estrogen. So do women who are taking hormone replacement therapy containing estrogen. And women who have their first child late in life or never become pregnant are exposed to more estrogen, since the hormone is lower during pregnancy and breastfeeding.[45,47]

Family history. Women with relatives who've had breast and/or ovarian cancer—including male relatives with breast cancer—are more likely to develop the disease. According to the ACS, a woman whose mother, sister, or daughter has had the disease has about double the risk.[45,47] In addition, having defects in two genes, called BRCA1 and BRCA2, makes you more likely to develop breast cancer. The genes suppress irregular cell growth; when they're altered, they don't do their job, and cancer can result.[45]

Obesity. Carrying around extra weight, particularly after menopause, raises your risk of breast cancer. Fat around the waist may be more dangerous than on the hips and buttocks in terms of breast cancer risk.

OH BOY, LEARN ABOUT SOY!

Soy foods are a good source of protein, fiber, and a type of phyto-chemical called isoflavone. Here's a rundown of what you'll find in common soy foods.

SOY PRODUCT	PROTEIN (G)	FIBER (G)	APPROX. ISOFLAVONES (MG)
Frozen edamame (1/2 c)	6	6	35
Black soybeans (1/2 c)	9	5	40
Yellow soybeans (1/2 c)	13	3	38
Soy nuts (1/2 c)	30	15	40
Roasted soy butter (2 Tbsp)	6	1	17
Soy flour, full-fat (1/2 c)	15	4	50
Soy flour, low-fat (1/2 c)	24	9	50
Tempeh (4 oz)	16	7	40
Tofu, firm (4 oz)	12	0	40
Soy milk (1 c)	8	0	40

Remember, your body fat produces estrogen, too, which can help dangerous cells in your breasts multiply.[45]

Excessive alcohol. Having more than one drink a day raises your risk of breast cancer.[45]

Food chemicals. Certain chemicals found in overcooked red meats can raise your risk of breast cancer and other types of cancer.[47]

Breast Cancer: Screening Methods

Genetic testing. You can be tested for alterations in the BRCA1 and BRCA2 genes through a blood test. If these genes are altered, you're three to seven times more likely to develop breast cancer. If you know you have these genetic alterations, you may find a greater motivation to adopt lifestyle changes and take other steps that can reduce your risk of the disease.[48]

Breast exam. This involves feeling your breasts—or having a health professional check them—for lumps or other abnormalities.[49]

Mammogram. This takes an x-ray of your breast to find tumors that are too tiny to detect with your fingertips.[49]

Magnetic resonance imaging (MRI). This method uses a magnet and radio waves to generate pictures of the inside of your breasts, which has been shown to be more sensitive in detecting tumors than mammography.[49]

Tissue sampling. According to the NCI, several methods of sampling cells and fluid from the breasts are being evaluated to see how well they can detect or predict breast cancer. These include extracting cells and fluid through a thin needle from the areola, which is the area around the nipple (fine needle aspiration); pulling fluid from the nipple with a suction device (nipple aspiration); and inserting salt water into the nipple, then drawing it back out to examine its contents.[49]

Ultrasound. Though this method is used to distinguish between different types of lumps (such as benign cysts and dangerous tumors), it is not used for routine screening because it does not consistently detect certain early signs of cancer, such as tiny deposits of calcium in the breast (microcalcifications) that can't be felt but can show up on a mammogram. Ultrasound is also used to examine lumps that are hard to see on a mammogram or in conjunction with another screening procedure, such as fine needle aspiration. An ultrasound examination involves spreading a thin coating of lubricant jelly over the area to improve conduction of the ultrasound waves. As sound waves are reflected back from the tissues within the breast, the wave patterns create a two-dimensional image of the breast on a computer screen for evaluation.[49]

Endometrial Cancer: Risk Factors

This is the fourth most common type of cancer in women. It begins in the endometrium, or lining of the uterus. It shares many of the same risk factors as breast cancer.

- Your age. The disease typically strikes in a woman's early sixties.[50]

- Exposure to estrogen. Early menstruation, late menopause, having few or no pregnancies in one's life, and excess body fat all set the stage for higher estrogen levels, raising the risk of the disease. So does estrogen replacement therapy. [50]

KNOW THE ABCS OF OMEGA-6s AND -3s

Omega-3s and omega-6s are different groups of fatty acids. Two of them are essential, which means our body doesn't produce them, so it's essential that we get them from our diet. Alpha-linolenic acid, or ALA, is an essential omega-3 found in flaxseed, flaxseed oil, and (in smaller quantities) walnuts, almonds, olive oil, canola oil, and wheat germ. It is found in much smaller amounts in dark green leafy vegetables. Many of us do not eat enough of these foods. Linoleic acid, or LA, is an essential omega-6 found in saturated animal fats, vegetable oils, margarines, nuts, and seeds. Most of us eat *too many* of these.

Other important omega-3s are *not* essential to our diet because our body converts them from essential ALA. DHA (docosahexaenoic acid) and EPA (eicosapentaenoic acid) are two nonessential omega-3s that offer many health benefits. There are also nonessential omega-6s that our body can make from linoleic acid.

At one time, omega-3s were abundant in our diet. Now that we eat more processed and fast foods, most of us have become deficient in this important nutrient. Cold-water fish such as salmon, mackerel, and herring are stellar sources. Omega-3s' many benefits include:

- Controlling the production of beneficial hormones that promote a diverse range of functions affecting bone and heart health, cancer risk, and much more

- Helping to slow the aging process

- Conferring heart-protective benefits, such as encouraging healthy cholesterol levels, reducing blood clotting, and preventing irregular heartbeat

- Possibly reducing the need for steroids in conditions such as rheumatoid arthritis or inflammatory bowel disease (IBD)

- Possibly delaying or even preventing the onset of Alzheimer's disease

- Promoting softer skin, thus possibly minimizing the appearance of wrinkles

A deficiency of omega-3s, on the other hand, can lead to loss of vision, concentration, attention, or memory, as well as contribute to depression and many of the problems associated with aging.

■ Other cancers. Women who have had breast or ovarian cancer may be at higher risk.[50]

■ Fatty foods. These may raise your risk of endometrial cancer, particularly foods high in saturated fat, such as red meat and full-fat dairy.[50]

Endometrial Cancer: Screening Methods

According to the NCI, there are no standard screening tests for endometrial cancer. However, the familiar Pap test that looks for abnormal cervical cells may point to endometrial cancer. An ultrasound image of the uterus can detect the disease, too. A health professional can also take a sample of endometrial tissue and have it examined for cancer cells if he or she has reason to suspect cancer.[51]

Reducing Breast and Endometrial Cancer Risk

In addition to the general rules for cancer protection from your diet, follow these specific suggestions to further reduce your risk of breast cancer.

Reduce omega-6 fatty acids. The American diet is way too high in omega-6 fatty acids, which are found in sunflower, safflower, corn, and soybean oils and are added to many processed foods. These fatty acids may encourage cancer growth, while omega-3 fatty acids (such as those found in salmon) may discourage it. Diets high in omega-6s are associated with increased risk of breast cancer.

Eating a healthier ratio of omega-6s to omega-3s may help protect you against breast cancer. According to a paper in a 2006 issue of the *Journal of Nutrition,* although the research is still limited, evidence suggests that as your ratio of omega-3s to omega-6s goes *up,* your risk of breast cancer goes *down.* Cut down on your use of oils rich in omega-6s and kick up your consumption of foods rich in omega-3s, such as flaxseed and cold-water fish.

Eat some soy. Research has indicated that the phytoestrogens, such as genistein, found in soy might help prevent breast cancer by blocking the effects of your own estrogen. And scientists have theorized that lower incidence of breast cancer in groups of Asian women might be due to the high amount of soy in their diets.

Soy is a nutritious source of protein, so it's a good idea to have several servings a week. Mark Messina, PhD, an expert on the health benefits of soy, recommends consuming about two servings of soy per day to provide 15 to 20 grams of soy protein and 50 to 75 milligrams of isoflavones. This amount is recommended on a daily basis to derive many of soy's health benefits.

Overall, the research is conflicting about whether soy can help prevent breast cancer. It may reduce your risk only a little, and it may be particularly helpful if you start eating it at a young age. When I worked in research at Cedars Sinai, the most common question my breast cancer patients asked was whether or not they could or should eat traditional soy foods. Even though soy's phytoestrogens can block your own estrogen from affecting your cells, these plant estrogens may also stimulate tumor growth or interfere with anticancer medication. If you've had breast cancer in the past or have it currently, talk to your doctor about whether it's safe for you to eat soy foods.

Research shows that phytoestrogens may play a role in reducing your risk of endometrial cancer. A California study from 2003 compared the diet habits of 500 women who'd had endometrial cancer with 470 women chosen at random. Those who ate the highest amount of isoflavones—which are found in soy—had about 40 percent less risk of endometrial cancer.[52]

Fill up on fiber. Some research makes fiber seem like a useful tool in the fight against breast cancer: Vegetarians (who get lots of fiber) have lower breast cancer rates compared with nonvegetarians, and a high-fiber vegetarian diet may reduce the levels of estrogen in your blood. However, big studies have found mixed results. One study that pooled the results of 12 previous studies found that increasing fiber by 20 grams daily can lower the risk of breast cancer by 15 percent. But other large studies, following thousands of women for years, didn't find a connection.

Still, fiber provides many other health benefits, and fiber-rich foods are full of nutrients and phytochemicals that work wonders in the body. Fiber also provides satiety, so eating more of it may mean that you eat fewer calories overall. Make sure you get at least 25 grams of fiber each day.

Get plenty of fat-free or low-fat dairy and calcium-rich foods. Some studies have shown an inverse relationship between calcium and breast cancer—meaning that more calcium is linked with a lower rate of breast

DIG INTO CALCIUM-RICH FOODS
FOR DISEASE PROTECTION

B e sure to work these common sources of calcium into your meals and snacks on a regular basis.

CALCIUM-RICH FOODS	CALCIUM CONTENT (MG)
Yogurt, plain, low-fat (1 c)	415
Calcium-fortified orange juice (1 c)	308–344
Milk, reduced-fat (1 c)	295
Sardines, with edible bones (3 oz)	270
Salmon, canned, with edible bones (3 oz)	205
Soy milk, fortified (1 c)	200
Almonds, dry roasted (1 oz)	97
Broccoli, raw (1 c)	90
Cottage cheese (½ c)	75

cancer. A 2002 study, analyzing data on more than 88,000 women, found that premenopausal women who ate more than one serving of low-fat dairy foods daily had about 30 percent less risk of breast cancer than women who ate fewer than three servings a month.[53]

In addition, research on populations has found that those with more exposure to ultraviolet light had lower risks of breast cancer. Your body produces vitamin D when you're exposed to a few minutes of sunlight each day, and you can also get it in your diet, especially from fortified dairy foods. Get two servings of low-fat or fat-free dairy foods each day.

Pour yourself some green tea. Lab studies have found that a component in green tea called epigallocatechin-3-gallate—or EGCG, for short—kills breast cancer cells and blocks cancer progression in animals. The component seems to halt cancer development in its very early stages, before it can even get started. This may be why research has linked green tea consumption with a lower risk of breast cancer.

Have you had your cup of green tea today?

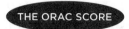

BREW A POT
OF THE CLOCK-STOPPING DRINK

As we're finding, some *Positively Ageless* foods that seem quite ordinary have extraordinary health benefits. For example, consider tea. Though we commonly think of tea as merely a familiar drink that can soothe or invigorate us, it's actually a powerful health enhancer and antiaging elixir.

Green or black, tea comes from the same plant. The distinction between the two is fermentation. Fermented tea leaves are black, a result of oxidized enzymes in the leaf. The potent concentration of antioxidants they contain is dependent on a variety of factors; most notably, the processing. Originally, researchers thought that fermentation caused lower antioxidant activity in black tea than green. But research is revealing that the difference is more qualitative than quantitative—in other words, the flavonoids that each contains are different.

GREEN TEA

Green tea is exposed to high temperatures immediately after harvesting, preserving the green pigment, which prevents the key antioxidant compounds, epigallocatechin (EGC) and epigallocatechin-3-gallate (EGCG), from being oxidized. Thanks to these flavonoids and other substances, green tea:

Colorectal Cancer: Risk Factors

This cancer arises in the colon, or large intestine. This is where digesting food travels after it leaves the small intestine. The last section of the colon is called the rectum—so these cancers are often called colorectal cancer. Most of the time, colorectal cancers develop over the course of years from abnormal growths called polyps. Factors that raise your risk of the disease include:[54,55]

■ Your age. The condition is more common after 50.

- Boasts cardioprotective benefits, including decreased cholesterol absorption, less clotting, and reduced oxidation of LDL cholesterol

- Suppresses cancer-cell activity in all stages of development; its most protective powers have been shown against stomach and colon cancers

- Boosts metabolism, as suggested by a study of EGCG; people who drank 3 or 4 cups of green tea daily burned an additional 80 calories per day

- Fights tooth decay with natural fluorine

BLACK TEA

Black tea's beneficial compounds are called thearubigens and theaflavins. In addition to rich flavor and color, they provide:

- More protection against skin cancers caused by ultraviolet radiation than green tea does

- Antibacterial and antiviral properties, such as killing the bacteria behind cavity-causing plaque.

TEA[1]	ORAC PER CUP
Green	2,951
Black	2,403
English breakfast	1,636
Earl Grey black	1,274

- Your race and ethnic background. African Americans and Jews of Eastern European descent are at higher risk.

- Family history. If close family members have had the disease, particularly before the age of 60, you're more likely to get it, too.

- Fatty foods. A diet high in animal fats raises your risk.

- Overweight. Carrying excess pounds can raise your risk of the disease.

- Smoking and drinking. Smoking makes you at least 30 percent more likely to develop colorectal cancer. Drinking alcohol excessively raises your risk, too.

- A sedentary lifestyle. Not getting enough physical activity puts you at higher risk of the disease.

Colorectal Cancer: Screening Methods

These tests can help you find out if you are in the early stages of colon cancer or, even better, if you have precancerous changes that should be removed before they turn dangerous.[56]

Fecal occult blood test. This provides a stool sample that a lab can analyze under a microscope for hidden—called occult—blood, a sign that something's amiss.

Sigmoidoscopy and colonoscopy. Both use a thin tube containing a light and a scope so your health care provider can examine your colon. A sigmoidoscopy views only your rectum and the bottom end of your colon; a colonoscopy looks at the entire length of the organ.

Barium enema. A special liquid is put into your rectum and coats the lining of your colon, which helps a subsequent x-ray make a more helpful image of the organ.

Digital rectal exam. Your health care provider feels the rectum with a gloved finger to check for growths or other abnormalities.

DNA stool test. According to the NCI, a new test being studied checks DNA in your stool for signs of genetic changes that could point to colon cancer.

Reducing Colorectal Cancer Risk

Get lots of fiber. Experts have speculated that fiber could help prevent colon cancer in a number of ways, including encouraging digested material to move more quickly, reducing the time that cancer-causing substances touch the colon; trapping and diluting cancer-causing substances; and encouraging growth of normal bacteria that help keep the colon healthy.[36]

Studies measuring the effects of fiber on large populations' colon-cancer rates have had mixed results. However, a European study involving 10 countries found that higher fiber intakes were associated with a 25 percent lower risk of colon cancer.[36] Be sure to get at least 25 grams of fiber from a variety of sources into your daily diet. Many plant-based foods that are high in fiber are rich in other nutrients that may help reduce your risk of cancer.

Cut down on meat. Red meat has been linked with an increased risk of colon cancer. One study that grouped the results of 13 other studies found that each increase of 3.5 ounces of meat eaten daily was associated with up to a 17 percent increase of colon cancer risk.[36] In addition, each increase of 0.88 ounces of processed meat eaten daily was associated with a 49 percent increase of risk! One deli sandwich may contain as much as 5 ounces of processed meat.[36]

Other studies have pointed to animal fat as a risk factor for colon cancer. Foods like red meat and whole-fat dairy foods are rich in saturated fat and cholesterol, which are also bad for your heart health. That's another good reason to stick to a diet that's heavy in vegetables, with the occasional chicken, turkey, or lean red meat as a side item, rather than vice versa.[36]

Get your dairy. Research has found calcium to be inversely related to your risk of colon cancer—in other words, as one goes up, the other goes down. Vitamin D also appears to be useful in reducing your risk of colon cancer.[36] Low-fat or fat-free milk, yogurt, and other dairy foods are rich sources of calcium and vitamin D. Make sure you get two servings of these foods each day, and choose other calcium-rich foods such as sardines, tofu, or broccoli when possible.

Find some folic acid. Studies of big groups of people have found that low folate intake is related to a higher risk of colorectal cancer. And research has shown that people who get supplemental folic acid have a 20 to 70 percent lower risk. Good dietary sources of folate (the form of the vitamin found in foods) include dark leafy greens, legumes, bananas, and broccoli. You can also find folic acid in some whole grain breads and cereals, which are specially fortified with the nutrient.

Stay active! Exercise helps keep digestive material moving along through your colon at a suitable pace, so harmful substances contained in the material have less time to interact with your colon. That's one more great reason to get moving for at least 30 minutes most days of the week.

chapter 3

DIGESTION: KEEP THINGS MOVING PROPERLY

As far as bodily systems go, your gastrointestinal system holds up relatively well as you get older. Although a number of digestive conditions tend to crop up more in the later years—and hormonal fluctuations at menopause can influence your digestion—your gastrointestinal organs don't generally lose much functioning simply due to age.[57] However, the conditions that do arise can be uncomfortable and even painful. They can also keep you from enjoying your activities and hamper your ability to eat a nutritious diet. That's not what healthy aging is all about.

Before we take a look at some common digestive complaints that you'll want to prevent, let's take a quick journey through a properly working gastrointestinal system (figuratively speaking, of course).

The Digestive System: Several Organs Forming One Route

The first stop along the digestive route is your mouth, though food doesn't stay here for long. Your teeth grind food into small particles and your saliva moistens it with enzymes, which begin to break down carbohydrates.[58]

Once you swallow, the food plunges down your esophagus toward your stomach. Waves of muscle action in the esophagus—called *peristalsis*—propel the food downward. A valve between the stomach and the esophagus opens to allow the material to enter. This hollow, muscular organ churns the food and mixes it with acid and more enzymes.

Eventually, the stomach releases its contents into the small intestine. Here the material encounters enzyme-rich fluid from the pancreas and another fluid from the liver called bile, which is stored in the gallbladder until needed.

These further break down carbohydrate, protein, and fat in the material.

The walls of your small intestine absorb the nutrients from the lique-fied food, and they're taken away through a network of blood vessels to your liver for processing. Fiber, which is indigestible, heads off to the colon, where it remains for a day or two. The colon absorbs extra fluid from the contents, and you expel the remaining material as stool.[58,59]

Problems in the System

Ideally, the foods and drinks you consume travel through your digestive system at a regular pace and in the right direction, and each organ pro-cesses the material without difficulty. But some problems that may be more likely to occur with age can occur throughout the system.

HEARTBURN AND GERD

The stomach is designed to handle its harsh digestive fluids without dam-age. The esophagus isn't supposed to touch them . . . but they can wind up there anyway. Sometimes the valve separating the bottom of the esopha-gus from the stomach doesn't seal tightly enough, allowing irritating acid to come into contact with the lining of the esophagus. This is called *reflux*. It causes heartburn (burning pain in the chest or throat) and a sour taste in the mouth.[60,619]

Occasional heartburn is annoying. When it happens more than twice a week or becomes persistent, it's a sign of a more serious problem called gastroesophageal reflux disease, or GERD, which you should discuss with your doctor. Persistent irritation can scar the esophagus and make it nar-row, creating swallowing problems. It may also cause changes in the cells in the esophageal lining, which can lead to cancer.[61] A number of control-lable factors can cause reflux or make it worse, including:[60,61,62]

- Obesity. The extra weight puts pressure against your stomach, pushing contents upward.

- Eating large meals. These fill up your stomach and take longer to pass into your small intestine.

- Eating certain foods. Some foods—including chocolate, mint, and anything fatty—can relax the muscles in the valve between the esophagus and stomach. This can minimize the barrier effect of the valve, leading to heartburn.

ULCERS CAN REALLY BUG YOU

Not too long ago, people attributed ulcers to stress and spicy foods. Though these factors can worsen the problem, we now know that peptic ulcers—little damaged spots on the lining of the stomach or beginning of the small intestine—are usually caused by bacteria.

Infections from a type of bacteria called *H. pylori*, which occur more often in people as they get older, allow harsh stomach acid to breach the mucous barrier that protects the stomach from its own contents. The acid causes an injured spot in the lining.

It's possible to confuse an ulcer with other forms of digestive upset. Symptoms include an aching sensation, typically a few hours after a meal or at night; pain relieved by antacids; and bloating. Your doctor can diagnose an ulcer by examining your stomach lining with a lighted scope on a long tube. *H. pylori* infection can be diagnosed with a simple blood test.

Treatment for ulcers typically includes a combination of drugs including antibiotics, medications to reduce stomach acid, and a drug to help protect the stomach lining from acid.[87]

Biomarkers for Heartburn and GERD

Doctors diagnose straightforward cases of heartburn and reflux by taking into account symptoms such as a burning pain in the chest, a sensation of food moving back into the esophagus, hoarseness, and an unpleasant taste in the mouth.[63,64] For more serious symptoms or problems unrelieved by lifestyle changes and medication—or if the doctor suspects complications—more complex tests include:[63,64]

- Inspecting the lining of the esophagus with a special scope

- Placing a sensor in the esophagus to measure acidity

- Having you swallow barium, which makes the outline of the esophagus show up better on an x-ray

Reducing Heartburn and GERD

Eat smaller meals. Putting less food into your stomach at one time means less material for your stomach acids to break down. Eat less at mealtime, but have more snacks. You'll have the same amount of food as usual, but divided throughout the day.

Shed excess pounds. If you're overweight, slimming down your abdomen can reduce pressure on your stomach, which pushes contents up into your esophagus. Wearing looser clothes and belts will also help lessen the pressure. Losing weight will make your clothes fit looser, too![65,66]

Eat your last meal well before bedtime. Acid in your stomach reaches its peak 2 or 3 hours after a meal. When you lie down, acid moves to the top of your stomach, where it can reflux into your esophagus more easily. So avoid eating within at least 3 hours of bedtime.[67]

Skip foods that worsen reflux. A number of foods can make heartburn and GERD more likely—and most don't play a significant role in a healthy diet, anyway. These include alcohol, fatty foods, peppermint, and chocolate, which may relax the valve between the stomach and esophagus; and coffee and (again) alcohol, which increase acid production.[67,66,65] Onions, garlic, tomatoes, and citrus are also linked to heartburn. These are nutrient-rich foods that you should cut out only if you have a good reason, so pay attention to whether you notice symptoms after eating these. If so, try them in smaller amounts. Cooked onions, garlic, and tomatoes may cause less heartburn pain than raw.

Stop smoking. The habit is also associated with worsened GERD, as it may increase stomach acid.[65]

LACTOSE INTOLERANCE

As you get older, your small intestine may produce less of an enzyme called lact*ase*. It acts on a sugar in dairy foods called lact*ose,* breaking it into smaller, simpler sugars that your small intestine can absorb. If undigested lactose heads on to your colon, the bacteria that live there break it down, producing gas and water, which trigger bloating and diarrhea. Symptoms— which also include cramps—begin 30 minutes to 2 hours after consuming the dairy food.[68,69] African Americans, Native Americans, and Asian Americans are more likely to have lactose intolerance than whites.[70]

Biomarkers for Lactose Intolerance

Common methods of diagnosing an inability to digest lactose include:

- A test in which you drink liquid containing lactose after fasting, then have several blood tests over the following hours to measure your glucose. If your glucose rises, that means your body was able to break the sugar down and digest it. If your glucose doesn't rise, it's a sign that the lactose didn't get into your bloodstream—hence, you're lactose intolerant.[71]

▓ A test in which you drink liquid containing lactose, then have the hydrogen in your breath measured. If undigested lactose gets to your colon, bacteria there ferment it and create hydrogen. Thus, hydrogen in your breath is a sign that you don't digest lactose properly.[71]

Treating Lactose Intolerance

One simple way to reduce symptoms of lactose intolerance is to avoid dairy foods. However, these are important sources of many nutrients, including calcium and vitamin D, which are crucial for preventing osteoporosis. If you do choose this route, make sure you get your daily calcium quota from other foods. Good sources include fortified whole grain cereals, collard greens, sardines containing bones, spinach, fortified orange juice, fortified soy milk, edamame (soybeans), turnip greens, black-eyed peas, and canned salmon with bones. Rather than cut out dairy altogether, however, try taking these steps to lessen the symptoms of lactose intolerance.

Eat a little at a time. Most people with lactose intolerance can handle 12 grams of lactose—the amount in a cup of milk—with minimal problems. Consuming dairy along with a meal will make it more tolerable, too, because it slows down the passage of lactose through your digestive system.[67]

Eat yogurt. The lactose in yogurt containing active bacterial cultures is easier to digest than the lactose in milk. Just remember to stick with low-fat or fat-free brands.[67]

Take supplemental lactase enzymes. If you don't have your own internal supply, the next best thing may be to get it elsewhere. Look for types of milk processed with lactase, which are designed to be more digestible. Or ask your pharmacist how to use over-the-counter lactase supplements to help you digest dairy foods more easily.[67]

GLUTEN INTOLERANCE

Another condition, called celiac disease, involves intolerance to gluten, a protein found in wheat, rye, oats, and barley. When a person with this con-

MEDICATION ALERT!

Your doctor can recommend a variety of over-the-counter or prescription medications to neutralize stomach acid or reduce its production in order to treat heartburn and GERD.

dition eats gluten, the immune system responds in a way that damages structures in the small intestine that absorb nutrients. Symptoms include gas, bloating, abdominal pain, fatigue, malnutrition, and weight loss.[72,73]

Although this condition generally appears in childhood, it can also crop up in later life. If women develop it in adulthood, it tends to be in their thirties. In adults, the condition is twice as common in women than men.[57]

Biomarkers for Gluten Intolerance

Your immune system produces antibodies against a wide range of things that it considers a threat, and sometimes it forms these against substances that shouldn't pose any danger—such as gluten. So, to diagnose celiac disease, doctors check a blood sample for specific antibodies created to confront gluten. If you have high levels of these antibodies after consuming gluten, your doctor will want to take a small sample of the lining of your small intestine to check for telltale signs of damage.[72,73]

Treating Gluten Intolerance

Unlike lactose intolerance, this problem really has just one solution with no alternatives: Avoid gluten. Even small amounts can cause intestinal damage in people with celiac disease, which may not cause noticeable symptoms.[74]

Since most diets rely heavily on grains containing gluten (wheat, rye, barley, and possibly oats)—and the stuff is used as an additive in so many foods—making this change takes careful concentration. It's beyond the scope of this book to discuss every food that's free of gluten, but in general the following grain foods will probably figure prominently in a gluten-free diet: rice flour, cornmeal, cream of rice cereal, rice wafers, cornmeal crackers, corn tortillas, popcorn, quinoa, and sorghum flour.[75]

In addition, check food labels to see if the food is called gluten free, and work with a dietitian familiar with this condition. Though health food stores used to be the sole source of gluten-free products, conventional supermarkets now offer an increasing variety of these foods in response to the growing awareness of gluten intolerances and allergies.[74]

GALLSTONES

As mentioned earlier, your liver produces bile—a liquid containing cholesterol and other substances—that's contained in your gallbladder until you need it to digest fat from the food in your small intestine. Then the fluid travels down a duct to your small intestine. However, this fluid can harden and form "stones." Most stones are made mainly of cholesterol. Your body may produce less bile as you get older, which could contribute to an increased risk of stones.[59] Being female also raises your risk.[57]

Most gallstones don't cause symptoms. If they're small enough, they travel unnoticed through the bile duct and into your small intestine. However, larger ones can get stuck in the duct and cause pain, nausea, vomiting, and indigestion. These blockages can be serious health threats because they can also block the ducts leading from the pancreas and liver, causing inflammations or infections.[59]

Eating too infrequently or eating too little fat—perhaps when dieting—may contribute to gallstone formation because the gallbladder doesn't empty as regularly. Insufficient physical activity may also be a factor. Exercise may stimulate hormones that cause the gallbladder to get rid of its contents more quickly, or the faster movement of food through the intestine triggered by exercise may keep the gallbladder working properly.[76]

Biomarkers for Gallstones

In many cases, gallstones that aren't causing symptoms are found during tests for other conditions. If you are having symptoms, common methods of diagnosing gallstones include making images of your gallbladder using an ultrasound device on your abdomen or with a CT machine, which uses x-rays to create a detailed image.[77,78]

Reducing Risk for Gallstones

Women who are older and overweight are looking at three factors for increased risk of gallstones. You can't do anything about the first two risk factors (being female is one of them), but you can change the third. A 2005 study of more than 8,000 women from cities around America found that the women who got the least amount of exercise were 59 percent more likely to get gallstones than the women who exercised the most. That's another good reason to rack up 30 minutes of physical activity most days of the week.[76]

A diet that's low in fat—particularly saturated and trans fats—may also reduce your risk. However, getting an adequate number of daily calories will help ensure a regular flow of fluid from your gallbladder—so if you need to lose weight, don't do it with crash dieting.[63]

CONSTIPATION

One of your colon's main jobs is to extract water from your stool so it's not wasted. If stool doesn't move rapidly enough, your colon may remove too much water. This leaves the material hard and dry, and it's more difficult to expel it during a bowel movement.[79,80]

Symptoms of constipation include having bowel movements fewer than three times a week, passing hard stools, or needing to strain. Many people report more problems with constipation as they get older, perhaps because contents may simply pass through the colon more slowly. But other causes that you can control may play a role, too.[80,57]

Physical activity stimulates your intestines to keep their contents pushed along their route. If your body doesn't get a lot of movement, your bowels may not, either. Not drinking enough fluids plays a big role. If your body senses that it needs more fluids because you're not drinking enough, it will try to remove more from the contents of your large intestine. A diet low in fiber—such as containing too few fruits, vegetables, and whole grains and too many processed foods—encourages constipation, too. Plenty of fiber attracts more water and keeps stool soft, bulky, and moving along its way.[57,79,80]

Biomarkers for Constipation

Your doctor may want to check if any medications you take may be causing your constipation or if other conditions, such as thyroid problems, may be contributing to sluggish digestion.[80]

Reducing Constipation

The tips for reducing constipation are similar to those for many other digestive ailments: lots of fluids, plenty of fiber, and regular exercise. Follow the *Positively Ageless* meal plans and recipes featuring fresh

PROTECT DIGESTION WITH BEANS AND LEGUMES

Beans and legumes may be inexpensive foods, but their antiaging benefits are priceless. They're excellent sources of folic acid, calcium, iron, potassium, zinc, and antioxidants. They provide steady energy because of their abundance of complex carbs, fiber, and protein.

However, some of the complex sugars they contain are hard to digest, which can lead to discomfort and gas. These sugars require special enzymes to break them down. If the enzymes are absent from your digestive tract, the sugars begin to ferment, causing intestinal distress and gas. So when preparing dried beans, soak them before cooking. This initiates the process of dissolving the complex sugars and minimizes their uncomfortable side effects.

In addition, supplemental enzymes are available over the counter to help you digest the complex sugars. They can be taken just before your first bite of beans. High heat inactivates the enzymes, so they cannot be added to beans during cooking.

Here's a listing of the antioxidant power in common beans and legumes, as measured in ORAC units.

BEANS AND LEGUMES (DRY) PER ¼ CUP	ORAC
Small red beans	6,864
Red kidney beans	6,630
Pinto beans	5,932
Black beans	2,091
Navy beans	1,287
Black-eyed peas	1,129

vegetables and fruits, whole grains, and beans. Drinking plenty of fluids will ensure that the fiber helps your stool move at a brisk rate through your colon. And getting adequate exercise most days of the week will help stimulate your colon to keep its contents moving along.

IRRITABLE BOWEL SYNDROME (IBS)

This condition is twice as likely to affect women as men. People most often visit their doctors with symptoms of IBS—which include cramping, bloating, and diarrhea or constipation (sometimes both)—between the ages of 30 and 50.[81,82]

According to the NIH, IBS isn't a disease—it's a cluster of symptoms indicating that the colon isn't working properly. The cause is unknown, but it's thought that during IBS the nerves and muscles that control the colon's function become extrasensitive. Since it's more common in women, hormonal changes may contribute to the problem.[82]

Working on ways to better handle stress may help quiet IBS symptoms. Plus, you can make many changes to your eating habits that should help. We'll discuss those later in this section.

Biomarkers for IBS

Your doctor diagnoses IBS based on your symptoms, though you may need tests such as a colonoscopy to rule out other intestinal problems.[82]

Treating IBS

Eat small, frequent meals. Digesting a large meal may trigger cramping and diarrhea. Try eating four or more small meals (or healthy snacks) during the day instead of three large meals.[82]

Experiment with problem foods. Foods that are more likely to contribute to symptoms include chocolate, alcohol, caffeinated or carbonated drinks, and fatty foods. Bloating and diarrhea can also result from sugar alcohols, such as sorbitol, which are used to sweeten low-calorie candies and other foods. Lactose intolerance can also appear to be IBS, so cutting down on dairy foods may relieve symptoms. If gas and bloating are a problem for you, reducing broccoli, cabbage, beans, and other vegetables that encourage gas may help.[82,85] Try eliminating each of these foods from your diet one at a time to see if you notice relief. It may help to keep a food diary to track what you eat and how you feel afterward. If you do cut out a fruit, vegetable, or source of calcium, be sure to eat more of an alternative food that provides the same nutrients.[82]

Eat plenty of fiber. If you're not getting enough fiber, start eating more vegetables, beans, whole grains, and fruits. Unfortunately, some of these foods may actually make gas and diarrhea worse. Slowly ramp up your consumption of fiber-rich foods over several weeks to minimize these side effects.[83]

Drink plenty of water. Adequate fluid helps keep your digestion working properly. Remember to limit or avoid sodas, coffee, and alcohol.[83]

Seek relief from stress. Stress can make symptoms worse. If you have issues that are causing stress in your life, invest time in finding healthy solutions or ways to deal with them. One good stress-relieving practice is regular exercise, which helps keep your digestive system working smoothly, too![82]

DIVERTICULOSIS AND DIVERTICULITIS

Sometimes pressure in your colon can cause weak spots to bulge outward, creating little hollow sacs that protrude from the outer wall of the organ. This is called diverticulosis, and by the age of 50, about one-third of the American population has it. Experts think that a low-fiber diet contributes to diverticulosis, since the problem is uncommon in areas of the world where people eat plenty of fiber. Lack of fiber contributes to constipation, which can lead to increased pressure within the colon.[57]

These pouches can become infected or inflamed, leading to a related condition called diverticulitis. Symptoms include pain in the abdomen—usually on the lower left side—and possibly fever, nausea, and chills. Diverticulitis can be a serious (even fatal) problem that causes infection and bleeding that may require surgical treatment.[84]

Dietary steps, particularly adding more fiber to reduce constipation, can make you less likely to develop diverticulosis. Other eating habits, which we'll discuss a bit later, may reduce your risk of diverticulitis, too.[85,84]

Biomarkers for Diverticulosis and Diverticulitis

Since diverticulosis typically doesn't cause symptoms, doctors often find it when checking your colon for other problems. To diagnose potentially serious diverticulitis, your doctor may run blood tests to look for signs of infection or make images of your colon with a CT scan.[85,84]

Treating Diverticulosis and Diverticulitis

Making sure that you eat 25 to 30 grams of fiber a day can help you avoid diverticulosis in the first place, according to the American Dietetic

Association.[86] This amount promotes normal bowel movements and helps prevent the development of diverticulosis. Eating a high-fiber diet rich in whole grains, vegetables, and fruits can reduce the risk of diverticulitis, too. These additional steps may also help prevent flare-ups if you have diverticulosis. If a flare-up does occur, a low-fiber diet usually is recommended until the area heals.

Drink plenty of fluids. An ample supply of fluids helps prevent constipation, and adequate fluid is vital when you're eating a high-fiber diet. Get at least 8 cups of water daily; you can substitute green tea, low-fat milk, or juice for some of that fluid.

Avoid itty-bitty edibles. Small foods like sesame and sunflower seeds, popcorn, and nuts can get stuck in diverticular pouches and create inflammation. If you have diverticulosis, the NIH recommends avoiding these.

Exercise. As in other conditions linked to constipation, exercising for at least 30 minutes almost every day will help ensure that you stay regular.

chapter 4

THE IMMUNE SYSTEM: STAY SAFE FROM INVADERS (AND YOURSELF!)

It's pretty easy to envision how your heart pumps blood as it beats day after day. You may know what your brain looks like, and you can probably picture how the organs of your digestive system process food.

Your immune system is not as easy to understand. This complex system is composed of different organs and tissues located throughout your body, along with an array of cells that they produce. These cells, in turn, produce hormones and other substances that help them communicate with each other, identify invaders that could harm your body, and serve as an elegant defense system to fight these invaders.[88]

As you age, your immune system becomes less efficient in certain ways. It may become less able to contain a threatening virus or emerging cancer cells. It may also turn aggressive and attack your own body, causing conditions like rheumatoid arthritis. Or a natural process of the immune system—inflammation—may contribute to a variety of age-related disorders, including heart disease and Alzheimer's disease.

Before we discuss how lifestyle changes can help keep your immune system in tune, let's learn a little more about how it works and how it can go astray.

The Immune System in Health and Sickness

One of the immune system's normal functions is to recognize and confront foreign invaders that don't belong in the body—like splinters, viruses, harmful bacteria, parasites, fungi, and cancer cells. The critical point here is that its normal function is to confront or attack *foreign* things, not cells that belong in your body.[88] The following are some of the more important cells in the immune system.

Lymphocytes: white blood cells that come in several varieties. B cells produce antibodies, which help fight foreign invaders, such as bacteria. The presence of these intruders, known as antigens, alerts the immune system. Antibodies then attach to the antigens, warning other immune system cells of their presence so they can respond to the threat, too.[88] T cells are lymphocytes that recognize antigen threats. "Helper" T cells coordinate the immune response, and "killer" T cells attack cells that have become infected or cancerous.

Phagocytes: white blood cells that "eat" microbes and other foreign invaders. When in the bloodstream, they're called monocytes; when they get into tissues, they're called macrophages.

Natural killer cells: These contain chemicals to take out invaders.

Cytokines: proteins that immune cells produce to communicate with each other and trigger certain activities. Some cytokines play a role in inflammation by bringing immune cells to the area to repair injuries or tackle foreign invaders.[88]

A streamlined process allows this network of immune cells to recognize legitimate threats, coordinate the appropriate response between different cells, then attack the problem and clean up afterward. Major immune problems that become more likely with age are:

Autoimmune diseases. Your immune system becomes less effective at telling the difference between your body's cells (which are *supposed* to be there) and harmful outsiders. The powerful defenses can go astray and attack your own body's cells and tissues. Sometimes the damage is subtle, and other times it is progressive and deadly.[89,90,91] More than 80 kinds of autoimmune diseases can develop, including rheumatoid arthritis and lupus.[89,90]

Inflammation. You're more prone to unwanted inflammation. Some researchers have called this inflamm-aging![92] Inflammation is actually supposed to be a helpful process. Your body responds to injuries and infections with a host of immune system cells and chemicals that increase bloodflow to the area, tackle invaders, minimize the damage, and clean it up. All this activity helps explain why an infected cut or a sprained ankle is red and warm.[93]

Sometimes, inflammation becomes chronic and is a source of damage, rather than a helpful function. At sites of smoldering inflammation, you'll find macrophages and cytokines encouraging inflammatory activity. Free radicals are also produced, which further fuels the fire.[94]

Inflammation is thought to play a role in many age-related conditions, including atherosclerosis and heart disease, Alzheimer's disease, vision-robbing age-related macular degeneration (AMD), and rheumatoid arthritis. In addition, chronic inflammation is associated with a number of kinds of cancer; it may play a role in the development of 15 percent of all cancer cases![94,95]

Less ability to fight cancer and infections. Age is a major risk factor for cancer, and other processes aside from inflammation are thought to play a role. For example, the aging immune system becomes less efficient at detecting cancer cells and nipping them in the bud.[91]

Certain infections become more common and more dangerous in older people, too, such as influenza, pneumonia, and infectious endocarditis, a heart ailment. These may be due to immune cells responding less efficiently to antigens or producing fewer antibodies when antigens are discovered.[90] Research has also found that monocytes and macrophages don't eat threatening invaders as well when you're older, and natural killer cells may perform more poorly.[92]

Biomarkers of Immune Impairment

A number of tests can shed light on how your immune system is functioning. Often, these are used to find out information on serious conditions including AIDS, certain cancers, heart disease, and autoimmune diseases. Tell your doctor if you think you should be tested for any of these conditions. Biomarkers for immune-related problems include:

C-reactive protein. As discussed earlier in the heart section, the presence of CRP indicates acute inflammation. Though this measure is used to assess flare-ups of rheumatoid arthritis and lupus, elevated CRP can also point to cancer or a variety of infections.[96]

Sed rate. The sedimentation rate—"sed rate"—measures how fast red blood cells, or *erythrocytes*, drift downward in a test tube containing a sample of your blood. When cells sink quickly, it's a sign that you have inflammation.[97,98] The sed rate cannot diagnose a specific condition but can indicate a variety of inflammatory conditions, including rheumatoid arthritis, lupus, and thyroid disease.

White blood cell count. If analysis of your blood sample indicates that the number of white blood cells is higher than normal, it may be a sign of infection, an inflammatory process in your body, severe stress, or leukemia. Your white blood cells may also be measured as part of a complete blood count, which also looks at red blood cells and hemoglobin.[99]

Measurement of T and B cells. A laboratory measures these immune system cells by analyzing a blood sample. A low T cell count may indicate a viral infection, an immune deficiency disorder, cancer, or simply aging, while an unusually high level could indicate several forms of cancer. Increased or decreased B cell counts may also mean cancer.[100,101]

The *Positively Ageless* Guide to a Healthy Immune System

Getting plenty of the following nutrients in your diet will help ensure that your immune system stays strong and ready to pounce on potential troublemakers, from viruses to mutated cells—and keeps its focus on your enemies and not your healthy cells, tissues, and organs.

Minimizing Autoimmune Diseases and Inflammation

Get plenty of omega-3s. Groups of people who eat a lot of fish—such as the Japanese and Greenland Eskimos—have lower rates of heart attacks and chronic inflammatory and autoimmune diseases. Antiaging fats called omega-3 fatty acids, found in seafood, seem to play a role.[102]

A balanced intake of omega-3s and omega-6s offers optimal health benefits. Ideally, the ratio of omega-6s to omega-3s should be less than 4 to 1; even better, 1 to 1. In other words, we should be eating closer to equal amounts of omega-3s and omega-6s.[102,103]

But, once again, that's very different from our traditional Western diet. The ratio of omega-6s to omega-3s in the typical American diet is about 18 to 1. The result: aging effects ranging from inflammatory disorders to increased risk for heart attack, stroke, and cancer. It's time we put omega-3s front and center in our diets to slow our aging clocks. The omega-3-rich

Positively Ageless diet can help you restore this balance and may even help to reverse disease processes.

Exactly how omega-3s discourage inflammation—and how omega-6s promote it—is complicated enough to make your head spin. When you eat an omega-6 called linoleic acid (LA), you use it for energy or convert it to a substance called arachidonic acid. This, in turn, can be converted into a number of proinflammatory chemicals.[102,103]

However, when you consume an omega-3 fat called alpha-linolenic acid (ALA), you might use it for energy or convert it to a substance called eicosapentaenoic acid (EPA). EPA competes with the processes that turn arachidonic acid into those inflammatory chemicals. When ample EPA is on hand, these processes convert it into relatively harmless products . . . and don't get around to the arachidonic acid. It's kind of like ensuring that your lawn is properly seeded and watered so grass fills out the yard and weeds never have an opportunity to grow.[102,103] Omega-3s are found in abundance in certain fish as well as in flaxseeds and some nuts and nut oils (see the sidebar on page 90 for specific amounts in different foods). The government hasn't established a recommended daily intake of omega-3s. However, experts suggest an amount anywhere from 1.5 to 4.5 grams of omega 3s each day.[104,105,106]

Shed pounds. Research has linked obesity with higher levels of CRP, a marker for inflammation. A number of weight-loss studies have found that losing just 10 pounds can lower your CRP by 10 percent. A 2006 study divided 47 overweight and obese adults into two groups, one of which received exercise and diet instruction and one that didn't participate in any lifestyle changes. The lifestyle-modification group lost weight, improved cholesterol levels, and enjoyed a "significant" drop in high-sensitivity CRP measurement.[107]

If you're carrying around too much weight, you may be fueling excess inflammation. Cut down your calories and bump up your physical activity.[108]

Get the right fats. Watching other kinds of fats in your diet—aside from the ratio of omega-6s to omega-3s—can help you reduce inflammation even further. Diets high in saturated and trans fats have been linked in studies to higher levels of inflammation biomarkers. In one study, the women who ate the most trans fat had 73 percent higher levels of CRP than women who ate the least.[108]

HOW DO YOU KNOW
IF YOU'RE DEFICIENT IN OMEGA-3s?

Though the guidelines are still emerging, a few laboratories are equipped to measure blood levels of omega-3 fatty acids. Because the science is still new, the FDA hasn't approved the testing, so your health insurance won't pay for it. Still, it's a measurement you might find worth knowing as you start living the *Positively Ageless* lifestyle.

The analysis measures omega-3 fatty acids (EPA + DHA) in your red blood cells (erythrocytes). The results reflect your dietary intake over a period of about 3 to 4 months, which is how long it takes to achieve a measurable change of omega-3 fatty-acid levels in your tissues. Some fatty-acid tests measure levels found in plasma, which is not as sensitive. This short-term measurement is more susceptible to variations in your recent diet, while erythrocyte measurements reflect long-term intake.

The best way to cut down on saturated fat is to eat less red meat and full-fat dairy products. To cut out a lot of trans fat—which is stuff you don't need in any amount—steer away from margarine and chips, cookies, and other processed baked goods. More and more of these foods nowadays are free of trans fats, but they still don't necessarily fit into the *Positively Ageless* antiaging plan.[108] Replace these fat sources with omega-3s—such as flaxseed and fish—and monounsaturated fats like canola oil.

If you drink alcohol, stick with red wine. It's not wise to start drinking alcohol for its health benefits, but research[109] has found an association between a daily glass of red wine and reduced inflammation.[18] Resveratrol, a compound in red wine, has exhibited an antioxidant effect against inflammatory free radicals. Compounds found in fruits, vegetables, tea, and spices have similar effects.

Get your antioxidants. A diet high in antioxidants may help protect you from inflammation. Studies have found that a high intake of fruits and vegetables reduces levels of CRP and a cytokine involved in inflammation called IL-6.[110]

A 2006 study of more than 600 older women found that higher blood

SERVE YOURSELF A HEAPING DOSE OF OMEGA-3s

You learned a lot about how omega-3s can help prevent cancer and quench the fire of inflammation. Your body can convert an essential omega-3 called ALA into EPA and DHA, or you can get EPA and DHA directly from your foods. The following chart summarizes the foods that will provide you with a sizable amount of omega-3 fatty acids. (The *Positively Ageless* recipes later in the book will also tell you how many grams of omega-3s they contain.) This number is a total of the ALA and EHA/EPA.

FOOD	ALA	EPA/DHA CONTENT
Pacific herring, baked (3½ oz)	0	1.2 g EPA/0.9 g DHA
Chinook salmon fillet, baked (3½ oz)	0	1.0 g EPA/0.7 g DHA
Anchovies (3½ oz)	0	0.8 EPA/1.3 g DHA
Farmed Atlantic salmon (3½ oz)	0	0.7 g EPA/1.5 g DHA
Greenland halibut fillet (3½ oz)	0	0.7 g EPA/0.5 g DHA
Sockeye salmon (3½ oz)	0	0.5 g EPA/0.7 g DHA
Wild coho salmon (3½ oz)	0	0.5 g EPA/0.5 g DHA
Flaxseed oil (1 Tbsp)	7.25 g	
Whole flaxseed (1 Tbsp)	4.4 g	

levels of the antioxidant mineral selenium and antioxidants called carotenoids were associated with a lower risk of death. According to the authors, these factors may help improve longevity by reducing oxidative damage and inflammation.[110]

Other anti-inflammatory substances found in plant foods include polyphenols (found in blueberries, blackberries, and raspberries) and quercetin (red grapes, broccoli, and red and yellow onions).

Keeping Your Immune System Strong

Make room for vitamin A. Some of your internal body parts interact constantly with the outside world and the health threats that it sends your way.

Your sinuses, lungs, mouth, stomach, and the rest of your digestive system are lined in a layer of cells called epithelial cells. These are situated close together and covered in a layer of mucus, making it hard for germs to penetrate your system.[88] One of vitamin A's most important jobs is keeping this epithelial barrier strong. When your diet is deficient in vitamin A, you can develop gaps between epithelial cells, allowing germs to slip through.[111]

The recommended daily allowance[112] of vitamin A is 2,333 IU daily for women. Vitamin A from animal foods is called *preformed vitamin A*. Because it is a fat-soluble vitamin, it is found in the fat of animal foods such as liver, whole milk, and some fortified food products. There are lots of reasons to limit our intake of animal products due to their high levels of saturated fats and cholesterol. But this form of vitamin A can also become toxic when the body stores too much of it.

A better place to get vitamin A is from colorful fruits and vegetables. This precursor form is called *provitamin A carotenoid*, which converts to vitamin A in our bodies. Provitamin A carotenoids are abundant in darkly colored fruits and vegetables such as cantaloupe, sweet potatoes, spinach, and carrots.

FOOD	SERVING SIZE	VITAMIN A CONTENT (IU)
Carrots, cooked, sliced	1/2 c	13,418
Spinach, cooked	1/2 c	11,458
Kale, cooked	1/2 c	9,558
Carrot, raw	7 1/2 in	8,666
Cantaloupe, cubed	1 c	5,411
Spinach, raw	1 c	2,813
Papaya, cubed	1/2 c	766
Mango, sliced	1/2 c	631
Peach	1 medium	319
Pepper, sweet, red, raw	1 ring, 3 in diameter × 1/4 in thick	313

See that you get enough C. Health experts have long known that vitamin C plays a crucial role in our immune health. Nobel Prize winner Linus Pauling began studying this micronutrient more than 4 decades ago, initially as a prophylactic for the common cold. In later years, he studied its value in fighting flu, infections, and diseases related to the aging process and observed the vitamin's high concentration in white blood cells. When these cells are low in vitamin C, the deficit is associated with poor immune function.[111]

Some enthusiasts of the vitamin have urged people to take megadoses to prevent or treat colds and other respiratory infections, but the evidence supporting this use is shaky.[111] Still, vitamin C is well known as a powerful antioxidant. Your immune system is especially prone to damage from oxidation, and one of the many ways vitamin C can help your immune system is by preventing free-radical damage to the DNA in your immune system's cells.[20] The RDI[112] for vitamin C is only 75 milligrams per day, but the *Positively Ageless* diet will provide much more than that. Good sources include the following foods.

FOOD	SERVING SIZE	VITAMIN C CONTENT (MG)
Guava	1 medium	165
Red bell pepper	½ c	95
Orange	1 medium	60
Broccoli, cooked	½ c	60
Strawberries	½ c	50
Papaya	½ medium	48
Green bell pepper	½ c	45
Grapefruit, white	half	40
Cantaloupe	½ c	35
Mango	1 medium	30
Tangerine	1 medium	25
Cabbage greens, frozen, boiled	½ c	25
Spinach, raw	1 c	15

Get plenty of vitamin E and selenium. Research [113,114] has found that when vitamin E is low, inflammation tends to be higher and the immune response to threats is diminished. Getting more in your diet helps reverse this problem—inflammation fades and immune health improves. Vitamin E is also a powerful free-radical-quenching antioxidant, helping to protect your immune system from oxidation.

Be sure to get at least 15 milligrams of vitamin E in your diet every day[112] from foods like the following:[111]

FOOD	SERVING SIZE	VITAMIN E (ALPHA-TOCOPHEROL) CONTENT (MG)
Wheat germ oil	1 Tbsp	20.3
Almonds, dry roasted	2 Tbsp	3.7
Sunflower seed kernels, dry roasted	2 Tbsp	3.0
Hazelnuts, dry roasted	2 Tbsp	2.2
Spinach, cooked	½ c	1.6
Broccoli, cooked	½ c	1.2
Peanuts, dry roasted	2 Tbsp	1.1
Kiwifruit, without skin	1 medium	1.1
Mango, peeled, seeded, and sliced	½ c	0.9
Spinach, raw	1 c	0.6

Selenium is also an important player in preventing free radical damage. This mineral is a component of glutathione peroxidase, an enzyme that's part of your body's natural antioxidant system. It helps prevent free radicals from forming—and vitamin E stops the chain reaction that results if free radicals begin damaging other molecules. It also stimulates the creation of T cells and encourages activity of your immune system's macrophages and natural killer cells.[111,115] Aim for 55 micrograms of selenium[112] every day. You'll find it in the following foods.

FOOD	SERVING SIZE	SELENIUM CONTENT (MCG)
Brazil nut, dried	one large	91
Cod, cooked	3 oz	32
Turkey, light meat, roasted	3½ oz	32
Chicken breast, skinless, roasted	3½ oz	20
Egg, whole	1 medium	14
Cottage cheese, low-fat 2%	½ c	12
Rice, brown, long-grain, cooked	½ c	10
Garlic, chopped	2 Tbsp	2.5

Think zinc. Many Americans aren't getting enough zinc in their diets or are barely getting enough to cover their needs. This mineral plays a role in many immune-system activities, and when your system runs short of it, you're more susceptible to infections. Evidence from many studies

ASK A CHICKEN FOR AN OMEGA-3 BOOST

Conversations about omega-3s in foods have traditionally focused on fish. But in recent years, an improved source of omega-3s has been finding its way into supermarkets and onto dinner tables: the egg.

You can now buy eggs containing extra omega-3s; they're produced by giving chickens a diet containing flaxseed. Flaxseed contains an omega-3 called ALA, and eggs from these hens contain extra ALA in the yolk.

One large egg enriched with ALA contains about 225 milligrams of omega-3, compared with 80 milligrams in a regular egg. As a result, the *Positively Ageless* diet encourages using omega-3-enhanced eggs in all your recipes and meals calling for eggs. They cost a bit more than regular eggs, but they're yet another source of a key antiaging nutrient that's too often scarce in our diets.

supports the importance of getting enough zinc. You'll find zinc in the following foods. Try to get at least 8 milligrams daily.[112]

FOOD	SERVING SIZE	ZINC CONTENT (MG)
Oysters, raw	3 medium	16.0
Pork tenderloin, lean only, cooked	3 oz	2.5
Yogurt, plain, low-fat	1 c	2.2
Yogurt, fruit, low-fat	1 c	1.6
Chickpeas, mature seeds, canned	½ c	1.3
Swiss cheese	1 oz	1.1
Milk, any kind	1 c	0.9
Chicken breast, skinless, roasted	half	0.9
Cheddar cheese	1 oz	0.9
Mozzarella cheese part-skim, low-moisture	1 oz	0.9
Cashews, dry roasted	2 Tbsp	0.8
Kidney beans, California red, cooked	½ c	0.8
Pecans, dry roasted	2 Tbsp	0.7
Mixed nuts with peanuts	2 Tbsp	0.55
Flounder or sole, cooked	3 oz	0.5
Almonds, dry roasted	2 Tbsp	0.5
Walnuts, black, dried	2 Tbsp	0.5

Get more B$_6$. This water-soluble vitamin has many effects on the immune system. It plays a role in the production of the amino acid cysteine, which is used to make glutathione. This substance, in turn, may help support the function of your T cells.[116] RDAs for B$_6$ increase for both men and women after age 50. From ages 19 to 50, women need 1.3 milligrams daily.[112] After 50, women need 1.5 milligrams daily. You'll find B$_6$ in the following foods.

FOOD	SERVING SIZE	VITAMIN B$_6$ CONTENT (MG)
Banana	1 medium	0.68
Garbanzo beans	$\frac{1}{2}$ c	0.57
Chicken breast, skinless	half	0.52
Pork loin, lean only	3 oz	0.42
Rainbow trout	3 oz	0.29
Avocado, sliced	$\frac{1}{2}$ c	0.20
Sockeye salmon	3 oz	0.19
Tuna, canned in water	3 oz	0.18
Wheat bran, crude or unprocessed	$\frac{1}{4}$ c	0.18
Peanut butter	2 Tbsp	0.15
Spinach, cooked	$\frac{1}{2}$ c	0.14
Sunflower seeds, kernels, dry roasted	2 Tbsp	0.12
Lima beans	$\frac{1}{2}$ c	0.10
Walnuts, English/Persian	2 Tbsp	0.07
Soybeans, green, boiled	$\frac{1}{2}$ c	0.05

Go for a probiotic boost. Health experts are putting a lot of focus on the use of probiotics to prevent and treat a variety of diseases. According to Sandra McFarlane, PhD, of the University of Dundee in Scotland, by the age of 60 the number of "friendly" bacteria populating the GI tract can be reduced by up to a thousandfold. Many scientists believe that this in turn can lead to an upset in the balance of the immune system, less resistance to infection, less tolerance to a variety of antigens, and an increase of allergic responses.

A poor diet that's high in fat, sugar, and white flour doesn't help you maintain an optimal GI environment and a strong immune system. Probiotics are live bacteria that offer health benefits when you consume them. Deliberately eating bacteria might seem odd, but many types of yogurt contain bacteria—referred to as "live cultures" on the label—and you probably don't give these invisible ingredients a second thought.

Some strains of probiotics are well known to enhance people's immune systems. Research has found that people who drank milk containing lactobacillus and bifidobacterium strains for 3 weeks had increased activity of phagocytes (immune cells that respond to threats by eating them). Supplemental probiotics in the diet may help address the decreased phagocyte activity that occurs with age.[117] There isn't an established RDA for probiotics, but excellent sources include yogurt, kefir, and miso, all part of the *Positively Ageless* pantry.

Hydrate yourself. Getting plenty of fluid is important for bringing nutrients and oxygen to your cells and carrying toxins away from them, which is generally important for good health. Make sure you drink at least eight 8-ounce glasses of water each day, in addition to a couple of cups of green tea; its EGCG has anti-inflammatory properties.[118]

Practice the other lifestyle improvements. Another benefit of regular exercise is an immune system boost. Exercise may help antibodies and white blood cells circulate more rapidly in your system; it reduces the stress-related hormones that may make you ill; and it causes your body temperature to rise, which may slow down bacterial growth and help you do a better job of fighting off bacteria.[119]

And if you smoke—stop already! If you don't, steer clear of other people's smoke. Research has found that long-term exposure to tobacco smoke causes your T cells to function poorly, which may explain why smokers are more likely to develop respiratory infections.[120]

chapter 5

FIGHT FATIGUE FOR A HIGH-ENERGY LIFE

Is your wrinkle count on the rise due to lack of sleep? Are you too tired for sex? If the only thing you want to do in bed is sleep, you're not alone. Feeling run-down and tired is very common; studies have shown that if you ask 100 people if they're fatigued, about 50 of them will say yes.[121]

More than 10 million people visit their doctors every year with concerns about fatigue, and women are twice as likely as men to mention this problem to their doctors. Complaints about fatigue reach a peak during the late teen years and early twenties (aren't young people supposed to be full of energy?) and again in the sixties and beyond.[121]

Fatigue can be caused by all sorts of minor lifestyle problems, including poor sleep habits, feeling overstressed, an unhealthy diet, and lack of exercise. A variety of medications can play a role, too.[122] However, fatigue is also a symptom of many medical conditions. Some are minor and some are quite serious. These include:[121,122]

- Allergies

- Anemia

- Cancer

- Coronary heart disease or congestive heart failure

- Depression

- Diabetes

- Food allergies

- Liver disease

- Sleep apnea

- Thyroid disorders

Another condition called chronic fatigue syndrome (CFS) is marked by severe fatigue that's not helped by resting, as well as muscle and joint pain, unrefreshing sleep, memory or concentration problems, and other symptoms. A diagnosis of CFS requires a prolonged period of fatigue—at least 6 months. The condition, which has unknown causes, is four times more common in women than men and seems to strike people most often in their forties and fifties.[123]

If you have extreme fatigue that's not getting better after a few weeks of rest and self-care, talk to your health care provider. You may need to have your medications reviewed to see if they're making you feel tired. You may also need further testing to find an underlying cause of your fatigue,[122] such as problems with your thyroid. This gland at the base of your throat produces hormones that regulate metabolism. When it doesn't create enough hormones—a condition called hypothyroidism—symptoms include fatigue, lethargy, and weakness. Women are at greater risk of this condition than men, and it becomes more common after 50. When the thyroid produces too much of a hormone—called hyperthyroidism—the problem can also result in fatigue.[125,126]

This section will cover ways to prevent and treat garden-variety fatigue that's due to controllable lifestyle factors. If your symptoms are the result of a serious medical condition, including CFS, talk to your doctor or a registered dietitian about ways to relieve your symptoms with dietary and other self-care steps in addition to medical treatment.

Biomarkers for Fatigue

Tests for fatigue may include the following to discern whether serious conditions may be playing a role in waning energy levels.[124,121]

- A complete blood count (CBC) to assess your red and white blood cells, which offers clues about anemia or infection

- Erythrocyte sedimentation rate to check for inflammatory conditions

- Blood tests to assess your thyroid's function

- Chest x-rays, tests of heart function, and tests for other potential conditions based on any other symptoms you have besides fatigue

The *Positively Ageless* Guide to Feeling Energetic

If you have a clean bill of health, but your energy account still feels bankrupt, the following diet and lifestyle fixes can give you the jump-start you need to stay up and running all day long.

Fill up with fiber. When your colon isn't moving its contents along speedily enough, you become constipated. And being constipated can make you feel sluggish and lackluster. Eating plenty of fiber, as you know, can help keep your heart healthy and cut your risk of colon cancer. It's great that fiber can help you sidestep those diseases, but it can be hard to appreciate the benefit of *preventing* problems year after year. However, when you notice a little extra spring in your step due to superior digestion, it's easier to understand how much good those 25 or more grams of daily fiber are doing for your health and your energy level.

Keep fueled with fluids. Your cells depend upon a river of fluid to bring them the oxygen and nutrients they require to function and to carry toxins away. When the fluid in your body dries up, your cells—which make tissues, which in turn make organs—don't work as well. In addition, fluid is necessary to keep all those high-fiber foods moving through your digestive tract. Keep a steady stream of water—and some green tea—flowing into your body during your waking hours. Set a water bottle on your desk at work. Take a drink whenever you walk through your kitchen or past a water fountain. Drinking a glass of water before each meal will also fill you up so you're inclined to eat less.

Get plenty of protein. Lack of protein can contribute to fatigue. In addition, your body needs a steady supply of protein to keep your muscles strong. When your muscles are weak, you may be dragging at the end of a day filled with chores and other physical activity. Be sure to get enough protein each day from lean poultry, soy foods, beans and legumes, and low-fat or fat-free cheeses and other dairy foods.

It's recommended that you get 30 percent of your calories from protein (and 45 percent from carbs and 25 percent from fat). To figure out how many grams of protein you need each day, follow this formula, which uses 1,500 calories as an example.

$$1{,}500 \times 0.30 = 450 \text{ calories from protein}$$

Then convert the calories to grams.

$$450/4 \text{ calories per gram} = 112.5 \text{ g of protein required each day,}$$
$$\text{which we'll round down to } 112$$

Now break it down to protein grams per meal and snack.

Breakfast	28
Snack 1	14
Lunch	28
Snack 2	14
Dinner	28

Keep your blood sugar steady. When you eat foods high in simple carbohydrates, like white pasta, cookies, and doughnuts, they convert rapidly to sugar, and in turn your blood glucose (also a sugar) jumps. Your pancreas then produces a rush of insulin so the glucose can enter your cells. Afterward, your blood sugar drops. If your sugar spikes and drops too suddenly, you can be left foggy-headed and tired.

A better way to go is to keep your blood sugar on more of an even keel. You can learn how to do this in the diabetes portion of the hormones section, starting on page 137. The basic points, though, are to:

- Eat small, frequent meals, rather than a few big meals. Make sure you eat a nutritious breakfast instead of going all the way to lunch without food.

- Choose mostly complex carbohydrates (like whole grains) rather than simple carbohydrates.

- Have some protein with each meal or snack. It helps slow the digestion of any carbs that you also eat. High-fiber *Positively Ageless* foods further enhance this effect.

Get plenty of B vitamins. The B vitamins all play roles in the many complex cycles and reactions that allow your body to turn food into energy. B vitamins are water-soluble, however, which means your body doesn't store them, so you need to steadily replace them. If you want to feel active and lively, you need to eat foods that provide an abundance and variety of B vitamins.

Drink only in moderation. Excessive alcohol can cause you to grow fatigued in many ways: It dehydrates you. It's a sedative. It disrupts your sleep. And it can cause B vitamin deficiencies.[122]

Pure alcohol contains about 7 calories per gram, which makes it nearly twice as caloric as carbohydrates or protein (both contain about 4 calories per gram)—and just below the 9 calories per gram that fat delivers. Additionally, your body burns alcohol calories first, before fat, carbs, or protein. That means it slows down the burning of fat. So if you want to lose weight or reduce excess body fat, keep your daily libations to a minimum. Again, aim for one drink a day, and don't have it within a few hours of bedtime, or it may disrupt your sleep.

Make sure you're getting enough iron. This mineral is a component of hemoglobin, the molecule in red blood cells that carries oxygen throughout your body. Deficiency of iron can cause fatigue.[127]

According to the National Library of Medicine, women are much more likely than men to have an iron deficiency. In fact, one out of five women is iron-deficient (and women who menstruate heavily are at extra risk due to blood loss).[127] But before you run out and grab a jar of supplements, keep in mind than too much iron can have a *pro*-oxidant and *pro*-aging effect. Check with your doctor before loading up on iron supplements.

The *Positively Ageless* diet should provide all the iron you need each day, plus it tastes much better than pills. The current RDA for iron for premenopausal women (ages 19 to 50) is 18 milligrams per day. For postmenopausal women (ages 50+), it's 8 milligrams per day.

Here are some foods that are good sources of iron.

FOOD	SERVING SIZE	IRON CONTENT (MG)
Soybeans, cooked	½ c	4.4
Spinach, cooked	1 c	3.7
Lentils, cooked	½ c	3.3
Pumpkin seeds, hulled, roasted	2 Tbsp	2.6
Bran muffin	1 medium	2.5
Garbanzo beans	½ c	2.4

(continued)

(cont.)

FOOD	SERVING SIZE	IRON CONTENT (MG)
Lima beans	½ c	2
Mackerel, canned, drained	3 oz	1.75
Pita bread, whole wheat	1 small	1.5
Lean ground beef	3 oz	1.4
Blackstrap molasses	1 Tbsp	1.2
Pork tenderloin, lean	3 oz	1
Lean ground turkey	3 oz	1
Oyster, raw	1	1
Pine nuts	2 Tbsp	1
Almonds, dry roasted	2 Tbsp	0.8
Sorghum flour	2 Tbsp	0.7
Shrimp, cooked	3 medium	0.44
Walnuts, chopped	2 Tbsp	0.4
Tomato, fresh, med	1	0.4

Exercise. Getting a workout might seem like it would just tire you out more—but it actually energizes you. When you're more fit, you're better able to handle the physical demands of your lifestyle. Exercise improves your mood, helps you handle stress better (depression and stress can leave you fatigued), and promotes better sleep. If you're not getting 30 minutes of exercise on most days, start working more deliberate physical activity into your schedule. It doesn't have to be 30 minutes at once—three 10-minute periods will work, too. Just don't exercise too close to bedtime; it can keep you awake.

Skip the caffeine. Sodas and coffee provide a temporary pick-me-up, but eventually caffeine's stimulation wears off, leaving you groggy again. So you reach for another, setting up a vicious cycle. And too much caffeine during the day can interfere with your sleep, setting you up for a fatigued tomorrow. Keep caffeinated drinks to a minimum, make green tea your "vice" of choice, and avoid highly caffeinated beverages during the late afternoon and evening. Here's a look at the amount of caffeine found in common drinks.

HOW CAFFEINE WORKS ITS MAGIC

The average American adult sips about 200 milligrams of caffeine a day, mostly from coffee. This is considered a moderate intake, and for most people it's not associated with any health risks. However, as little as 200 milligrams can make some people feel nervous and anxious. In addition, caffeine can increase heart rate, cholesterol levels, blood pressure, and anxiety—so it may not be advisable for everyone.

Caffeine is similar in structure to adenosine, a chemical found in the brain that slows down its activity. Since the two compete, the more caffeine you drink, the less adenosine is available up to a point. That's why caffeine temporarily heightens concentration and wards off fatigue.

The caffeine in green tea is surrounded by tannic acid compounds, which slow its release into the bloodstream. This effect, in addition to an overall lower caffeine level, results in fewer feelings of agitation or jitters that you sometimes get from coffee.

BEVERAGES AND OTHER PRODUCTS	SERVING SIZE	CAFFEINE CONTENT (MG)
Coffee, brewed	8 oz	137
Black tea, brewed	8 oz	65
Green tea	8 oz	50
Iced tea, black, instant	8 oz	47
Espresso	2 oz	42
Dark chocolate, bittersweet	1 oz	20
Natural unsweetened cocoa powder	1 Tbsp	12
Decaf green tea	8 oz	5
Decaf coffee, brewed	8 oz	2

Practice good sleep hygiene. Along with avoiding exercise, alcohol, and caffeine near bedtime, the National Sleep Foundation offers these tips for getting better sleep.[128]

■ Go to bed and wake up on a regular schedule, even on the weekends. Sleeping late on some days will throw off your body's internal clock.

HOT CHOCOLATE: A TASTY TREAT THAT DOES YOUR BODY GOOD

Ounce for ounce, cocoa beans are perhaps the richest source of antioxidants. Cocoa powder has a higher concentration of antioxidant polyphenols than any other chocolate product—it contains nearly twice the amount found in dark chocolate bars and four times that in milk chocolate bars. But it *doesn't* have all of the added pro-aging fat and sugar.

Cocoa's abundance of polyphenols is acidic, which means the antioxidant numbers are reduced when cocoa powder is alkalized. Dutch process cocoa is a method that adds alkali during processing to create consistent color, flavor, and texture. To ensure that you get a product with no added alkali—and the most antioxidants—choose "natural" when shopping for cocoa powder.

However, natural cocoa powder is high in starch, which makes it difficult to dissolve in liquid. To prevent lumps, add cold liquid to dissolve the powder in recipes. This helps separate the starch particles so lumps won't form. Try the *Positively Ageless* Hot Chocolate recipe on page 277. Sources for natural cocoa powder are found on pages 352 and 353.

CHOCOLATE AND COCOA[3]	ORAC PER TBSP
Natural cocoa powder	4,100
Dutch cocoa powder	2,000
Unsweetened chocolate, grated	1,986

- Do something relaxing before bedtime. Avoid stimulating yourself with exciting movies or aggravating yourself by paying bills.

- Keep your bedroom cool, dark, and quiet, and use the room only for sleeping and sex.

- Finish dinner at least 2 hours before bedtime. A full belly can keep you from settling comfortably into bed, and it can contribute to heartburn.

Also, if you feel sleepy and tired during the day, you may have sleep apnea. About 18 million Americans have this condition, in which tissues in your throat block your airways while you sleep, causing you to stop breathing, perhaps hundreds of times per night.[129] People with apnea frequently awaken to resume breathing, though they may not even remember it. Your bed partner may notice that you snore heavily or stop breathing. Other symptoms include morning headaches and falling asleep easily during the day.[129]

If you think you may have this problem, discuss it with your health care provider. To treat apnea, doctors often recommend a special machine that provides pressurized air through a mask over your nose and mouth to keep you breathing while you sleep.[129]

chapter 6

THE *POSITIVELY AGELESS* PROGRAM FOR AGE-PROOFING YOUR VITAL FUNCTIONS

At the end of each weekly section, you'll find an overview of specific tips to follow to incorporate the *Positively Ageless* diet into your lifestyle. These tips are broken down into stages. "Make One Change" is a list of easy-start changes. If you can only make one change per week, pick one from this list. "Quick Start" includes tips and strategies that are important but may take a bit longer to incorporate into your life. Suggestions you should follow for maximum antiaging benefit are listed in "Young for Life."

In addition, we've included a week's worth of meal plans that utilize the *Positively Ageless* ingredients. You'll find recipes for many of these menu items in the recipe section toward the back of the book.

The RDIs for various vitamins and micronutrients listed throughout this book are the minimal amounts required to avoid deficiencies and prevent chronic disease. For optimal antiaging nutrition, a daily omega-3 supplement and a potent multivitamin are recommended. Please see Shopping Resources (page 351) for specific recommendations.

Make One Change

If you feel able to make only one change in your life, pick it from this list. Research has shown these to be the most important strategies for slowing the aging clock.

Lose the cigarettes! In addition to substantially raising your risk of cancer, smoking helps form those distinctive wrinkles around your lips. If you're still smoking, make an appointment with your doctor to discuss how you can quit most easily. Prescription medications may help with nicotine withdrawal. Also, many state health organizations and the American Lung Association offer cessation hotlines, programs, and other services to help you quit.

Get a face-lift—for your kitchen. The contents of your fridge and cupboards mirror your health. If your shelves are loaded with sugar and white stuff—chips, crackers, microwave popcorn packets (with oil and "flavorings")—and your freezer is filled with ice cream treats, it's time to take out the garbage. Remember, the prize for eating white stuff, processed foods, and soft drinks is a ticket on the Wrinkle Express. Toss the "fogy food" and make room for your new best friends. The prize for eating *Positively Ageless* foods is a slow ride to a healthy longevity.

List it! Buy a magnetic shopping list and keep it on your refrigerator. Constantly update it with items you need for your next trip to the supermarket. Use the *Positively Ageless* pantry starting on page 108 to select your choices. This may seem like a given, but I am underscoring this for those of you who will find most of the *Positively Ageless* foods new to your kitchen. Until you familiarize yourself with them and really start to enjoy them (and appreciate their benefits), it's like starting over. You're shopping in a new way for the first time, and you really do need to rethink (and forget) your old habits.

Measure it. If portion sizes are your downfall, invest in a few tools to help you get a handle on this. If you like to cook, you probably have measuring cups and spoons on hand already. Additionally, invest in a food scale to weigh foods for consistency. After measuring your foods for a week or so, you'll be able to make fairly accurate estimates by eye. What you learn at home will guide you when you dine out, too. You'll know how much to eat and how much to wrap up and take home. Food scales range from a few dollars to $30 or more.

Unstick it. Since you'll be minimizing your use of added fats, be sure that you have a couple of great nonstick sauté pans on hand. One large pan is perfect for stir-fries or cooking for a crowd. A small one is ideal for making an omelet or to sauté a piece of chicken or fish for a solo meal.

Buy a basket. It's time to make fruit more accessible. Keep the basket in a convenient place, such as near the entry door or kitchen, so it's easy to pick up a healthy antiaging snack when hunger strikes. Plus, the vibrant colors will be a constant reminder to continually replenish your antioxidant levels.

CLOCK-STOPPER'S PANTRY

The following nutrient-dense, omega-3-rich, antioxidant-packed foods should provide the backbone of your meal ingredients. Use this section to help you compose your shopping list each week.

Vegetables

Artichokes

Asparagus

Avocados

Beets

Bell peppers

Broccoli

Brussels sprouts

Cabbage

Carrots

Collard greens

Corn

Eggplant

Garlic

Ginger

Kale

Mushrooms

Mustard greens

Onions

Peppers

Pumpkin

Radicchio

Romaine lettuce

Spinach

Squash

Sweet potato

Swiss chard

Tomatoes

Watercress

Fruits

Apples

Apricots

Bananas

Blackberries

Blueberries

Cherries

Cranberries

Dried plums

Grapefruit

Grapes and raisins

Kiwifruit

Lemons

Limes

Mangoes

Melons

Oranges

Plums

Pomegranates

Raspberries

Strawberries

Whole Grains and Seeds

Brown rice

Buckwheat/kasha

Bulgur wheat

Flaxseed

Millet

Oats

Pumpkin seeds

Quinoa

Steel-cut or rolled oats

Sesame seeds

Sorghum flour

Stone-ground cornmeal

Sunflower seeds

Whole wheat flour

Wild rice

Beans and Legumes

Black beans

Black-eyed peas

Fava beans

Garbanzo beans (chickpeas)

Kidney beans

Lentils

Peanuts

Pinto beans

Red beans

White beans

Soy Foods

- Edamame
- Miso
- Soybeans
- Soy milk
- Tofu

Unsalted Nuts

- Almonds
- Brazil nuts
- Cashews
- Hazelnuts
- Pecans
- Pine nuts
- Pistachios
- Walnuts

Dairy (preferably organic)

- Kefir
- Low-fat and fat-free milk
- Low-fat and fat-free yogurt
- Low-fat and fat-free cheeses, including ricotta and cottage cheese

Lean Proteins

- Chicken (organic, free-range skinless white meat; non-hormonally raised, if possible)
- Nonhormonally raised beef (lean beef cuts include eye of round, sirloin tip, top round, bottom round, top sirloin, flank steak)
- Pork tenderloin (occasional)
- Turkey (skinless white meat)

Omega-3 Eggs

Omega-3-Rich Fish

- Anchovies
- Herring
- Mackerel
- Salmon
- Sardines
- Tuna

Antioxidant-Rich Spices and Fresh Herbs

- Cinnamon
- Cloves
- Cocoa powder (natural, un-sweetened)
- Cumin
- Curry powder
- Dill
- Garlic
- Ginger
- Lavender
- Mint
- Mustard
- Onions
- Oregano
- Parsley
- Rosemary
- Saffron
- Sage
- Thyme
- Turmeric
- Vanilla

Sweeteners

- Agave nectar
- Brown rice syrup
- Dark honey (such as buckwheat)
- Sorghum syrup

Beverages

- Beer
- Black tea
- Green tea
- Milk, organic fat-free or 1 percent
- Red wine
- Soy milk (unsweetened)
- Water
- White wine

Count 'em. Figure out your calorie requirements (see the formula on page 30), and if have you have a few pounds to lose, remember that your calories going out through physical activity must be greater than your calories coming in through antioxidant-filled food and drink.

Schedule it. If you haven't had a medical checkup in a while, it's time to call your doctor. Prepare for the visit with a list of any new symptoms or concerns that have developed since your last visit.

Quick Start

These strategies are a little more involved, but the benefits will reflect the additional effort you're spending. They'll provide a jump-start for measurable results in a short period of time.

Go organic. If you can afford to buy all organic food, do it. You'll trim a lot of pesticides and other unwanted chemicals from your diet. At the very least, budget for organic dairy products and eggs.

Load up on antioxidants. When you shop with your *Positively Ageless* list in hand, you can more easily restock your antiaging arsenal with wholesome foods and ingredients, and you'll be less likely to buy the junk you used to eat. These are your most important purchases. What you put in that shopping cart now predicts your health and longevity later. Once you know where to find all you need in the supermarket and local health food stores, you'll be set. You won't have to go scouting again.

Go nuts. Stock up on a variety of nuts to keep on hand for snacking, all the better if they're still in the shell. They'll be fresher, plus having to crack them will keep you from eating too many *and* you'll burn a few extra calories in the process. Remember that nuts are a source of healthy fats, omega-3s, and vitamin E. One solitary Brazil nut packs more than 100 percent of your daily requirement for age-busting selenium.

Bag it—tea bags, that is. Stock up and experiment with different blends and find your favorite way to prepare it. Hot or iced; with lemon, a slice of ginger, or a few mint leaves; just don't forget the incredible antioxidant bang in this powerful libation. Aim for a cup each day. We'll gradually increase this amount by Week Four.

Fiber up! Go slow with improving your fiber intake, though. It will take a week or so for your body to adjust to more fiber, so aim for at least 3 cups of fruits and vegetables a day, mostly veggies. (We'll work up to 4

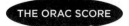
GO CRAZY FOR NUTS

For years, many women have considered nuts forbidden foods based on their fat content. However, given their protein content and other components, they're actually quite nutritious.

Along with antioxidant vitamin E, nuts contain essential fats such as omega-3s. Brazil nuts are a powerhouse of selenium, a mighty antioxidant. Nuts also provide cholesterol-lowering effects. Alpha linolenic acid (ALA), particularly in walnuts, converts to omega-3s, which promote decreased levels of harmful cholesterol.

Because they're high in fat, nuts and nut oils become rancid if exposed to light and heat. For optimal shelf life, keep nuts stored in airtight containers in the freezer.

Here's an overview of the antioxidant content in nuts, measured in ORAC units.

NUTS	ORAC PER 2 TBSP
Pecans	2,548
Walnuts	1,923
Hazelnuts	1,370
Pistachios	1,130
Almonds	633
Peanut butter	549
Peanuts	450
Cashews	284
Macadamias	240
Brazil nuts	202
Pine nuts	102

cups a day by Week Four.) And be sure your grain choices are whole grains. These foods will provide the antioxidants to keep those free radicals at bay and anti-inflammatory compounds to boost your immune system.

Drink up. If you're not already doing so, increase your water intake to about 8 cups a day, especially if the *Positively Ageless* fiber recommendations exceed your "normal" fiber intake, which they probably do. If you don't already have one, buy an inexpensive 2-quart pitcher just for your daily water intake. Fill it each night before bed, and be sure you've emptied it during the course of the next day. If you're a bottled water drinker, hang on to your bottles to count each day, or record them in your journal throughout the day to be sure you've met your quota.

Focus on 3s. Get your ratio of omega-6s to omega-3s back on track. Have two or three servings of fish this week. Also try some of the ALA-rich plant food sources. Sprinkle flaxseed on your cereal and in your yogurt, or mix a few tablespoons in your whole grain recipes. Try using flaxseed oil or walnut oil to replace some of the oil in your favorite vinaigrettes. Snack on raw walnuts, and be sure to add some dark leafy greens to your salads. Watercress and purslane are especially high in ALA, and soybeans are an excellent plant source of omega-3s. A salad with Tomato Ginger Vinaigrette (page 283) will provide a healthy dose.

Do dairy. Whether it's milk on your cereal, yogurt for snacks, or cottage cheese with a salad, go for two servings of organic low-fat or fat-free dairy each day. They're great sources of lean protein, calcium, and (in the case of yogurt) probiotics for a healthy GI tract.

Drink safely. If you enjoy alcohol, limit yourself to one a day and choose red wine. I like to call red wine my Stop the Clock!tail. Yes, white wine is antioxidant-rich, but red is even more potent. Remember that most antioxidants are concentrated in plant pigments; since red wine is fermented with the skins, it contains more antioxidants.

Spice it up. Put away the saltshaker, and try a few new herb and spice combinations. They add layers of flavor and an antioxidant bang. Sweet spices such as cinnamon and ginger can also satisfy cravings and, when added to tea or fruit, may eliminate the need for supplemental sweeteners. Review the herb and spice list on page 274, and be sure to keep your cupboard well stocked.

Experiment. The *Positively Ageless* pantry includes a large number of fresh fruits, vegetables, whole grains, beans and legumes, nuts, and seeds. Try two new items each week to expand your repertoire. Between the pantry, the recipes, and the eating plans, you should find enough variety to keep you and your family interested and engaged well beyond the introductory 4 weeks of the program.

Grab your tools. A chef's knife, paring knife, and sharpening steel are indispensable now, especially with all of the fresh produce that will be brightening your kitchen. A citrus planer is a quick and easy way to remove the zest from your citrus fruit before you peel it. (The zest is the brightly colored outer covering of the fruit, and the peel is the whole of the skin.) Since 53 percent of the vitamin C is in the layers of the peel, why not add the zest to vinaigrettes, salads, tea, or water?

Steam it. A steamer allows you to cook chicken, fish, or veggies without added fat. For extra flavor, steam over broth instead of water. Better yet, use green tea to create steam. We're going all-out creative to put the greatest number of antioxidants in every bite you take.

Take a step—toward exercise. Even if it's just to find your sneakers or join a gym, get the ball rolling toward establishing an exercise program. This week, start off with 10 minutes twice a day. Whether it's walking or cycling, do something to get moving. We'll be building on this each week.

Young for Life

This list of strategies is for those of you who are ready for a major lifestyle intervention. While you'll need to spend a bit more effort enacting these good habits, the payoff can be a dramatic, lasting impact on your health.

Book it. Begin planning times for your meals and snacks. It may take a couple of weeks to find a system that works for you, but by Week Four, you'll have your *Positively Ageless* schedule memorized. Timing is important to maintain not only a steady stream of energy and even blood-sugar levels but constant antioxidants, too. Remember, some of them stay in your system for only 4 to 6 hours, so the key is regular replenishment. A schedule will help provide this. If your weight is an issue, small meals at regular intervals will make you less inclined to gorge at mealtime because you haven't eaten in so long.

Journal it. Buy a small notebook or journal and start tracking what you eat. Keep it in your desk, your handbag, your backpack, or wherever is handiest or most convenient for you. Whether or not you're watching your weight, a food journal may be helpful in the beginning for meeting the weekly goals of the *Positively Ageless* program. It will help you identify when you eat certain things, allowing you to learn from your eating patterns. Take notes throughout the day because it's easy to forget an unplanned snack or tasting. Find a routine, a favorite place, and a time to record what you eat in your journal.

Jot it down. If you have some work to do to reach your target weight, it may behoove you to keep a food *and* exercise journal. Remember, you must burn off more calories than you take in to lose weight. Recording your input and output can help you stay on track. And if you overdo it with too many calories one day, you can make up for it the next with extra exercise or less food.

Get quizzical. Take the Cardio Quiz on page 38 to measure your risk for heart disease. During your physical, discuss your *Positively Ageless* plans with your MD to ramp up your focus on exercise, low cholesterol and saturated fat, high omega-3s, and increased fiber.

Feel them. Check your breasts: A significant number of women detect early signs of breast cancer by checking themselves each month. The American Cancer Society's Web site at www.cancer.org offers helpful instructions on the best way to do this.

Get physical. Depending on your overall health, you should have a physical exam every 1 to 5 years from age 30 onward. After 65, you should have an exam annually. The tests your health provider orders will depend on your history. Generally, your work-up will include a blood pressure check, a blood test, and sometimes urinalysis. Ask your doctor which biomarker exams may be beneficial to you. Be sure to record all values in your journal to serve as your baseline. You can track your progress over weeks, months, and years.

Here's an overview of specific tests.

Colon screening: You should have a test for colorectal cancer at age 50 if there is no family history of the disease. If you've had unusual symptoms or this runs in the family, you should be tested earlier. Your doctor will tell you whether you need a colonoscopy, a sigmoidoscopy, or a stool sample.

Fasting blood sugar test: You're at risk for type 2 diabetes if you are overweight, have a family history, or had gestational diabetes during pregnancy. If you are at high risk, have a fasting blood sugar test by the age of 35 and every 3 years after that.

Mammogram: A woman over 40 should have a mammogram annually. Women at risk for breast cancer should get mammograms even earlier. If possible, schedule your exam at the same location and using the same machine to aim for the most accurate results. If you're taking hormone replacement therapy (HRT), ask your doctor about temporarily discontinuing your meds just before the test to get a better picture of what's going on in your breasts. (HRT can make your breast tissue more dense, so it's more difficult to read the mammogram.)

Pap test and pelvic exam: You should have these tests to check for cervical cancer and other disorders starting at age 18 (earlier if you're sexually active). Some doctors advise checks only every other year if the results are negative. After age 65, you should have a Pap smear every 1 to 3 years if your test results are negative for 3 years in a row.

STD testing: If you are sexually active, you should have a test for chlamydia, HIV/AIDS, and other sexually transmitted diseases. Ask your doctor about the new human papillomavirus (HPV) vaccine, which may be helpful in preventing cervical cancer.

Thyroid test: At age 35 and every few years after that, the blood panel your doctor orders may include a test for your level of thyroid-stimulating hormone (TSH). If you have any personal or family history of autoimmune disease but have previously tested for normal TSH, your doctor may suggest further tests to check levels of two thyroid hormones, free T4 and free T3, and thyroid antibodies. If you have any signs of thyroid disease, you need to have your thyroid hormone levels tested regularly—once or twice a year.

chapter 7

EAT SMART,
LIVE LONG MENUS

Positively Ageless Menus Week One

The *Positively Ageless* menu plans are based on an average of 1,200 calories per day. If your calorie needs are a little higher (or lower), you can adjust accordingly. Adding a glass of 1 percent milk, 6 ounces of fat-free yogurt, one pear or a large apple, or a glass of red wine with dinner will each provide an additional 100 calories.

Positively Ageless **recipes** are listed in bold and designated as one serving size.

The two snacks can be scheduled between meals, or have one between meals and one after dinner.

DAY 1

1,246 calories; 28 grams fiber; 6,820 milligrams omega-3s

BREAKFAST

1 ounce lox

1 soft-cooked omega-3 egg

1 slice **Whole Grain Bread** (page 306) toast or 2 flax crackers with 1 tablespoon **Easy Blueberry Jam** (page 288)

½ grapefruit

8 ounces green tea with a slice of ginger or water

MID-MORNING SNACK

¼ cup fat-free cottage cheese with ¼ cup cherries and 1 tablespoon slivered almonds

8 ounces water

LUNCH

Baby Spinach Salad (page 314)

½ medium apple, sliced

8 ounces water or fat-free milk

MID-AFTERNOON SNACK

¼ cup plain fat-free yogurt topped with 1 tablespoon **Mango Butter** (page 286) and 1 tablespoon ground flaxseed

¼ cup blueberries

8 ounces green tea or water

DINNER

Grilled Salmon with Almond Pomegranate Sauce (page 320)

⅓ cup steamed brown rice or wild rice

1½ cups salad (dark-green leafy lettuce with 1 tablespoon **Tomato Ginger Vinaigrette**) (page 283)

1 pear

8 ounces water or green tea with mint

DAY 2

1,212 calories; 35 grams fiber; 2,750 milligrams omega-3s

BREAKFAST

Breakfast Polenta with Berries and Vanilla (page 267)

½ cup fat-free milk or soy milk

2 slices (1 ounce) nitrate-free turkey bacon

¼ cup yogurt with 1 teaspoon chopped fresh mint and 1 tablespoon ground flaxseed

8 ounces green tea with a slice of ginger or water

MID-MORNING SNACK

¼ cup fat-free ricotta cheese with ½ teaspoon vanilla, ¼ cup raspberries, and 1 tablespoon slivered almonds

Mint tea or water

LUNCH

1 cup **Red Bean Mole Soup** (page 300)

2 cups dark green leafy salad with 1 tablespoon **Tangy Mustard Dressing** (page 281)

¼ cup sliced strawberries

8 ounces water

MID-AFTERNOON SNACK

2 tablespoons **Zippy Hummus** (page 294) and 1 teaspoon flaxseed served with ½ cup celery and jicama sticks

8 ounces water or iced green tea with lemon

DINNER

4 ounces poached or grilled salmon with 1 tablespoon **Miso Marinade** (page 287)

5 roast or steamed asparagus spears

⅓ cup steamed bulgur or brown rice

½ cup fresh raspberries or 1 (2-inch) wedge cantaloupe

4 ounces red wine

8 ounces **Zinger Green Tea** (page 271), water, or fat-free milk

DAY 3

1,170 calories; 27 grams fiber; 1,880 milligrams omega-3s

BREAKFAST

Cheesy Vegetable Frittata (page 262)

⅓ cup sliced strawberries

¼ cup fat-free vanilla yogurt

8 ounces green tea or water

MID-MORNING SNACK

Bran Yogurt Muffin (page 264)

8 ounces ginger tea or water

½ apple

LUNCH

4 ounces grilled chicken breast with 2 tablespoons **Barbecue Sauce** (page 285)

1 cup salad (dark green leafy lettuce, cherry tomatoes, and edamame, dressed with 1 tablespoon extra-virgin olive oil and fresh lemon juice to taste)

1 peach or pear

8 ounces iced green tea or water

MID-AFTERNOON SNACK

⅓ cup fat-free cottage cheese with ⅓ cup salsa

2 Brazil nuts

8 ounces spring water

DINNER

10 medium poached or grilled prawns with ¼ cup **Curried Tomato Dipping Sauce** (page 280)

1 cup wilted baby spinach with garlic, black pepper, and olive oil

⅓ cup steamed brown rice

¾ cup diced watermelon with fresh mint

8 ounces water with fresh lime or green tea

DAY 4

1,231 calories; 27 grams fiber; 1,600 milligrams omega-3s

BREAKFAST

Baked Eggs in Savory Turkey Cups (page 266)

1 slice **Whole Grain Bread** (page 306), toasted

½ cup fresh blueberries

8 ounces green tea, water, or fat-free milk

MID-MORNING SNACK

1-ounce slice smoked salmon with 1 Wasa Crispbread or 2 flax crackers

1 kiwifruit

8 ounces iced green tea or water

LUNCH

Spanish Meatball Soup (page 303)

1 sliced tomato with cider vinegar and cilantro

¼ cup fresh raspberries

8 ounces iced white or green tea or water

MID-AFTERNOON SNACK

Smoothie made with ⅓ cup kefir, 1 teaspoon ground flaxseed, and ¼ cup sliced strawberries

8 ounces water

DINNER

Moroccan Fish Stew (page 328)

1 cup spinach salad with ¼ cup cherry tomatoes, dressed with 1 tablespoon extra-virgin olive oil and fresh lemon juice to taste

½ peach or pear

4 ounces red wine

8 ounces water or mint tea

DAY 5

1,217 calories; 28 grams fiber; 2,800 milligrams omega-3s

BREAKFAST

Old-Fashioned Breakfast Sausage (page 259)

³/₄ cup fat-free milk or soy milk

¹/₂ cup old-fashioned oatmeal

¹/₄ cup sliced strawberries

8 ounces green or white tea or water

MID-MORNING SNACK

¹/₃ cup fat-free vanilla yogurt mixed with ¹/₂ apple, diced, and 1 tablespoon chopped walnuts

8 ounces mint tea or water

LUNCH

Southwest Salmon Burger (page 324) served on baby spinach with ¹/₄ avocado and ¹/₄ cup cherry tomatoes

1 medium orange

8 ounces iced green tea with lemon or water

MID-AFTERNOON SNACK

1 (2-inch) cantaloupe wedge wrapped with ¹/₂-ounce slice turkey breast, drizzled with 1 teaspoon flaxseed oil

8 ounces water or green tea

DINNER

3 ounces grilled chicken breast with 1 tablespoon **Miso Marinade** (page 287)

¹/₂ medium artichoke, steamed

1 cup salad (dark green leafy lettuce dressed with 1 teaspoon extra-virgin olive oil and fresh lemon juice to taste)

¹/₂ cup fresh raspberries

8 ounces water or mint tea

DAY 6

1,160 calories; 31 grams fiber; 2,470 milligrams omega-3s

BREAKFAST

Omelet (1 whole omega-3 egg plus 1 egg white) with ½ ounce smoked salmon, 1 teaspoon fresh dill, and 4 cherry tomatoes

⅓ cup fat-free vanilla yogurt with 1 cup fresh blueberries

8 ounces green tea or water

MID-MORNING SNACK

1 medium apple

4 **Indian Olives with Citrus and Panch Puran** (page 292)

1 rye Wasa Crispbread or 1 flax cracker

8 ounces water or mint tea

LUNCH

Italian Vegetable Soup (page 302)

Whole Wheat Pita Chips (page 295) or Wasa Crispbread

Rich Cocoa Sorbet (page 342)

8 ounces water or green tea

MID-AFTERNOON SNACK

¼ cup fat-free plain yogurt with 1 tablespoon chopped pistachios and ¼ cup diced kiwifruit

8 ounces water or iced tea

DINNER

3 ounces grilled salmon with fresh lemon

Arthur's Tomato Salad (page 311)

1 cup roasted Brussels sprouts with 2 teaspoons slivered almonds

1 plum

4 ounces red wine

8 ounces green tea with mint or water

DAY 7

1,223 calories; 30 grams fiber; 3,390 milligrams omega-3s

BREAKFAST

1 hard-cooked omega-3 egg

Creamy Almond Kasha (page 261)

1 cup fresh blackberries or blueberries

8 ounces green tea with lemon or water

MID-MORNING SNACK

Mini sandwich: 1 ounce sliced roast turkey or chicken with 1 tablespoon **Watercress Sauce** (page 289) on 1 whole grain cracker or ½ slice **Whole Grain Bread** (page 306)

8 ounces water or iced tea

LUNCH

4 ounces wild poached salmon with fresh lime

1 sliced tomato with 1 tablespoon fresh basil and 1 tablespoon balsamic vinegar

½ cup wild rice

1 cup diced honeydew melon

8 ounces fat-free milk, water, or iced tea

MID-AFTERNOON SNACK

Mango Mint Smoothie (page 269)

8 ounces water

DINNER

4 ounces grilled chicken with 1 tablespoon **Tangy Mustard Dressing** (page 281)

1 cup sautéed spinach or escarole with ½ cup sliced mushrooms

Spaghetti (Squash) with Basil-Cress Pesto (page 334)

1 medium tangerine

8 ounces green tea or water or fat-free milk

AGE-PROOF YOUR HORMONES AND YOUR MIND

Aging gracefully means sailing into a healthy future with the confidence to chart your own course. In this section, we'll discuss more serious conditions that are key signs of the aging process, like diabetes, stroke, and Alzheimer's disease—and the simple choices you can make to lower your risks for them.

We'll also unravel the mysteries of menopause. This inevitable era can be the best or worst of times. Understanding what happens and why can help you make the most of your best years yet.

chapter 8

DIABETES: A CONDITION WITH MANY AGE-ROBBING CONSEQUENCES

On the surface, diabetes may not sound particularly threatening: In essence, your blood sugar is too high. But this one problem generates a ripple effect that can cause many serious consequences that lead to disability or an early death. Diabetes may be the ultimate *pro*aging condition. As a result, preventing diabetes—or maintaining good control over your blood sugar if you have diabetes—is crucial for living a long, healthy life.

Age is a major risk factor for type 2 diabetes. According to the National Institutes of Health, only 2.4 percent of people between the ages of 20 and 39 have the condition. Between ages 40 and 59, the number leaps to 10.1 percent. And after age 60, prevalence more than doubles to 21 percent.[1]

Certain ethnic and racial groups are at greater risk of diabetes. African Americans are 80 percent more likely to develop the condition than whites of a similar age. Mexican Americans are 70 percent more likely to develop it than whites, and Native Americans are 2.2 times more likely.[2]

Your family history also raises your risk; if you've had a parent or sibling with diabetes, you're more likely to have it. You can't do anything about the extra risk posed by your age, ethnic or racial background, or family history. However, as you'll learn, many other risk factors for developing diabetes fall under your control. First, though, let's look at what causes diabetes and a condition called prediabetes that can lead up to it.

What Is Diabetes?

After you eat a meal or a snack, your body converts most of your food into glucose, its primary source of fuel. The glucose gets into your blood-stream—where it's known as blood sugar—so it can be delivered to your body's cells, which use it to generate the energy they need to work properly. However, the sugar can't just slip into the cells on its own. Insulin, a hormone produced by your pancreas, is required to allow the sugar to enter the cells in your muscles, liver, and fat stores. Think of insulin as a key that unlocks the cells for the blood sugar.[3]

Diabetes occurs in three main forms.

- Type 1 diabetes usually develops early in life. The body's immune system turns against the pancreas and destroys cells that make the hormone insulin. A person with type 1 diabetes must supplement the body's own insulin supply.

- Gestational diabetes develops during pregnancy due to hormonal shifts or a deficiency of insulin, and it usually goes away after childbirth.

- Type 2 diabetes is the most common type, accounting for 90 to 95 percent of diabetes cases. The pancreas produces insulin but perhaps not enough, and the body cannot properly utilize the insulin that is made. The pancreas pumps out more insulin in response but eventually tires out and produces even less. People with type 2 diabetes may be able to manage the condition by diet and exercise alone, but some patients require oral medications and/or insulin to keep blood sugar under control. The advice in this chapter will focus on preventing and treating type 2 diabetes with lifestyle changes because this type of diabetes is so common, and diet and exercise are so helpful in reducing its impact.

As we get older, our body fat tends to increase and our muscle mass tends to decrease. This makes our muscles less sensitive to insulin, meaning we need to produce more of it to achieve the same result. This is called poor insulin sensitivity, which leads to poor glucose control. Body fat stored around the midsection is more of a risk factor than fat on the hips and thighs.

When you have type 2 diabetes, glucose builds up in your bloodstream. That's not good—high glucose can cause a number of serious problems, including: [3,4]

- Increasing the deposits in your arteries found in atherosclerosis, which can lead to heart disease and stroke.

DON'T LET DIABETES
CATCH YOU OFF GUARD

Millions of people in America have type 2 diabetes but don't even know it. Like high blood pressure, diabetes may not have any outward symptoms. Prediabetes and insulin resistance usually don't, either. That's why getting tested at age 45, or even earlier if you have certain risk factors, is a good idea. Sometimes, however, the body does offer clues that you have diabetes. If you notice any of these symptoms, talk to your doctor.

- Increased urination

- Increased thirst

- Fatigue and increased hunger

- Sudden or unintentional weight loss

- Vision problems

- Poor wound healing

Heart attack and stroke are the main causes of death in people with diabetes. Diabetes also raises the risk of high blood pressure.[4,5]

- Damaging the tiny blood vessels in your retinas, which line the insides of your eyes, causing blindness. Diabetes also makes you more likely to develop cataracts (cloudiness in the clear lenses in the front of your eyes). These also cause visual impairment or blindness.[6]

- Damaging the tiny "filters" within your kidneys due to high glucose and high blood pressure. Your kidneys are responsible for filtering wastes out of your bloodstream so they can send them out in urine, while holding on to valuable protein so it doesn't escape your body. Diabetic damage to your kidneys causes wastes to build up in your system and protein to be lost in your urine.[7]

- Creating foot problems by causing nerve damage that prevents you from feeling blisters and other injuries, so they go untreated, and reducing bloodflow to your feet through your arteries. High glucose in your blood encourages infections, and poor blood circulation means injuries heal slowly and poorly. People with poorly controlled diabetes are at risk of related complications that can ultimately lead to surgical removal of toes, feet, or lower legs.[8]

Those are just some of the main complications of uncontrolled blood sugar. Diabetes also increases your likelihood of developing gum disease and tooth loss, digestive problems, and sexual difficulty (for women as well as men). Plus, having high glucose sets the stage for the formation of damaging AGEs—advanced glycation end products—which you learned about on page 10.

Having too much insulin promotes storage of body fat, increases triglyceride and cholesterol levels, and elevates blood pressure. It also raises levels of chemicals that are responsible for inflammatory responses. Diabetes is even linked to a greater risk of Alzheimer's disease.

This is a sizable burden of disease, loss of functioning, and threat of early death. It's no wonder that keeping your blood sugar under good control is mandatory if you want to enjoy good health in your later years. The good news is that:

■ Type 2 diabetes typically takes plenty of time to develop, which gives you ample opportunity to stop it before it becomes a full-blown condition.

■ It's often controlled with diet and lifestyle change.

Let's take a look at a condition called prediabetes, which serves as a warning signal for type 2 diabetes.

Prediabetes: A Chance to Stop the Problem in Its Tracks

More than 54 million American adults have prediabetes: Their blood glucose is higher than normal but not enough to warrant a diagnosis of diabetes. It's a sign that your body is not responding well to its insulin, which experts call insulin resistance. According to the National Institutes of Health (NIH), most people with prediabetes will develop the full-blown disease within 10 years if they don't take steps to reduce their risk.[9]

People with insulin resistance and elevated blood glucose often are overweight—especially around the belly—and have high blood pressure, high LDL cholesterol, and low HDL cholesterol.[9] You may remember from the heart section that all of these signs point to a problem called metabolic syndrome, which raises your risk not just of diabetes but also cardiovascular disease.[9]

Odds are good that you won't notice any symptoms from prediabetes (or possibly even full-fledged diabetes). As with high blood pressure, you frequently can't feel or see that anything's amiss, so the NIH recommends routine testing for insulin resistance or prediabetes once you turn 45. This helps ensure that you catch blood sugar problems early in their development. It's particularly important to be tested if you're older than 45 or overweight.[9]

Even if you're not yet 45, talk to your doctor about being tested if diabetes runs in your family; if you have low HDL cholesterol or high triglycerides (a type of blood fat) or high blood pressure; or if you have had gestational diabetes or are a member of an ethnic or racial group at high risk of diabetes.[9]

If tests indicate that you're at risk, here's the good news: Simple steps can have a powerful influence in staving off the disease. Once again, *you* can help control whether you'll go down the path toward diabetes (and all these scary complications) or whether you'll step out of harm's way.

A major study from the NIH called the Diabetes Prevention Project found that people can cut their risk of developing diabetes by 58 percent. That means slicing your risk by more than half! The risk-lowering tools are concepts in the *Positively Ageless* program that you've already learned will improve your health.

Biomarkers of Prediabetes and Diabetes

The following tests are commonly used to diagnose prediabetes and diabetes and to keep an eye on the potential complications from these conditions.

Fasting glucose test. With this test, you abstain from eating for at least 8 hours. Your health care provider then takes a blood sample (usually first thing in the morning). Ideally, your blood glucose will be relatively low because you haven't eaten in a while. If your glucose is less than 100 milligrams per deciliter of blood (mg/dL), your blood sugar is normal. If it's between 100 and 125 mg/dL, you have prediabetes and, according to the NIH, you've likely had insulin resistance for some time. If it's 126 mg/dL or higher—and it's confirmed with a follow-up test—you're considered to have diabetes.[9,10]

Oral glucose tolerance test. You also prepare for this test by fasting overnight. The next day, you drink an extremely sweet liquid in your health care provider's office and provide a blood sample 2 hours later. This test is less common, but it may be helpful in determining diabetes in people who show symptoms but have normal blood sugar levels when fasting.[10] If your blood sugar is less than 140 mg/dL, it's normal. If it's between 140 and 199 mg/dL, you're considered to have "impaired glucose tolerance," or prediabetes. You probably have had insulin resistance a while and are at greater risk of diabetes. A readout of 200 mg/dL or higher is a sign of diabetes, though it needs a follow-up confirmation.[9,11]

At-home glucose monitoring. Maintaining good control over your glucose is crucial for avoiding complications when you have diabetes. Depending on your individual circumstances, you may need to test your glucose daily or even more frequently. Testing is a simple process that involves pricking your finger, forearm, or thigh, then placing a drop of blood into a meter that gives you a readout of your blood glucose. If you have diabetes, talk to your health care provider about what kind of testing schedule you should follow and how to properly measure your blood sugar.[12,13]

Glycated hemoglobin test. Also known as the HbA1c, this test looks at your hemoglobin, a protein in red blood cells. Hemoglobin survives for about 4 months, and, during its life span, glucose in your bloodstream latches on to it. When you have excess glucose, it attaches to more of your hemoglobin. So this test shows how well you've controlled your glucose over the past few months, rather than day to day and at one point in time. According to the American Diabetes Association, in people *without* diabetes, the HbA1c would reveal that about 5 percent of their hemoglobin is glycated. If you have diabetes, you'll want to keep this number under 7 percent. If it rises to 8 percent or above, it will require that you change your diet, exercise program, and/or medication regimen to bring your blood glucose back down to a safer level.[12,14]

Other tests. If you have diabetes, you'll need to have your eyes, feet, and kidneys checked regularly for signs of damage. Blood and urine tests can tell your doctor how your kidneys are functioning. Talk to your doctor about what sort of schedule you should follow to be screened for diabetes complications. In addition, even if you only have prediabetes, your doctor will want to monitor your blood pressure, cholesterol, and other risk factors for heart problems.

The *Positively Ageless* Guide to Preventing and Treating Diabetes

These lifestyle recommendations shouldn't take the place of your health care provider's advice. If you're at risk of developing diabetes—or you already have it—follow your doctor's recommendations for medications and other treatments for your particular needs. A registered dietitian who is a CDE—a certified diabetes educator—is an expert who can steer you in a healthy direction. Meanwhile, the following are general goals to pursue if treating or avoiding diabetes is a priority for you.

Lose weight. In the Diabetes Prevention Project mentioned earlier in this chapter, researchers helped a group of people with prediabetes, whose average BMI put them into obesity territory, lose at least 7 percent of their body weight. The people in the weight-loss group cut an average of 450 calories a day, and their daily calories from fat dropped to about 28 percent of total calories. They were also urged to get 150 minutes of moderate exercise, such as brisk walking, each week. That translates to 30 minutes of physical activity, 5 days per week. As mentioned earlier, these people cut their diabetes risk by more than half![15]

The most important rules for weight loss apply to managing diabetes, too. Remember these:

1. Plan your meals, your snacks, and your exercise time. Don't just trust that they'll happen on time, on their own.

2. Start each day with breakfast. No skipping meals—period.

3. Include fruit and/or vegetables with each meal.

4. Include protein with each meal and snack.

5. Be physically active. It may take a little trial and error, but you must find a sport or activity that you *love to do*. You'd better like your bicycle, swimsuit, or dancing shoes, because you'll be spending a lot of time together.

(continued on page 137)

CONSULT THE BMI CHART TO ASSESS THE RISK FROM YOUR WEIGHT

To get a sense of whether your body weight poses a risk to your health, experts use a simple number called the body mass index, or BMI. Your BMI is determined with a formula using your height and weight.

Figuring it out using the formula requires a calculator. An easier way is to consult the chart below. Find your height on the left-hand side, then run your finger along the row until you find your weight. The number at the intersection of your height and weight is your BMI.

Height	Weight (lb)										
4'10"	86	91	96	100	105	110	115	119	124	129	134
4'11"	89	94	99	104	109	114	119	124	128	133	138
5'	92	97	102	107	112	118	123	128	133	138	143
5'1"	96	100	106	111	116	122	127	132	137	143	148
5'2"	99	104	109	115	120	126	131	136	142	147	153
5'3"	102	107	113	118	124	130	135	141	146	152	158
5'4"	105	110	116	122	128	134	140	145	151	157	163
5'5"	109	114	120	126	132	138	144	150	156	162	168
5'6"	112	118	124	130	136	142	148	155	161	167	173
5'7"	116	121	127	134	140	146	153	159	166	172	178
5'8"	120	125	131	138	144	151	158	164	171	177	184
5'9"	123	128	135	142	149	155	162	169	176	182	189
5'10"	126	132	139	146	153	160	167	174	181	188	195
5'11"	130	136	143	150	157	165	172	179	186	193	200
6'	134	140	147	154	162	169	177	184	191	199	206
6'1"	138	144	151	159	166	174	182	189	197	204	212
6'2"	141	148	155	163	171	179	186	194	202	210	218
6'3"	145	152	160	168	176	184	192	200	208	216	224
6'4"	149	156	164	172	180	189	197	205	213	221	230
BMI	18	19	20	21	22	23	24	25	26	27	28

The BMI doesn't factor in body composition (how much fat and how much muscle you have), but it will give you a sense of what your healthy weight should be. For example, if you're very muscular and athletic, your BMI may overestimate your health risks. But in general, if you fall into the overweight category—and even more so if you're obese—your weight puts you at higher risk of diabetes, heart disease, stroke, unhealthy cholesterol, and other problems. Try to work your way down to a weight that would put you in the "normal" category.

Underweight: Less than 18

Normal: 18–24

Overweight: 25–29

Obese: 30–34

Very obese: 35–39

Extremely obese: 40 and above

138	143	148	153	158	162	167	172	177	181	186	191
143	148	153	158	163	168	173	178	183	188	193	198
148	153	158	163	168	174	179	184	189	194	199	204
153	158	164	169	174	180	185	190	195	201	206	211
158	164	169	175	180	186	191	196	202	207	213	218
163	169	175	180	186	191	197	203	208	214	220	225
169	174	180	186	192	197	204	209	215	221	227	232
174	180	186	192	198	204	210	216	222	228	234	240
179	186	192	198	204	210	216	223	229	235	241	247
185	191	198	204	211	217	223	230	236	242	249	255
190	197	203	210	216	223	230	236	243	249	256	262
196	203	209	216	223	230	236	243	250	257	263	270
202	209	216	222	229	236	243	250	257	264	271	278
208	215	222	229	236	243	250	257	265	272	279	286
213	221	228	235	242	250	258	265	272	279	287	294
219	227	235	242	250	257	265	272	280	288	295	302
225	233	241	249	256	264	272	280	287	295	303	311
232	240	248	256	264	272	279	287	295	303	311	319
238	246	254	263	271	279	287	295	304	312	320	328
29	**30**	**31**	**32**	**33**	**34**	**35**	**36**	**37**	**38**	**39**	**40**

WHOLE GRAINS PROVIDE AN ANTIOXIDANT KICK

If you assume that fiber is the only thing that grains have going for them, think again. There are plenty of reasons to love whole grains: They're versatile, inexpensive, and surprisingly easy to prepare, plus they have amazing flavors and textures. Although whole grains lack the vibrant colors that proclaim the antioxidant punch of many fruits and vegetables, they do contain polyphenols, carotenoids, and phytosterols. This translates to antiaging power on par with many fruits and exceeding most vegetables.

Barley, brown rice, bulgur, corn grits, whole wheat couscous, millet, rolled oats, oat bran, wild rice, and sorghum flour are part of the *Positively Ageless* pantry; so are pasta and cereals, breads, and crackers that list "whole wheat" or a whole grain as the first ingredient on the label.

Watch out for the term "enriched," however. It's usually a sign that a food like bread or pasta is low in fiber because it's made with processed flour, meaning the nutrients have been stripped out and then replaced synthetically. Unless a bread or pasta is made from whole wheat, its fiber content is no different than the enriched version, which is loaded with carbohydrates but not much else.

Below you'll find the antioxidant content of common whole grains.

GRAIN PER 1/4 C	ORAC
Sorghum flour	9,378
Wheat germ	4,205
Cream of wheat	1,376
Ground flax	1,184
High-fiber cornmeal	1,147
Wheat bran	855
Whole wheat flour	570
Cracked wheat	420

Protect your heart. Since prediabetes and diabetes put you at higher risk of heart disease, it's important to follow the steps that can help lower your blood pressure and LDL cholesterol. You'll find these recommendations in the heart section starting on page 46. In general, though, you should lower your daily sodium intake to no more than 2,400 milligrams, and eat lots of fruits and vegetables and a few daily servings of low-fat dairy products to help treat or prevent blood pressure. To encourage healthy cholesterol levels, reduce your saturated fat calories to 10 percent of your daily calories (7 percent may be even more helpful); minimize (ideally, eliminate) trans fats; and shift your fat intake to monounsaturated fats such as olive oil and canola oil and omega-3 fats from cold-water fish and flaxseed. Regular exercise and weight loss will help both your blood pressure and your cholesterol profile.[16]

Studies have also suggested that a diet high in saturated fat can decrease your insulin sensitivity (which is a bad thing), and trans fats may contribute to developing diabetes. Unsaturated fats, on the other hand, are associated with a lower risk of diabetes.[17]

Eat to keep your blood sugar steady. Throughout this book, I've been beating the drum about the importance of keeping your blood sugar and insulin levels steady rather than letting them soar, then crash, over and over again. That's obviously important if you have diabetes or prediabetes, though you don't have to monitor every last bite of carbohydrates, like you might think. A concept called glycemic index (GI) ranks foods by how quickly their carbohydrate content turns into glucose, and a concept called glycemic load is a combination of a food's GI and the amount of carbohydrate in its serving size. You can take a look at the lists of foods and their GIs on page 138.

In terms of preventing diabetes, a few large studies have found that people with the highest-GI diets were more likely to develop diabetes—but other large studies found no relationship.[17] So it's best to use the glycemic index as a general concept to guide your choices.

- If you have a choice between a starchy vegetable and a vegetable with a low GI, go with the one that'll raise your blood sugar less.

- Have whole fruit (which contains fiber) rather than juice.

- Eat whole grain instead of simple carbs like white sugar and white flour.

(continued on page 140)

GLYCEMIC SCALES RATE FOODS' EFFECT ON BLOOD SUGAR

We've talked a lot about keeping your blood sugar steady. Two common scales can give you information about how quickly foods will affect your blood sugar: the glycemic index and the glycemic load.

The glycemic index (GI) tells you how rapidly a carbohydrate turns into glucose in your body. One drawback is that it doesn't tell you *how much* carbohydrate a specific food contains. Thus, the GI for a food is the same, regardless of portion size. For example, a tablespoon of honey and a cup of honey have the same GI. So just because a food ranks high in GI doesn't always mean that it will raise your blood sugar level rapidly.

The glycemic load (GL), however, also takes into account a food's available carbohydrates, which provide energy, like starch and sugar (so it excludes fiber). The GL measures the effect of a food's GI multiplied by its available carbohydrate content in a standard serving; thus, it is a more realistic measure of the food's potential to raise blood sugar. The glycemic load of honey, for example, is based on the serving size.

Some research says that high GLs may put you at risk for disease.[21,22] The general principles of this idea should be considered when you're making food choices, especially if you're overweight or have prediabetes or a strong family history of diabetes.

If you don't fall into one of those categories, monitoring GL is not as important from day to day. If you're following the *Positively Ageless* plan, you can be certain that most of your food is loaded with fiber and on the lower end of the GL range (with the exception of some of the sweeteners and desserts).

At some times, you might actually benefit from a high-GL food. Reach for a high-quality higher-glycemic food before a workout to fuel your muscles. You'll regain your energy and feel refreshed faster.

On the opposite page is a list of the glycemic index and glycemic load of common foods. When referring to the list, keep in mind that:

- Low GI = 55 or less
- Medium GI = 56–69
- High GI = 70 or more

- Low GL = 10 or less
- Medium GL = 11–19
- High GL = 20 or more

FOOD[23]	SERVING SIZE	GLYCEMIC INDEX	GLYCEMIC LOAD
Cornflakes	½ c	119	13
Baked potato, without skin	1 medium	85	29
Pretzels	1 oz	83	18
Rice cakes	3 small	82	4
Banana	1 medium	77	19
Sweet potato, baked with skin	1 small	77	15
Doughnut, cake	4 in	76	36
French fries	5 oz	75	39
Popcorn, plain, microwaved	1½ c	72	5
Plain bagel	3 oz; 1 medium	72	36
White rice	½ c	72	15
Parsnips	½ c	69	7
Sugar	1 Tbsp	68	9
Pineapple, diced	½ c	66	6
Raisins	2 Tbsp	64	10
Sweet corn, cooked	½ c	60	10
Brown rice syrup	1 Tbsp	55	12
Honey	1 Tbsp	55	9
Apple with peel	1 medium	54	9
Orange juice	4 oz	53	6
Brown rice, cooked	½ c	50	10
Chickpeas, cooked	½ c	47	8
Agave nectar	1 Tbsp	46	7
Green grapes	½ c	46	6
Orange	1 medium	42	6
Pinto beans, cooked	½ c	39	5
Barley, cooked	½ c	36	8
Fat-free milk	1 c	32	4
Soybeans, mature, cooked	½ c	20	1
Almonds	2 Tbsp	0	0
Cauliflower	½ c	0	0
Bok choy	1 c	0	0
Celery	1 medium stalk	0	0

- Eat lots of fiber throughout the day to slow down your absorption of carbs.

- Have four or five small meals and healthy snacks instead of three large meals. If you do indulge from time to time in something that's not on the *Positively Ageless* plan, have a bowl of Chocolate Almond Pudding (page 338) instead of a whole box of cheap cookies.

Get plenty of chromium. This is an essential mineral—meaning that our bodies don't produce it, so it's essential we get it from our diet. Chromium helps metabolize fat and carbohydrates. It's also important in insulin metabolism, so a deficiency can raise your blood sugar. Some research has found that chromium supplements may help control blood sugar, but more studies need to be done to demonstrate that chromium is helpful for people with diabetes. A small study reported in 2006 divided 37 people into two groups; one group received a diabetes drug for 6 months, and the other got the drug plus a chromium supplement. Those who took chromium had significantly better insulin sensitivity and glucose control.[16,18]

The daily recommended intake for chromium[19] is 25 micrograms per day, dropping to 20 micrograms after age 50. Because research is still emerging, there is not a higher chromium recommendation for people with diabetes. People taking medications for diabetes should ask their doctor before supplementing with chromium. Good dietary sources of chromium include:

FOOD	SERVING SIZE	CHROMIUM CONTENT (MCG)
Broccoli, cooked	1 c	21.9
Whole grain cornmeal	1/4 c	10
Barley, dry	1/4 c	6
Edamame, shelled	1/2 c	2.8
Lean flank steak	4 oz	2.7
Egg	1 large	2
Brown rice, cooked	1/2 c	0.4

Stay moderate with alcohol. Low to moderate alcohol use—that's up to one drink a day for women—may actually *reduce* your risk of developing diabetes. If you do have diabetes already, drinking moderately with food has been shown to have no significant effect on blood sugar or insulin levels.[16,17] Remember, though, that alcohol is high in calories, and excessive use causes a lot of health problems. If you don't drink already, don't start simply to possibly lower your risk of diabetes.

Skip smoking. It shouldn't come as a surprise that smoking makes you more likely to develop diabetes. It has been linked to higher glucose levels and may increase your insulin resistance. One large study found that women who smoked more than 25 cigarettes a day were 42 percent more likely to develop diabetes than women who had never smoked.[17]

Get plenty of sleep. Research has linked chronic insufficient sleep with a higher risk of developing diabetes. A large German study from 2005 found that women who had trouble sleeping had nearly double the risk of developing type 2 diabetes.[20] Lack of sleep may throw appetite-regulating hormones out of whack, leading you to eat more. It may also alter your blood sugar and insulin levels.

chapter 9

MENOPAUSE: NAVIGATING "THE CHANGE" WITH HEALTH AND HAPPINESS

Unlike the other topics in this book, menopause isn't a disease or an ailment that contributes to the aging process. It's merely a time when the hormonal processes that supported fertility and reproduction in your younger years wind down, and a new phase in your life begins.[24]

Menopause isn't something you need to "cure," but it does represent a time in your life when your diet and exercise habits become even more important. Some of the changes that come with menopause, such as not dealing with monthly periods or worrying about getting pregnant (once you've gone a year with no periods), may be welcome.[24,25]

Other changes that often occur may be aggravating, like difficulty sleeping, forgetfulness, hot flashes, and moodiness. Other changes pose more serious health threats. The ovaries drastically reduce estrogen production at menopause, which puts your bones at greater risk of osteoporosis. This hormonal change also seems to be why your risk of heart disease climbs.[26] In addition, at this time of life, a woman's body shape tends to change, with weight gain and fat accumulating around the belly. The risk of diabetes goes up, too—which, as you know, sets the stage for still other health problems.[26]

It's common nowadays for women to live one-third of their lives—or even more—after menopause. Making simple lifestyle changes can help you cope with the relatively minor symptoms that tend to develop around this time . . . and will help ensure that you have plenty of healthy years to enjoy during the next phase of your life. I haven't personally entered this time in my life (though it's likely something I'll get to experience in the near future), but my friends have begun talking about it. And they're finding plenty to like about menopause!

"The joys of menopause are not having periods any longer!" says my good friend Robin. "I also have found that there's an innate 'wisdom'—for lack of a better word—that comes with menopause. Finding depth and meaning in my relationships with those around me, loving myself even more, and really embracing this *change* to the next chapter of my life are causes for celebration."

Let's *all* celebrate this phase in our lives with good health!

What Is Menopause, Anyway?

Menopause isn't just a single event; it's more of a process or transition. It's defined as going 12 consecutive months without a period, and the absence isn't explained by pregnancy, breastfeeding, or other causes.

Once this has occurred, you enter the postmenopausal phase. In America, women reach natural menopause at 51, on average. Induced menopause, on the other hand, may occur earlier. This is brought on by factors such as surgery to remove the ovaries or, sometimes, chemotherapy and radiation for cancer treatment. Genetics can also bring on menopause early; sometimes, trauma or stress induces a very early menopause.[27]

The phase leading up to menopause—called perimenopause—may last several years. During this time, the ovaries' production of estrogen and progesterone, the hormones that control ovulation and menstruation, fluctuates. Common symptoms of perimenopause include irregular periods, hot flashes, and sleep problems. You can still get pregnant during perimenopause—a fact that has surprised many women who became late-in-life moms.[27,24]

Common Symptoms of Menopause

Some complaints, such as untimely hot flashes, are notoriously associated with the onset of menopause. But not all women experience the same symptoms nor to the same degree. Some find menopause to be mild and/or barely noticeable. If any of these symptoms are problematic for you, jot them down to discuss with your physician at your next checkup.

Menstrual changes. Irregular periods occur because of changing levels of estrogen and progesterone and decreasing ovulation. Each of us has a unique pattern to her periods and a personal "norm." As menopause approaches, however, periods may become irregular. Bleeding may be lighter or heavier than usual and may last for fewer days or for more. Your periods may be closer together or missed altogether. When these changes begin, start a journal and record dates, duration, and symptoms.

Hot flashes. Also called flushes, these are common among women at this time. They typically last a few minutes and cause a feeling of heat or burning, followed by profuse sweating—which can really disrupt your sleep during the night. Changing estrogen levels appear to affect the body's central thermostat, causing flashes of heat.[26]

Skin changes. During menopause, the skin becomes thinner and less elastic, leading to sagging and wrinkles, particularly on the face, neck, and hands. These changes may be due to the loss of estrogen. Also, tissue changes and dryness in the vagina may make intercourse uncomfortable.[26]

Achy joints. Many women report stiffness or achy joints, though studies have yet to find a link between these symptoms and "the change." However, we do know that lower levels of estrogen contribute to bone loss, and this may affect cartilage, too. Exercise may help alleviate these symptoms, but be sure to see your doctor if joint pain persists.

Weight gain. Here's one major change that *isn't* thought to be caused by the hormonal shifts: increased body fat. Weight gain—particularly around the midsection—is likely due to decreased physical activity, loss of muscle, and eating too many calories.[26] As you'll see later, studies have shown that lack of exercise is a major contributor to the diminished muscle mass that often strikes in the later years. When you lose muscle, you burn off fewer calories—thus, you're likely to put on pounds of fat.

Memory loss, lack of concentration, migraines, and depression. There seems to be an association between these symptoms and menopause, though research has not illuminated a clear role for changing hormone levels. Having the blues could be hormonally related since estrogen is thought to help neurotransmitters (brain chemicals) work better. Some women also become depressed about the changes they are experiencing in their bodies. Depression is not a given with menopause, but if it does persist, be sure to inquire whether medications may be necessary. Ideally, this will be temporary and also relieved by exercise and proper food choices.

Loss of libido. Stress and relationship problems can certainly contribute to a loss of desire, but internal changes may also be to blame. Fatigue and physical changes related to hormonal fluctuations can make your sizzle fizzle. Loss of desire is not unusual, but it's probably temporary. Ask your health care provider about having your hormone levels tested.

Palpitations. Sometimes a heart palpitation or flutter is experienced along with hot flashes. Although this may be associated with the ebb and flow of changing hormone levels, be sure to mention it to your doctor. Dropping hormone levels during menopause are also associated with more serious health threats that crop up around this time.

Heart disease. Among young adults and people in early middle age, heart disease is more of a worry for men. But at this time of life, women's risk starts to rise, and at the age of 70, women catch up with men in terms of heart disease risk. After 55, women are more likely to die of heart disease than any other cause. Lower estrogen is associated with higher LDL and lower HDL cholesterol. Also, a balanced combination of estrogen and progesterone may have protective effects on the heart, so when they decline, so does the benefit they confer.[26]

Osteoporosis. As you'll learn in the musculoskeletal section, bones aren't static, unchanging body parts. Structures within them are constantly breaking down existing material and building new bone. Ideally, these processes work together proportionally so that the breaking down doesn't exceed the building up. Estrogen plays a role in these processes, and as it dwindles around menopause, your bones may become progressively weaker and more fragile. If you develop osteoporosis, minor bumps or falls can cause broken bones that require a painful recovery and can lead to disability.[26] Sometimes the bone is so weak, it actually breaks *first*, causing a fall. This is often the case with broken hips among the elderly.

You might think that because low estrogen contributes to many menopause-related conditions, taking supplemental estrogen would be a good treatment. Indeed, for years doctors readily prescribed estrogen (along with a form of progesterone for women who hadn't had their uteruses removed; estrogen alone in these cases can contribute to uterine cancer) because hormone therapy *can* help protect your bones and relieve hot flashes and vaginal dryness.[28] However, this treatment became much less appealing in 2002, after a major study was stopped early because hormone therapy was associated with an unacceptably high risk of breast cancer, heart attacks, strokes, and blood clots.[28]

The NIH now recommends you talk with your doctor before using hormone therapy for hot flashes to make sure the benefits outweigh the risks in your particular case. It's a very subjective matter, and hormones are a very complicated issue. This is no time for self-diagnosis or self-medicating.

For preventing osteoporosis, lifestyle changes and bone-building medications are recommended before hormone therapy. The NIH also urges that you not take hormone therapy for heart protection. If you need estrogen to treat vaginal dryness, the NIH recommends local estrogen applications instead of system-wide estrogen. In addition, if you do use menopausal hormone treatments, the NIH suggests that you use the lowest dose possible for the shortest period of time necessary.[28]

Hormone therapy is only one of many steps you can take to treat and prevent menopause-related problems. A lot of lifestyle changes will help you protect yourself from heart disease and osteoporosis and can ease the symptoms of hot flashes.[28]

Biomarkers for Menopause

In general, your health care provider will confirm that you're in perimenopause based on symptoms such as hot flashes and menstrual changes. Once you've gone 12 months without a period, your postmenopausal years have begun.

However, tests that monitor several hormones may be helpful in some cases. One of these is follicle-stimulating hormone (FSH). Your pituitary gland produces this hormone, which makes your ovaries produce estrogen. As menopause approaches, the pituitary gland makes more FSH in an attempt to coax the ovaries into producing estrogen. Thus, several tests showing that your FSH is high can help determine that you're in menopause.[27,24]

The *Positively Ageless* Guide to Managing Menopause Symptoms

Your doctor can prescribe a number of medications to help you handle menopause-related problems, including a short course of hormone therapy for hot flashes (if the risks of replacement hormones aren't too steep in your case), antidepressants or antianxiety drugs for mood swings, medications to preserve bone density, and drugs to reduce the risk of heart disease and treat high blood sugar, if necessary. However, living a menopause-friendly lifestyle—a *Positively Ageless* lifestyle—may help you navigate through these problems with less need for medication.

Keep control of your diet. After age 40 or so, as perimenopause begins or approaches, it becomes time to "be much more vigilant" about how you eat, says Pamela Peeke, MD, MPH, an expert in developmental endocrinology and metabolism and author on women's issues. At midlife, many women tend to not move their bodies as much as they did through either deliberate exercise or the active lifestyles they had when they were younger and raising kids. As you'll learn later in this book, as we get older, our bodies tend to lose the muscle that provides firmness and burns off calories. Even if your weight doesn't change, you may add fat as you lose pounds of muscle. The result can be a "menopot"—the term Dr. Peeke has coined to describe a little mound of fat on the lower belly. "Women after 40 have to be exquisitely aware of the fact that food is not only delicious and nutritious, but it becomes a medicine cabinet that will allow them to attain and maintain their health and keep it going for a heck of a lot longer time," she says. Her suggestions include:

Eat every few hours. This book has already discussed why it's important to spread your daily calories over numerous meals and snacks—it keeps your blood sugar steady and provides a constant stream of antioxidants. Always have your refrigerator and pantry stuffed with nutritious choices so you don't miss a chance to feed some nutrients into your system.

Skip the refined sugar. Avoid the white stuff like processed snacks full of sugar and bleached flour. Get your carbs from whole grains, beans, fruits, and vegetables. You'll feel better in general, and you'll help protect yourself from insulin resistance.

Get plenty of protein. Have your protein-rich foods throughout the day instead of just eating a sizable portion at supper. Protein helps you feel full, so you're less likely to snack on junk, and it supports your muscles.

Keep your heart in mind. In addition to those suggestions, make all the other changes you need to help protect yourself from the rising risk of heart disease. The tips in the heart section of this book, starting on page 37, may be worth a reread, but in general, remember to:

- Eat lots of fruit and vegetables, and go light on salt and sodium to keep your blood pressure from getting high. You may find that once you get filled up on vegetables, grains, and fruits, you won't have room for the less healthy things!

- Steer clear of saturated and trans fats, and emphasize monounsaturated fats to maintain healthy cholesterol levels.

- Eat plenty of salmon and other cold-water fish for their heart-healthy omega-3s.

- Get 30 minutes of exercise most days of the week. And fit in little bits of exercise whenever you can, like taking the stairs instead of the escalator or elevator at the mall or spending part of your lunch hour going for a walk instead of sitting down with friends.

Protect your bones. You'll find an entire section about preventing osteoporosis starting on page 190. Keep these bone-protecting tips in mind.

- Get more calcium and vitamin D. At the age of 50, your calcium requirement climbs to 1,200 milligrams a day. Vitamin D, which helps your body make the most of that calcium, also plays an especially important role at this point in your life. You need between 400 and 800 IU each day, according to the National Osteoporosis Foundation. It's best to get these nutrients in your diet (and vitamin D from a few minutes of sun exposure daily), but ask your doctor whether you'd benefit from supplements. You can find calcium in dairy foods, broccoli, almonds, and fortified orange juice and cereal. Good sources of vitamin D include fortified dairy foods, egg yolks, and saltwater fish.[9]

- Certain forms of exercise are especially helpful for building bone strength: weight-bearing exercise and resistance training. Weight-bearing exercises are those in which your own body weight creates impact, like jogging, walking, and dancing. Swimming and bicycling, by contrast, aren't weight bearing. The vibrations that go through your bones each time your feet strike the ground encourage better bone density. Resistance training is muscle-building exercise, such as lifting weights, which also strengthens your bones. Make sure to include these types of exercise in your regular fitness routines.

Eat soy. Soy foods contain a rich supply of isoflavones, which are chemicals that work like estrogens but more weakly. They fit into estrogen receptors on your cells, kind of like a key in a lock. If you don't have much estrogen, the phytoestrogens can help play the role of estrogen in bodily processes. If you do have a lot of estrogen, however, phytoestrogens can block the effects.[29]

Asian women may have fewer hot flashes because they generally eat a soy-heavy diet. Some studies—but not all—that looked at soy and hot flashes found that soy isoflavones are associated with fewer of these problems.[30,31] In addition, osteoporosis is reportedly less common among Asian women than Western women. Research shows that soy foods may help protect bone density.[29,32] In her book *Body for Life for Women,* Dr. Peeke recommends soy foods such as soy burgers and "crumbles," soy milk, and edamame to help prevent hot flashes, as well as for their possible effects in reducing vaginal dryness, helping preserve bone density, and other health benefits.[33]

Protect your mood. Deficiencies in B vitamins and omega-3 fatty acids may contribute to depression.[34,35,36,37] Take a B-complex vitamin daily to cover any potential deficiencies, and, again, eat several servings of fish weekly, and work flax and flaxseed oil into your diet for their omega-3s.

Take simple steps to reduce hot flashes. According to the NIH, avoiding caffeine and spicy foods may help cut down on hot flashes. Other helpful steps include dressing in layers (so you can remove clothing as you heat up) and keeping your bedroom cool at night.[28] And consider my friend Robin's suggestion: Keep a fan in the bedroom year-round that you can direct at yourself so it doesn't bother your bedmate.

USE OIL TO GIVE YOURSELF A DOSE OF ANTIOXIDANTS

Olive oil contains small but potent amounts of antioxidant polyphenols called tyrosols, which are not found in other common foods. One in particular, called hydroxytyrosol, is thought to have the highest free radical–scavenging capacity. Additionally, olive oil:

- Has compounds that promote increased HDL and a better total cholesterol profile
- Contains vitamin E, an antioxidant that works against free radicals and promotes oxidative balance

Extra-virgin olive oil is considered to be the highest quality, while fine virgin, semifine, refined, and pure olive oil are other grades, in descending order of quality.

Extra-virgin olive oil does not withstand high cooking temperatures, but it is the preferred choice of oil for an uncooked dish such as a salad or a dressing where its assertive flavor can shine. Nonvirgin olive oils, such as semifine, refined, or pure olive oil, stand up to higher temperatures and are the preferred choice for cooking.

Don't use aerosol cooking spray—make your own. Spray bottles are available in health food and kitchen-supply stores and can be filled with your own fresh oils as needed. For regular baking and sautéing, fill the spray bottle with a mild-flavored oil.

Store cooking oils in a cool, dark place for up to 4 months. Because they're composed of highly unsaturated fats, they will turn rancid within several months after opening. Buying a large bottle is not the best option if you use oil infrequently. When in doubt of your oil's freshness, throw it out and open a new bottle. One tablespoon of rancid oil can ruin the flavor of an entire recipe.

OIL PER 2 TABLESPOONS	ORAC
Extra-virgin olive oil	322
Peanut oil	29

chapter 10

STRESS: LET OFF STEAM TO PROTECT YOUR HEALTH

When's the last time you had to protect your kids or your loved ones from a wild animal? Do you frequently have to flee from sudden threats to your life?

Odds are good that you haven't had to do any of these things lately. But our bodies are still set up with an ancient alarm system that kept our ancestors alive long, long ago. In those days, the fight-or-flight response allowed them to quickly get ready to confront danger or run from it.[38]

The body's nervous system and hormonal processes prompted the following changes to prepare our ancestors for action.[38]

- Increased heart rate

- Raised blood pressure

- Raised blood sugar to fuel muscles for activity

- Made blood more likely to clot, in case of injury

- Diverted bloodflow from the digestive tract to the muscles

Even though our modern world tends to be a much safer place than our predecessors faced (at least for most of us, barring natural disasters and wars), our bodies still apply this same fight-or-flight reaction to common, routine sources of stress, like arguments with boyfriends, spouses, or kids; deadlines at work; traffic jams; or long lines at the supermarket.[38] Stress can be acute, such as when you get worried or upset over one event that soon passes—rushing to get to an important meeting on time, for example. Or it can be chronic, such as when taking care of an ailing parent, feeling trapped in an unpleasant relationship, or being deeply in debt.[38]

Sometimes even good events can be stressful, like getting married or going on vacation. Stressful events don't have to be major, either. An important factor in how they affect you is how you perceive them. Some people stay calm even during big problems, while others get worked up over every little issue.[38]

Frequent stress, whether it's acute bouts or a chronic grind, can cause a variety of health problems, from minor to serious. A condition called post-traumatic stress disorder (PTSD)—in which you go through a scary situation, and then relive it in your mind over and over again—can also cause lasting and harmful health effects.[38]

Making some changes to your diet can help protect you from the ill effects of stress, and shifting the way you deal with your surroundings can also turn down your stress level—key steps to protecting your body from the harmful and cumulative effects of stress. Stress can be a major contributor to many major diseases that have a pro-aging effect on the body, so a key antiaging strategy is to manage it effectively. Before we get to specific tips, though, let's take a quick look at what occurs in your body during stress.

Stress Hormones Can Wreak Havoc on Your Health

When you're confronted with a stressful situation, the pituitary gland in your brain—called the master gland because it can affect so many hormonal processes—produces a hormone called ACTH. This hormone prompts the adrenal glands atop your kidneys to produce other hormones, including adrenaline and cortisol, which prepare you for fighting or fleeing.[38,39]

You learned in the immune system section that inflammation can be a good process when it's directed at the right target in controlled doses, but when it rages out of control, it harms your body. Stress hormones work the same way. When you really need them to outpace a mean dog while you're bicycling, stress hormones are great. But when they keep flooding your system over and over again, they can cause illness.[39,40] Adrenaline contributes to elevated cholesterol, increased blood clotting, and atherosclerosis. As you already learned, these are factors that help create clogged arteries and heart attacks.[40]

Elevated cortisol contributes to all kinds of health-harming issues. It causes fat to accumulate around your midsection—a risk factor for heart disease and diabetes. It increases insulin resistance and keeps your cells from taking in glucose. And it impairs your immune system, making you more likely to get sick.[40]

These are big health problems that can keep you from enjoying a long, healthy life. But stress also contributes to problems that are less serious but can rob you of your quality of life, such as:[40]

- Tension headaches

- Temporomandibular joint syndrome (TMJ), which causes jaw pain

- Migraines

- Indigestion

- Diarrhea

- Irritable bowel syndrome

- Weight loss

- Weight gain

- Insomnia

All these potential consequences of stress add up to some powerful influences on how healthy you'll remain as you age. But they're not the only ways that stress can affect health.

A common reaction to stress is to eat. And the foods we reach for when we're wound up aren't typically turkey sandwiches and low-fat yogurt. We grab chocolate bars and bags of chips from the vending machine, we guzzle sodas, and we dig our spoons into pints of gourmet ice cream. These "comfort foods" that we unconsciously feed ourselves are too often foods that have little place in the *Positively Ageless* plan. So part of the plan for handling stress is to learn to reach for healthier choices when pressure builds.

Some of us react to stress by not eating at all, which only makes us feel worse. It's important to try to reestablish regular meal patterns with healthy choices even when we're not up to it. Eating snacks or small portions of the regular *Positively Ageless* fare is better than nothing at all.

The *Positively Ageless* Guide
to Stress Reduction

The *Positively Ageless* eating plan *is* an antistress diet. It gives you B vitamins, antioxidants including vitamin C, and all the other nutrients you need to fortify your immune system when stress beats it down. It also protects your other organs from the threats that stress poses.

If you're chronically under stress, the processes going on in your body are tilting you toward not only a dampened immune system but diabetes, heart disease, and other problems, too. It's especially crucial that you make a priority of getting good fats and lots of fruits and vegetables in your diet and eating small meals throughout the day. In addition, these steps will help.

Eat breakfast. Studies have shown that eating breakfast can lower levels of cortisol, the stress hormone.[41] Though food may be the last thing on your mind when you're feeling topsy-turvy, it's the first step to starting your day on a positive note.

Avoid caffeine. Often we reach for sodas or coffee when we're feeling the pinch. But caffeine's a stimulant, and when it wears off, you can be left foggy-headed, tired, and less able to deal with stressful situations. If you need a flavorful pick-me-up, try a cup of herbal or decaffeinated green tea.

Drink water. Hydration brings oxygen and nutrients to tissues, including the brain. This can provide energy and help us think more clearly, too.

Skip the alcohol. Drinking in response to stress is not a healthy way of coping with pressure—and becoming dependent on alcohol just adds more problems to your life. It may help you feel better temporarily, but alcohol is a depressant and may make you feel even lower. Stress is one of the worst reasons to pour yourself a drink.

Keep wholesome snacks on hand. You probably know what types of situations cause you to feel the pressure of stress: challenges at work, traffic jams on your commute, and paying bills at home. These are the times when you may long for candy, chips, mashed potatoes with butter, fried chicken, and other comfort foods from days past. Keep plenty of *Positively Ageless* foods handy so that you can reach for them instead. Bring a bag of trail mix, dried berries, nuts, or healthy cereal to munch on during rush hour. Keep low-fat yogurt in your workplace refrigerator. Tea bags are portable and offer a variety of flavors to suit your mood. Keep them everywhere—your purse, desk, and car, plus a big supply at home.

Exercise. Exercise is a great stress reliever. It can serve as a form of meditation, and it helps you sleep better so you're more refreshed and ready to face the next day. Some forms of exercise are particularly good at reducing stress; namely, yoga and tai chi, especially in a communal setting so you can interact with other people. Look for classes in your area at gyms, the YMCA, or community centers.

For those times when you just can't leave the house, buy a yoga or Pilates video and follow along. Even if you don't go for these relaxing activities, make sure to devote half an hour to your favorite exercise on most days. The best part about exercising to relieve stress is that it elicits a need to drink water and a desire to eat healthier foods. A great workout or brisk walk rarely leaves you craving junk food or thirsty for a cocktail.

Think positively. If you have a tendency to "go to the dark side," keep a stress rubber band loosely on your wrist. When you have a negative thought, snap the rubber band. That's a reminder to think positively.

Practice stress relief. Regular prayer, meditation, guided visualization (which is like organized daydreaming), and deep breathing have powerful relaxation qualities. Making time to do one of those can help lower your stress levels in general, and, when you're caught up in a stressful situation, allow you to quickly regain a sense of control. Check your local bookstore or library for books on these stress-relieving activities.

Explore your reactions. Remember, stress isn't just a matter of outside events that happen to you—it also comes from how you react to these events. Consider keeping a "stress journal," in which you take a few minutes each day to write down unpleasant events, how they made you feel, how you reacted to them, and how you could react differently next time.

Get organized. Sometimes taking half a day or even a couple of hours to get affairs in order can greatly alleviate feelings of being overwhelmed. Organize your finances, file away paperwork, or update your calendar and appointments. Make a schedule to do this regularly so you'll always feel on top of it, rather than feeling overwhelmed by the weight of *it* on top of you.

Laugh. Go see a comedy show, rent a film, or call a funny friend. Laughter should be a part of every day. It releases tension and minimizes stress.

Walk your dog. If you don't have a pet, consider getting one. The therapeutic benefits of pets have gained recognition in recent years. Pets provide a consistent source of comfort and love. They accept us unconditionally and elicit a nurturing response. Research has shown that pet ownership can reduce stress-induced symptoms, including high blood pressure. A study conducted at UCLA found that dog owners required much less medical care for stress-induced aches and pains than non–dog owners.

Stay in touch. Feeling stressed and/or depressed often makes us want to isolate ourselves. This is especially dangerous when you live alone. Pick up the phone and call a friend or relative. Make plans for a movie or a walk. Stay connected to the people who love and support you.

chapter 11

STAY SAFE FROM STROKE DAMAGE

Your brain is a greedy organ. Though it weighs only about 3 pounds—about 2 percent of the average person's weight—it takes in roughly one-quarter of all the blood that your heart pumps out.[42] Each pulse of blood that reaches your brain delivers a new batch of oxygen and glucose that your billions of neurons depend upon for survival. If anything interrupts this constant supply of fuel, the neurons will die.[43]

That's what a stroke is—an interruption of blood to your brain. These events are a major source of death and disability. According to the American Heart Association (AHA), once you've had a stroke, you have three possible outcomes.[44]

- You may die. Twenty-four percent of strokes are fatal.

- You may be left with a permanent disability. This happens to 15 to 30 percent of people who survive their strokes.

- You'll get better or have only a mild disability, which occurs in 50 to 70 percent of stroke survivors.

Depending on the severity of the stroke and where it strikes the brain, the resulting disability can involve paralysis; memory loss; vision problems; swallowing difficulty; and trouble speaking, reading, or comprehending speech. In addition, strokes are thought to be the second-most common cause of dementia (Alzheimer's is the first). A series of tiny strokes that don't cause serious problems nevertheless can cause mental changes that accumulate into dementia.[45]

Most strokes have a lot in common with heart attacks, leading some experts to refer to strokes as brain attacks. And the steps that you've learned will help protect you from heart disease will do double duty, helping your brain stay safe from stroke, too!

KNOW THE SIGNS OF A STROKE

If you notice any of these signs of a stroke, call 911 or seek emergency medical help immediately. Quick treatment can reduce the risk of serious consequences.[52]

- Sudden numbness or weakness in your face or an arm or leg, particularly on one side
- Sudden confusion or difficulty speaking or understanding speech
- Sudden difficulty seeing
- Sudden dizziness, difficulty walking, or trouble balancing
- Severe headache with a rapid onset and no known cause

In addition, if you think that someone else might be having a stroke, ask the person to do the following actions:

- Smile.
- Raise both arms.
- Speak a simple sentence.

If he or she can't do them, a stroke may be to blame. Call 911.

How Lifestyle Changes Can Prevent Strokes

Strokes typically come in two forms. The most common is an *ischemic* stroke, accounting for about 88 percent of the events. These occur when something blocks the flow of blood through an artery feeding the brain. This "something" may be a buildup of plaque (from atherosclerosis) in an artery or a blood clot that's formed in or near the brain or traveled through an artery from elsewhere in the body. Or the two can combine to block the flow of blood through an artery.[44,46]

The other main type of stroke is a *hemorrhagic* stroke. This occurs when an artery ruptures, allowing blood to leak into the brain tissues.

This starves one part of your brain of blood and may cause more damage if the leaking blood builds up pressure on surrounding brain tissue. High blood pressure may also play a role in hemorrhages.[44,46]

You may be inclined to think that your heart and brain are distant organs, so what threatens the health of one isn't necessarily a danger for the other. That isn't the case. The blood vessels that feed your heart and your brain are part of one big system. Imagine if you had problems with the water pipes in your home: Gunk was building up within the pipes throughout the house, and stray clumps of material occasionally flowed into your home from the water company. These problems might mean that water would stop flowing to your kitchen sink, the bathtub upstairs, or the faucet outside. You wouldn't consider these to be separate issues but complications of the same underlying causes. By getting a plumber to help you treat and prevent buildup in the pipes and calling the water utility so it would keep clogs from flowing into your home, you'd reduce the chances of blockages in all your fixtures. You want to make sure you take the same steps to keep the arteries, or "pipes," to your brain healthy and free from obstruction.

The *Positively Ageless* Guide to Preventing Strokes

For detailed information on how to follow the principles of a heart-healthy diet that protects your brain, refer back to the tips in the heart section starting on page 37. In short, though, remember to:

Keep your blood pressure low. This will help lower your risk of hemorrhagic strokes and help cut down on atherosclerosis, one of the processes that underlie ischemic strokes.[47] To help lower blood pressure, eat a diet rich in potassium—fruits and vegetables are a great source—and low in sodium. Cut down on processed foods and toss out your saltshaker. Exercising regularly, avoiding smoking, and keeping your weight at a normal level are important for good blood pressure, too. Finally, hold your alcohol consumption to one drink a day.

Keep your LDL low and your HDL high. Keeping your cholesterol in check is an important step toward preventing atherosclerosis.[47] This means limiting saturated fat, such as in red meat and full-fat dairy, and emphasizing healthier oils such as olive, canola, and flaxseed. Cut out trans fat, found in processed baked goods. And eat your fish! The omega-3s in salmon,

(continued on page 162)

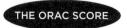
THE ORAC SCORE

DO A LITTLE MATH TO ESTIMATE
YOUR STROKE RISK

The following formula can help women who are 55 or older determine their risk of having a stroke during the next 10 years. If you discover that you're at high risk—or your risk is simply higher than you'd like it to be—the knowledge may inspire you to make dietary and other lifestyle changes that will lower your risk. Also ask your doctor if you'd benefit from medications to lower your blood pressure or cholesterol.[53]

This formula comes from the National Institutes of Health. First add up points based on your age and blood pressure and whether you have diabetes or cardiovascular disease, smoke, and/or have had two particular heart conditions. Then find your 10-year probability of having a stroke.[53]

AGE	POINTS
55–56	+0
57–59	+1
60–62	+2
63–64	+3
65–67	+4
68–70	+5
71–73	+6
74–76	+7
77–78	+8
79–81	+9
82–84	+10

SYSTOLIC BLOOD PRESSURE (UNTREATED)	POINTS
95–106	+1
107–118	+2
119–130	+3
131–143	+4
144–155	+5
156–167	+6
168–180	+7
181–192	+8

SYSTOLIC BLOOD PRESSURE (UNTREATED)	POINTS
193–204	+9
205–216	+10

SYSTOLIC BLOOD PRESSURE (TREATED)	POINTS
95–106	+1
107–113	+2
114–119	+3
120–125	+4
126–131	+5
132–139	+6
140–148	+7
149–160	+8
161–204	+9
205–216	+10

DIABETES	POINTS
No	0
Yes	+3

CIGARETTES	POINTS
No	0
Yes	+2

CARDIOVASCULAR DISEASE	POINTS
No	0
Yes	+2

HISTORY OF ATRIAL FIBRILLATION	POINTS
No	0
Yes	+6

DIAGNOSIS OF LEFT VENTRICULAR HYPERTROPHY	POINTS
No	0
Yes	+34

(continued)

(cont.)

YOUR POINTS	10-YEAR PROBABILITY	YOUR POINTS	10-YEAR PROBABILITY	YOUR POINTS	10-YEAR PROBABILITY
1	1%	10	6%	19	32%
2	1%	11	8%	20	37%
3	2%	12	9%	21	43%
4	2%	13	11%	22	50%
5	2%	14	13%	23	57%
6	3%	15	16%	24	64%
7	4%	16	19%	25	71%
8	4%	17	23%	26	78%
9	5%	18	27%	27	84%

sardines, and some other fish may help protect you from stroke. A diet rich in fiber (especially soluble fiber) also helps reduce bad cholesterol, while regular exercise helps both lower your LDL and raise your HDL cholesterol.

Limit dietary cholesterol. If you're at high risk of vascular disease, you should limit yourself to 200 milligrams of dietary cholesterol daily. If you're not at high risk, you can have 300 milligrams daily. You won't find dietary cholesterol in plant foods—only animal foods like egg yolks, meat, and some seafood, including shrimp.[50]

Eat your antioxidants. You learned earlier that LDL cholesterol in artery walls can become oxidized by free radicals, which contributes to the accumulation of immune-system cells and other substances during the process of atherosclerosis. Eating foods high in antioxidants like vitamin C and vitamin E will help protect you.[50]

Taking single antioxidants in supplement form isn't the answer, though. Different kinds of fruits and vegetables contain a tremendous variety of antioxidants and phytochemicals that work in concert to protect you. Nutrition experts have barely scratched the surface of knowing what these food components do individually, let alone in teams. Blueberries alone contain more than 300 different plant chemicals.

Antioxidants often provide the color, scent, and flavor in fruits and vegetables, so going for an ever-shifting palette of colors will offer the variety you need for steady protection from free radicals while keeping your menus delicious and interesting.[50]

INTENSE FLAVORS CAN BRING
INTENSE BURST OF ANTIOXIDANTS

Many cultures consider garlic, ginger, and onions the "trinity" of core seasoning ingredients. A small amount of these distinctive ingredients can add large layers of flavor to nearly any recipe. But their healing powers transcend flavor and texture.

Check out the antioxidant power, measured in ORAC units, of these *Positively Ageless* allies.

THE ORAC SCORE

FOOD	SERVING SIZE	ORAC
Ginger	2 Tbsp	1,781
Onion, red, raw	½ c	917
Onion, yellow, raw	½ c	823
Garlic, raw	2 Tbsp	330

Prevent diabetes damage. Reducing your risk of diabetes—or carefully controlling your blood sugar if you have the condition—will make you less likely to have a stroke.[47] The damage that high blood sugar does to your blood vessels encourages atherosclerosis. As said before, maintaining a healthy weight and getting regular exercise can help you prevent or treat diabetes. Eating several small meals throughout the day, including protein with each meal and snack, and focusing on complex carbohydrates rather than processed "white" carbs will help keep your blood sugar stable.

Reduce homocysteine. Having high levels of the amino acid homocysteine in your blood is associated with a higher risk of stroke. Its harmful effects include damaging the lining of your arteries and encouraging blood clots.[50,51] You can lower your homocysteine levels by raising your vitamin B_6, B_{12}, and folate (also known as folic acid) levels. Doing so can help protect you from its harmful effects.[50,51] For food sources that supply an ample amount of these B vitamins, check the list in Week One on page 95.

chapter 12

ALZHEIMER'S: ENJOY A FIT MIND AND BODY IN YOUR BOOMER YEARS AND BEYOND

The number of people who live to an old age will swell dramatically in coming decades. That's great news in terms of improving your chances of living a long life. Unfortunately, as more people live to their eighties, nineties, and beyond, the number of people affected by Alzheimer's disease is expected to skyrocket, too. That paints a more troubling picture of what old age will hold for many people.[54]

The numbers are startling. Right now, about 4.5 million Americans have Alzheimer's. By 2050—a not-so-distant time in which quite a few baby boomers will still be alive—that number may more than triple to 16 million, according to the Alzheimer's Association.[54]

As you progress through your later years, the chance that you'll develop Alzheimer's will rise steeply. Fewer than 1 percent of people in their early sixties have the condition. After the age of 65, the number rises to 10 percent. And almost every other person who's 85 or older has Alzheimer's![54]

This disease is cruel to the people it strikes and heartbreaking for their families and loved ones. Though occasional memory slips are very normal as we get older, Alzheimer's symptoms typically begin with increasing forgetfulness. People have trouble with simple, everyday tasks; struggle to find words; and get lost in familiar settings. They may behave inappropriately and show sudden mood swings. In later stages, people with Alzheimer's can no longer recognize their families or function independently.[54]

The goal of *Positively Ageless* living is to reap the rewards of a lifetime of healthy choices: You arrive in your later years unburdened (or less burdened) by major health complaints. You're able to treasure a rich array of experiences with a sharp mind and a strong body.

Obviously, many health conditions can interfere with that goal, and Alzheimer's is the most significant threat to your ability to think clearly in your senior years. Although experts still don't know exactly what causes Alzheimer's—and even less about how to prevent it—the evidence is accumulating that the same sensible steps that can prevent heart disease and cancer may also help protect you from this tragic memory-robbing disease.

What Is Alzheimer's?

The physical signs of the disease that Dr. Alois Alzheimer noticed in a female patient a century ago are still the focus of interest with researchers today: clumps and jumbles of protein in the brain called plaques and tangles.[55]

Your brain contains 100 billion nerve cells called neurons. These allow you to process information, store memories, communicate, and do the other things that you consider "thinking."[54,56] Plaques are dense clumps formed from bits and pieces of a protein called beta-amyloid that accumulate between neurons. Tangles are made of twisted fibers of a protein called *tau* within the neurons. Normally, this protein provides structure to internal components in the neurons; when they become tangled, the cell doesn't work right or dies.[54,56]

According to the Alzheimer's Association, it's normal to develop plaques and tangles with age, but people with Alzheimer's get a lot more, and they show up in specific areas of the brain.[54] Experts still aren't sure what causes these spots of damage. However, they now suspect that the plaques outside the neurons can play a role in the development of the cell-damaging tangles within the neurons.[56]

You can't do anything about your age to reduce your risk of Alzheimer's. Nor can you do anything about your family history, which is another risk factor: Having close relatives with the disease means you're at least twice as likely to develop it. But some risk factors may be changeable. Here are some other features that are thought to be involved in Alzheimer's that you may find interesting, now that you've already learned so much about preventing them.[54]

Oxidation. The plaques of beta-amyloid are thought to contribute to oxidation, or free-radical damage within the brain. Experts think that antioxidants may play a helpful role in interfering with this process. Some studies looking at large groups of people support the idea that antioxidant vitamins C and E may help delay the development of Alzheimer's. A 2004 study that followed more than 3,000 elderly people found that taking supplemental vitamins E and C lowered the risk of Alzheimer's by more than 60 percent.[57,55,58]

Inflammation. Experts also believe that plaques contribute to inflammation in the brain, which causes the death of neurons. A number of studies of large groups of people have linked the use of anti-inflammatory drugs with a lower risk of Alzheimer's. It's too early to say that foods that discourage inflammation will keep you safe, but a diet rich in these foods may lower your risk.[55]

AGEs. Early laboratory research shows that advanced glycation end products (AGEs) may contribute to the development of plaques and tangles. These substances, which are a combination of glucose and protein, are thought to play a role in a wide variety of diseases of aging. As you may remember from page 10, these are formed in your body (particularly when you have high blood glucose); they can enter your body from smoking; and you also ingest them in foods, particularly those high in saturated fat and fried or broiled meats.[59]

Risk factors for cardiovascular disease. Although Alzheimer's disease accounts for the majority of cases of dementia—which brings memory loss and difficulty thinking—the next most-common type of dementia is called vascular dementia. This is caused by small strokes, which are blockages or ruptures in blood vessels feeding the brain.[54]

Vascular (blood vessel) disease may also contribute to Alzheimer's. Experts still are unclear about the connection between the two, but vascular problems could lead to Alzheimer's, or they could interact with Alzheimer's to make it worse.[66] A number of factors that raise your risk of vascular disease are also associated with a higher risk of Alzheimer's: diabetes, high cholesterol, high blood pressure, smoking, high homocysteine levels, and being overweight. Living a heart-healthy, diabetes-preventing lifestyle may also protect your mental functioning in later life.[60]

Biomarkers for Alzheimer's Disease

A skin test in the initial stages of development may one day allow detection of Alzheimer's at early onset. Though there is a vital need for an early biomarker, according to the Alzheimer's Association, there's currently not a particular test that proves that a person has the disease. However, a doctor can diagnose dementia by asking a patient questions and observing her responses, behaviors, and mood.

A variety of blood and urine tests can rule out other conditions that might cause mental confusion, like diabetes, liver disease, and thyroid problems. A doctor can also create an image of a person's brain with a CT scan (computerized tomography) or MRI to rule out strokes, tumors, and other causes of symptoms.[54] A skilled health care provider familiar with the condition can also diagnose the condition by looking for its specific symptoms.

The *Positively Ageless* Guide to Preventing Alzheimer's

Eat like the Mediterraneans do. Research has linked certain foods, nutrients, and other food components to a lower risk of Alzheimer's or a slower decline in mental functioning. These include fish, vitamins C and E, flavonoids, unsaturated fat, certain B vitamins, and moderate alcohol use—all a part of the *Positively Ageless* eating plan. On the other hand, other studies haven't found a relationship between many of these factors and Alzheimer's risk or cognitive functioning.[61]

However, we don't live on a steady diet of particular nutrients—we eat many different things that work synergistically to influence our health. In 2006, a team of researchers from Columbia University in New York City published their findings about the possible influence of the so-called Mediterranean diet on the risk of Alzheimer's. People in the Mediterranean region have traditionally eaten lots of vegetables, fruit, grains, beans, and olive oil; quite a bit of fish; a moderate amount of alcohol (usually wine); and a relatively low amount of dairy, meat, and saturated fat. A lot of evidence has linked this eating style to a lower risk of cardiovascular disease, cancer, and dying in general.[61]

The researchers followed more than 2,200 New Yorkers without dementia for several years. These people were, on average, in their late seventies; during the course of the study, 262 of them developed Alzheimer's. The researchers divided the participants according to how closely they adhered to the eating habits of the Mediterranean diet: high, medium, or low adherence.[61] The people who most closely followed the Mediterranean diet were 40 percent less likely to develop Alzheimer's than the group whose diet least resembled that of the Mediterraneans![61]

A lesson from this study is that you shouldn't focus on individual food elements to prevent Alzheimer's (at least, based on today's knowledge of the disease). Instead, make sure you constantly eat a wide variety of plant foods—all those fruits and veggies, grains, beans, and good-for-you oils you've been reading about in these pages—to ensure that your body receives a steady stream of all their health-protecting nutrients. Make cold-water fish a major supply of your protein.

Reduce your risk of cardiovascular disease. Just as the foods you eat work in concert to keep you healthy, the systems in your body depend upon the support of each other to maintain health.

Where your cardiovascular system goes, your mind may follow. It's becoming more evident that people at risk of heart disease and stroke could face an extra-high risk of developing Alzheimer's. In turn, people are more likely to develop cardiovascular disease if they have diabetes—which has also been linked to Alzheimer's.

You just can't get away from the importance of the steps for maintaining your cardiovascular health. These aren't pat suggestions that support an abstract notion of "health"; they play very specific roles in regulating your body's interlinked chemical processes to ensure that they work properly.

- Exercise regularly.

- Keep your weight at a healthy level.

- Avoid tobacco smoke—yours and other people's.

- Eat unsaturated fats and fish high in omega-3s.

- Eat foods high in folate to lower your homocysteine levels.[62] Good dietary sources of folate include dark leafy greens, legumes, bananas, and broccoli. Homocysteine, a major risk factor for cardiovascular disease, was found to be a "strong, independent factor for the development of dementia and Alzheimer's disease" in a 2002 study in the *New England Journal of Medicine*. As homocysteine levels rise, so does the risk of these conditions, the study reported. (See the B_6 chart on page 95.)

Keep your brain active. "Exercising" your brain may help it develop and maintain connections between neurons that are important for protecting your mental faculties as you age. In other words, if you don't use it, you may lose it.[63] Ways to maintain your mental sharpness include:

- Constantly learning new things. Check out library books about unfamiliar subjects. Watch educational TV programs that challenge you to think about new topics.

- Do crosswords, sudoku, and other puzzles every day.

- Be a perpetual student. Take classes at your local college or community center.

- Memorize short lists of objects—such as items on your shopping list—and bring up old memories and try to remember details.

- Combining social activities with your mental challenges can be especially helpful in warding off dementia. A Swedish study from 2002 that started tracking more than 1,000 seniors for nearly a decade found that those who engaged in frequent social activities had roughly 40 percent less risk of developing dementia.[64] Join a book club or other club, volunteer for organizations that get you out of your home, and travel to see new places.[65]

The *Positively Ageless* Program for Age-Proofing Your Hormones and Mind

At the end of each weekly section, you'll find an overview of specific tips to follow to incorporate the *Positively Ageless* diet into your lifestyle. These tips are broken down into stages. "Make One Change" is a list of easy-start changes. If you can only make one change per week, pick one from this list. "Quick Start" includes tips and strategies that are important but may take a bit longer to incorporate into your life. Suggestions you should follow for maximum antiaging benefit are listed in "Young for Life."

In addition, we've included a week's worth of meal plans that utilize the *Positively Ageless* ingredients. You'll find recipes for many of these menu items in the recipe section toward the back of the book.

Make One Change

If you feel able to make only one change in your life, pick it from this list. Research has shown these to be the most important strategies for slowing the aging clock.

Lose the white stuff! This age-robber is insidious—sugar and refined flour are hidden in everything from condiments to cereal. *Positively Ageless* includes lots of homemade condiments (and cereals!) for this reason. Make some **Miso Marinade** this week (recipe on page 287). Patrol your kitchen as a label detective, and make your kitchen come clean of these pro-aging foods.

Fiber up. Not only will this help you feel full so you eat less and stay regular, but more fiber will keep your blood sugar even. "Good" sources of fiber have at least 2.5 grams per serving; excellent have at least 5 grams per serving. Check the labels in your pantry and your shopping cart this week and aim for at least 4 grams per serving.

Go for grains. Whole grains increase satiety, raise fiber, and promote regularity. Choose whole grains for bread, cereal, and baking ingredients. For more tips, see the *Positively Ageless* pantry on what to choose (and what to lose) on page 108.

Bean out. Stock up on dried beans and lentils, and always keep a couple of cups cooked and in the fridge to sprinkle on a salad or add to your entrée. Cooked lentils have a whopping 8 grams of fiber per half cup, and black beans have 7 grams.

Berry up. Make berries a part of your breakfast and dessert routine. Blueberries contain compounds that promote better memory retention. They also have tons of fiber and more antioxidants than most fruits and vegetables. Stock up on fresh berries; when they're out of season or prohibitively expensive, buy frozen.

Hold the caffeine—especially if stress or insomnia are big issues for you. Switch to green or herbal teas by the cup. Whip up a batch of **Zinger Green Tea** (page 271) to keep in the fridge for a cool refresher, and stash extra green tea bags in your purse and glove box and at work. See the sidebar on caffeine on page 103.

Track it. If you suspect you're on the edge of crossing over to menopause, start keeping a menstrual diary. (See On the Web on page 350 for a diary template.) Record the dates, duration, and intensity of your periods.

You can even include physical, emotional, behavioral, and eating patterns that you observe. As time progresses, it will be easier to discuss with your doctor and discern when things started and what action plan to take for your optimal comfort.

Quick Start

These strategies are a little more involved, but the benefits will reflect the additional effort you're spending. They'll provide a jump-start for measurable results in a short period of time.

Test it. If you suspect you've met the first few criteria of perimenopause (see page 143), take a home test to measure your FSH. If it's positive, discuss the results with your health care provider to decide on your "next steps." See the On the Web on page 350 for home test kit details.

Pop it! Though I am a very strong advocate of meeting nutrition needs through food, menopause is a crucial time when your body is being taxed and needs to be well nurtured and nourished. If you're having trouble eating a balanced diet or getting enough fish, or if you just don't like fish or flax, now's the time to consider taking a good multivitamin and/or omega-3 supplements. See the Shopping Resources on page 351.

Savor soy. Traditional soy foods are stellar sources of vegetable protein and also confer mild estrogenic effects, just when your body's turning off the tap. Moderate amounts can help promote cardiac health and preserve bone mass. Try roasted soy nuts for a high-protein snack, or use calcium-fortified soy milk instead of dairy in smoothies and other recipes as inventive ways to introduce this valuable legume to your diet.

Find your groove. If you're having trouble sleeping or making time for exercise, you can still switch your schedule around this week to find out what works best for you. If insomnia is a concern, you may want to work out earlier in the day, and be sure to have your second snack before dinner instead of after. A gradual boost in exercise can only mean good things—for your weight, your muscle, your bones, your mood, and your sleep! A routine schedule also helps regulate your hormones to control your insulin and your appetite.

Step up to the scale. Last week a food scale; this week a *you* scale. A calibrated scale will track your progress. Be sure to choose a scale with a zeroing mechanism. See the Shopping Resources on page 351 for body-fat scales.

Walk, run, swim, shake it, or stretch it. It's time for more exercise this week; aim for 30 minutes a day. Your real program starts next week, so by then, let's get the motivation, soreness, and "don't have a thing to wear" issues out of the way. Snacks are really important now; don't forget to include protein with every meal and snack.

File it. If you're overwhelmed or having problems with memory or clarity, set aside a half day to organize your paperwork. It may take a few sessions to find your way, but putting everything in its place will clear your office space as well as your head. Set aside at least an hour a week to stay on top of it from now on so it won't topple you. With your home and your things organized, it will be easier to keep your thinking on track.

Cool down. If you're experiencing hot flashes, find a small fan to keep by your bed (and maybe one for near your desk at work).

Make some memories. If you're having problems with depression, isolating yourself is the worst thing to do (though it's often the easiest). Pick up the phone and make plans to join a friend for a meal, tea (green tea!), or just a great conversation. Strive to put aside any grudges or anger you may have and focus on the positive. Seeking professional help is a sign of strength, not weakness. Optimism and positive thinking help stop the clock!

Laugh it up. Rent a funny film, see a comedy show, or call a funny friend. Laughter is healing and cathartic. There's no biomarker at this point, but studies show that laughter can definitely stop the clock. In the words of Norman Cousins, a prominent author and world peace advocate, "Laughter is inner jogging."

Rub down. Need a reason for a massage? Look no further. Massage—along with yoga, hot baths, and meditation—is an excellent way to achieve deep relaxation, clear your mind, and induce restful sleep.

Young for Life

This list of strategies is for those of you who are ready for a major lifestyle intervention. While you'll need to spend a bit more effort enacting these good habits, the payoff can be a dramatic, lasting impact on your health.

Make time for a visit. Depending on the results of your menstrual journal or any personal or family issues with diabetes, Alzheimer's, or depression, you may need to schedule an appointment with your physician or an endocrinologist to discuss menopause or blood sugar issues. If you had positive results from a home FSH test, be sure to share them with your doctor.

Assess it. Take the test for stroke risk on page 160. For further information, see On the Web on page 350.

Play games. If you're not already participating in an organized sport, consider joining a team or club for softball, walking, running, hiking, or cycling. Not only will the scheduled get-togethers motivate you to increase your allotment of exercise, you'll also meet new acquaintances and make new friends.

Stretch your social circle. Start a new tradition, whether it's entertaining guests for Sunday suppers or exploring a new restaurant with a friend once a month. Step back and take a good look at your socializing patterns. If they're really humdrum (or worse yet, nonexistent), it's time to expand your horizons.

Find peace. Set aside 20 minutes each day to pray, meditate, or do yoga or deep-breathing exercises. Fill your heart and your mind with positive thoughts and energy.

Catch some z's. Spend a half day doing a makeover on your bedroom. Whether it's new pillows, linens, room-darkening shades, or a night-light, make your space conducive to restful sleep. Try to take an invigorating catnap each day for renewed energy and clarity so the last part of the day is as full and enjoyable as the first half. And be sure you get enough sleep. Burning the candle at both ends has cumulative effects. It *will* catch up with you.

Sign up. Become a lifelong learner. Whether it's history, cooking, or Japanese paper folding, keeping your mind active not only makes you more attractive but gives your brain the same type of workout that your body is now enjoying. Think young to stay young.

chapter 13

EAT SMART, LIVE LONG MENUS

Positively Ageless Menus Week Two

The *Positively Ageless* menu plans are based on an average of 1,200 calories per day. If your calorie needs are a little higher (or lower), you can adjust accordingly. Adding a glass of 1 percent milk, 6 ounces of fat-free yogurt, one pear or a large apple, or a glass of red wine with dinner will each provide an additional 100 calories.

Positively Ageless **recipes** are listed in bold and designated as one serving size.

The two snacks can be scheduled between meals or one between meals and one after dinner.

DAY 1

1,243 calories; 37 grams fiber; 1,330 milligrams omega-3s

BREAKFAST

½ cup cooked old-fashioned oatmeal topped with ¼ cup fat-free yogurt, ⅓ cup blueberries, and 1 tablespoon slivered almonds

8 ounces hot green tea or water

MID-MORNING SNACK

1 hard-cooked omega-3 egg

Jicama sticks and **Zippy Hummus** (page 294)

8 ounces iced green tea

LUNCH

Asian-Style Fish (page 319)

½ cup brown basmati rice

1 pear

8 ounces green tea with ginger

MID-AFTERNOON SNACK

⅓ cup fat-free ricotta cheese with ¼ cup raspberries and 2 teaspoons chopped pecans

8 ounces water or green tea

DINNER

Lebanese Kebabs (page 322) with **Tangy Mustard Dressing** (page 281)

1½ cups salad (dark green leafy lettuce dressed with 1 tablespoon vinaigrette)

1 cup mixed berries

8 ounces green tea or fat-free milk

DAY 2

1,182 calories; 33 grams fiber; 1,550 milligrams omega-3s

BREAKFAST

Omelet made with 1 omega-3 egg plus 1 egg white, 6 halved cherry tomatoes, basil, and 2 tablespoons sautéed onion

$\frac{1}{2}$ grapefruit drizzled with 1 tablespoon **Pomegranate Syrup** (page 282)

$\frac{1}{2}$ whole grain muffin or bagel

8 ounces white or green tea or water

MID-MORNING SNACK

2-inch wedge honeydew

2 ounces thinly sliced turkey breast

4 almonds

8 ounces water

LUNCH

Green Tea Miso Soup (page 297)

$1\frac{1}{2}$ cups salad (dark green leafy lettuce dressed with 1 tablespoon extra-virgin olive oil and fresh lemon juice to taste)

$\frac{1}{2}$ cup black raspberries

8 ounces iced green tea with lemon or water

MID-AFTERNOON SNACK

Smoothie with $\frac{1}{2}$ cup kefir, $\frac{1}{4}$ cup almond milk, and $\frac{1}{4}$ cup sliced strawberries

8 ounces water or green tea

DINNER

4 ounces boneless, skinless grilled chicken breast

Wild Rice with Radicchio and Dried Cherries (page 309)

Steamed artichoke with lemon

Spicy Strawberry Frozen Yogurt (page 337)

8 ounces mint tea or water

DAY 3

1,173 calories; 29 grams fiber; 1,430 milligrams omega-3s

BREAKFAST

Breakfast wrap made with small whole grain tortilla, 3 egg whites scrambled with 2 tablespoons fat-free refried black beans, 2 tablespoons salsa, and 1 tablespoon grated low-fat Cheddar

¼ cup diced melon plus ¼ cup blueberries

8 ounces fat-free milk or iced green tea

MID-MORNING SNACK

Nutty Chocolate Shake (page 270)

8 ounces water or green tea

LUNCH

4 ounces grilled tofu or chicken breast

Rainbow Radicchio Slaw (page 315)

1 peach

8 ounces iced green tea with lemon or water

MID-AFTERNOON SNACK

Almond Berry Bar (page 346)

8 ounces water or mint tea

DINNER

Sesame Turkey Stir-Fry with Cabbage and Green Beans (page 326)

1 cup cherry tomatoes sprinkled with 1 teaspoon vinaigrette, 1 teaspoon ground flaxseed, and 1 tablespoon chopped parsley

½ medium apple, sliced

4 ounces red wine

8 ounces white tea with ginger slice or water

DAY 4

1,211 calories; 32 grams fiber; 1,930 milligrams omega-3s

BREAKFAST

2 egg whites scrambled with 1 ounce smoked salmon and 1 teaspoon chopped chives

1/4 cup **Positively Ageless Flax Cereal** (page 260) with 1/2 cup sliced strawberries and 1/4 cup fat-free yogurt

8 ounces green tea or water

MID-MORNING SNACK

1 ounce sliced turkey, 1/4 avocado, and 1 tablespoon **Watercress Sauce** (page 289) on 1 Wasa Crispbread

8 ounces iced green tea or water

LUNCH

4 ounces grilled tofu with 1 tablespoon **Miso Marinade** (page 287)

1/2 cup brown rice

1 medium kiwifruit, sliced

8 ounces water

MID-AFTERNOON SNACK

1/2 cup fat-free cottage cheese with 1 teaspoon flaxseed and 1/2 medium apple, chopped

8 ounces water or iced tea

DINNER

3 ounces roast skinless chicken breast

Sweet Potatoes with Onion Confit (page 333)

1 cup steamed broccoli

1 cup fresh raspberries

8 ounces water or chamomile tea

DAY 5

1,172 calories; 31 grams fiber; 5,100 milligrams omega-3s

BREAKFAST

Omelet made with 1 whole omega-3 egg, 1 egg white, $\frac{1}{4}$ cup chopped roasted yellow bell pepper, 2 tablespoons sautéed red onion, $\frac{1}{2}$ teaspoon chopped thyme, and 1 teaspoon olive oil

1 cup fresh blueberries with 1 teaspoon ground flaxseed and $\frac{1}{2}$ teaspoon ground cinnamon

8 ounces green tea or water or fat-free milk

MID-MORNING SNACK

$\frac{1}{2}$ cup fat-free plain yogurt with 1 tablespoon **Mango Butter** (page 286) and 1 chopped Brazil nut

8 ounces iced tea or water

LUNCH

3 ounces grilled lean turkey burger

Salad with 1 cup mixed greens, 1 cup watercress, $\frac{1}{2}$ cup cherry tomatoes, and 1 tablespoon **Tomato Ginger Vinaigrette** (page 283)

$\frac{1}{2}$ cup fresh blackberries

8 ounces green tea or water

MID-AFTERNOON SNACK

1 ounce sliced chicken or turkey breast

4 almonds

$\frac{1}{2}$ apple

8 ounces water

DINNER

3 ounces grilled flank steak

Cumin-Spiced Bulgur and Lentils (page 308)

1 cup Swiss chard sautéed with $\frac{1}{4}$ cup sliced shiitake mushrooms, 1 teaspoon olive oil, 1 teaspoon chopped garlic, and fresh lemon

$\frac{1}{2}$ medium pear, sliced and drizzled with 1 teaspoon dark honey and sprinkled with 1 teaspoon chopped hazelnuts

8 ounces green or white tea or water

DAY 6

1,225 calories; 35 grams fiber; 2,060 milligrams omega-3s

BREAKFAST

1 poached omega-3 egg

Bran Yogurt Muffin (page 264)

2 pieces lean nitrate-free turkey bacon

$\frac{1}{2}$ cup fresh raspberries

8 ounces hot green tea or water

MID-MORNING SNACK

Pinolillo (Spanish Chocolate Shake) (page 273)

2 tablespoons roasted soy nuts

LUNCH

3 ounces thinly sliced roast pork tenderloin

Barley Risotto with Wilted Greens (page 305)

$\frac{1}{2}$ cup sliced tomatoes

$\frac{1}{2}$ cup black raspberries

8 ounces iced green or white tea or water

MID-AFTERNOON SNACK

3 medium asparagus spears wrapped with $\frac{1}{2}$ ounce smoked salmon

8 ounces iced tea with lemon and mint or water

DINNER

3 ounces grilled sea bass

$\frac{1}{2}$ medium artichoke, steamed

Black-Eyed Peas with Garlic (page 332)

4 ounces red wine

1 nectarine

8 ounces green or white tea or fat-free milk

DAY 7

1,227 calories; 27 grams fiber; 3,080 milligrams omega-3s

BREAKFAST

1 omega-3 egg plus 1 large egg white scrambled with 1 tablespoon chopped green onion, 2 tablespoons chopped bell pepper, and 1 ounce lean turkey

½ slice **Whole Grain Bread** (page 306), toasted

½ cup blueberries with ¼ cup fat-free yogurt and 1 teaspoon ground flaxseed

8 ounces green or white tea with fresh lemon or water

MID-MORNING SNACK

Orange and Blueberry Compote in Green Tea–Ginger Syrup
(page 344) and 2 tablespoons fat-free ricotta cheese

8 ounces green tea or water

LUNCH

3 ounces poached salmon topped with ½ cup halved cherry tomatoes, 1 tablespoon chopped black olives, and 1 teaspoon minced basil

2 cups baby lettuce and arugula salad with 1 tablespoon vinaigrette and 3 sliced olives

Chocolate Almond Pudding (page 338)

8 ounces green tea or water

MID-AFTERNOON SNACK

1 ounce sliced smoked turkey

4 walnuts

½ medium apple

8 ounces water

DINNER

3 ounces chicken breast baked with 1 tablespoon **Miso Marinade**
(page 287)

Gingered Edamame with Fire-Roasted Tomatoes (page 331)

1 cup sliced mushrooms sautéed with 1 tablespoon chopped shallots, 1 tablespoon chopped parsley, and 1 teaspoon olive oil

½ cup chopped cantaloupe

8 ounces green tea with mint or water

MUSCLES AND BONES: STRONG IS SEXY

Just as the right food choices help keep our hearts and internal organs vital and healthy, so can the right exercise keep us active and strong. Our musculoskeletal system plays a pivotal role in determining how youthful and active we are. Weakened bones can lead to disability. Out-of-shape muscles can rob us of independence in our later years—while contributing to excess fat now. As you begin the 28-day plan to start aging gracefully, be sure to devote as much attention to exercise as you do to your diet.

chapter 14

STRONG BONES SUPPORT A HEALTHY BODY

Your bones have a few important characteristics that may seem surprising. They give your body structure and support and help you move, but that's not their only job. First of all, your bones also act as a bank that stores calcium, which your body uses for a variety of chemical processes. The mineral helps your nerves send messages and helps your muscles contract, among many other functions. What most people don't realize is that calcium levels in the bloodstream are tightly controlled and do not vary with diet, so that just because your blood levels are normal, it doesn't mean you are taking in enough. When you don't get enough calcium in your diet, your body "withdraws" it from your bones.[1,2]

Second, your bones aren't stable and unchanging. Tiny cells called osteoclasts within your bones are constantly removing old bone, and their counterparts called osteoblasts are laying down a sort of scaffolding for new bone to form. For your bones to stay strong and healthy, the activity of these cells must stay balanced.[2,3]

Bone mass peaks in young adulthood, and after age 30 or so, it starts to dwindle as it breaks down faster than it's being replaced. For a while around menopause, bone loss in women goes even faster,[4] and bones can become fragile and weak. When you look at bone from a healthy young person under a microscope, it looks like a dense honeycomb with thick walls. However, the bones of a person with osteoporosis look more like a lace curtain.[2]

If your bones become thin, your journey through healthy longevity will become more difficult. According to the National Osteoporosis Foundation (NOF), 10 million Americans are thought to have osteoporosis, and another 34 million have low bone mass that puts them at risk of the condition. Although osteoporosis chiefly affects women, men can get it, too.[5]

CHECK YOUR MEDICINE CABINET FOR THESE BONE-ROBBERS

Certain medications, especially when taken in large doses or over long periods of time, are associated with bone loss. Don't stop taking medications or reduce your dose on your own, but if you're concerned that any medications may worsen your risk of weakened bones, discuss this with your doctor. Drugs linked to bone loss include:[3]

- Oral or injected forms of glucocorticoids (also called corticosteroids), which are used for a variety of conditions, including allergies, asthma, and arthritis
- Thyroxine, a thyroid medication, when taken excessively
- Long-term use of certain anticonvulsant drugs
- Heparin, an anticlotting drug
- Drugs that suppress the immune system

Osteoporosis can cause any bone to grow weak enough that it breaks, but it most often leads to fractures in the back, hips, and wrists. A broken bone may be the first sign that you even have a problem! According to the NOF, at least 1.5 million fractures each year in America are due to osteoporosis. Even a bump or a simple fall can cause a brittle bone to break. Sometimes you won't know *what* caused it.[5]

Broken bones cause pain and disability, of course, but those aren't the only consequences of osteoporosis. If your mobility is limited because of a fracture, your muscles can quickly weaken due to lack of movement. Deterioration of the bones in the spine also contributes to the stooped posture and decreased height seen in some elderly women. This is not painless, either—it hurts!

Osteoporosis may also make you want to limit your activities because you're worried about injuring yourself. That may mean fewer hikes with your spouse or less vigorous playtime with your kids or grandkids. These are the things that increase the quality of your life! And osteoporosis may make exercise worrisome if you're anxious about injuries. Exercise helps ward off or treat a variety of major illnesses, and osteoporosis is no exception. Being physically active is important for bone health; you may simply need to take extra precautions if your bones are already weak.[5;1;6]

It's *much* better to plan ahead and prevent weak bones than it is to deal with them once the problem has started. Let's take a look at some of the factors that can make osteoporosis more likely to strike you, so you can take the right steps to fortify your protection.

Factors That Put You at Risk for Osteoporosis

Understanding the risk factors of osteoporosis can inspire you to take action now to prevent this condition. However, even if you aren't in a high-risk category, you can still develop osteoporosis, so it's wise for *all* women to examine their lifestyles to ensure that they're protecting themselves. According to the National Institutes of Health (NIH), these factors (in addition to being female) increase your risk of the condition.

Your age. As you get older, the chance that your bones will become weaker rises.[4]

Your racial and ethnic background. White and Asian women are at the highest risk. African American and Hispanic women have a lower risk, but they can certainly develop the condition, too.[4]

Menopause. Estrogen appears to directly affect your bones, thus playing a role in protecting them from osteoporosis. The hormone seems to do this by influencing the activity of your bone-building osteoblasts and your bone-erasing osteoclasts. Of course, estrogen supply dwindles in menopause. During your last few years of perimenopause (the time before menopause) and the first few years of your postmenopausal life, bone loss occurs at a particularly quick pace. If you go through menopause early, either naturally or due to surgery or cancer treatment, your risk goes up, compared with women your age who haven't gone through menopause yet. Hormone therapy inhibits loss of bone, and research has associated it with fewer fractures. However, hormone therapy brings on other risks, as discussed in Chapter 2, so it's not the answer for everyone.[4,7,3,8]

Your body size. Women with small, thin frames are more likely to develop osteoporosis. Women of menstruating age who have stopped having periods—called amenorrhea—are also at risk. This condition is often

THIN ISN'T IN, AS FAR
AS YOUR BONES ARE CONCERNED

As the saying goes, you can't be too rich or too thin. We'll let you discuss that first one with your accountant, but we know that being too thin really can be a bad thing for your health, including your bone mass. Women who are "small boned" or thin are at greater risk for osteoporosis. What's the cutoff? Research associates a higher risk of osteoporosis with a body weight of less than 127 or a body mass index (BMI) of less than 20. (You can calculate your BMI using the table on page 134.)[22]

associated with athletic women who work out hard, keep their weight and body fat low, and eat poorly. Women with exercise-induced amenorrhea may have lower bone mass.[4,9]

Family history. Like your age and your ethnic background, family history is one of the risk factors for osteoporosis that you cannot change. Because mothers and daughters often have similar body types, if one family member has osteoporosis, other family members have an increased risk.

Your diet history. If you've consumed too little calcium and vitamin D in your life, you're at increased risk of osteoporosis. Having anorexia, an eating disorder in which you eat too little, also makes you more likely to have weak bones. Conditions that reduce your absorption of nutrients—such as inflammatory bowel disease—can keep you from making use of all the calcium in the food you eat, too.[4]

A sedentary lifestyle. A lack of exercise and other physical activity puts you at added risk.[4]

Smoking and drinking. Research shows that women who smoke lose bone at a faster rate and have lower bone density than women who don't smoke, although experts don't know exactly *how* smoking affects your bones. In addition, excessive alcohol use reduces bone formation. Plus, it impairs your coordination so you're more likely to fall and sustain an injury.[4,10]

Medications. Certain medications for diseases—including arthritis, asthma, and thyroid problems—can cause bone loss. See the sidebar on page 186 for more details. You shouldn't stop taking medications or change your regimen without talking to your doctor, but it's a good idea to discuss any possible effects that your medications may have on your bones.[4]

Biomarkers for Osteoporosis

Your doctor may recommend a test of your bone mineral density as a way to determine the strength of your bones. It can identify osteoporosis or even a milder level of bone loss leading up to it, called osteopenia.[11] Bone density testing is performed for people at risk of the condition, including:[12]

- Those with a family history of osteoporosis, osteopenia, or certain fractures

- People with low body weight

- People who have had a previous fracture, particularly after menopause

- Women who are simply postmenopausal and concerned about osteoporosis

Several different procedures can measure bone density. One technique, called DEXA (dual energy x-ray absorptiometry), is a popular method because it is highly accurate. This test can measure bone density in your forearm, hip, spine, and total body. The test takes less than half an hour as the machine scans your body slowly from head to toe. (Pregnant women should not undergo this test.) However, since the equipment is very expensive, the test is also costly, though it's sometimes covered by insurance. DEXA provides results based on whether your bone mineral density is above or below average and lets you know if your bones are normal or if you have osteoporosis or osteopenia.[13] This test helps you and your doctor decide which steps to take to prevent future problems if you're still okay or how to treat you if your bones are already weak. Follow-up testing can determine whether your efforts are working sufficiently.

Another method to identify weakened bones is an ultrasound bone densitometer, a portable machine sometimes found in drugstores and at health fairs. This method is affordable and fairly accurate. However, it's not as thorough as the DEXA. It takes a measurement near your heel, where there is a high percentage of the kind of bone most affected by osteoporosis. The results are used to predict future risk of fracture.

In addition to these scans, your doctor may recommend blood and urine tests to help point out the causes of any bone loss that's found. These measure factors including your calcium and vitamin D levels, thyroid function, and estrogen, which point to how fast your bones are building up or breaking down.[12]

The *Positively Ageless* Guide to Bone Protection

The following lifestyle steps have proven helpful in preventing and treating osteoporosis. However, if you already have osteoporosis or weakened bones, talk to your doctor about how to fit self-care into a comprehensive program, along with possible bone-building medications.

Get plenty of calcium. This point can't be drilled in enough: You must keep your bones well stocked with calcium throughout your life! Teens who are pregnant or breastfeeding should aim for 1,300 milligrams daily—or more. During adulthood, you need[14] 1,000 milligrams of bone-building calcium daily. Once you hit the age of 50, your daily needs jump to 1,200 milligrams. Calcium supplementation may not build bone in menopausal women, but combined with a good diet (including fluoride and vitamin D) and weight-bearing exercise, it can minimize bone loss.

Ideally, you'll meet your calcium needs as part of your *Positively Ageless* diet. The traditional sources of calcium in the American diet are dairy foods, and consuming fat-free or low-fat milk, cheese, and yogurt will help you meet your quota. But plenty of other foods that belong in a healthy diet also supply lots of calcium: leafy green vegetables, canned wild salmon or sardines that contain edible bones, and fortified beverages such as soy milk and orange and grapefruit juices. Half a cup of raw tofu delivers 260 milligrams of calcium. In addition, fruits and vegetables contain components that help you absorb calcium from your diet.

In addition, it's a good idea for many women to take supplemental calcium to ensure that they're protected. If you suspect that your diet falls short of meeting your calcium needs, consider a supplement. See the sidebar for information on how to properly use supplements.[4]

Get plenty of vitamin D, too. Vitamin D acts as calcium's very special assistant in protecting your bones. It helps your intestine absorb calcium

USE CALCIUM SUPPLEMENTS TO THEIR GREATEST ADVANTAGE

Simply tossing back a randomly chosen calcium supplement won't necessarily give you the most helpful dose of bone protection. Keep in mind the following tips.[9,21]

- The main forms of calcium in supplements are calcium carbonate and calcium citrate. The carbonate form is cheaper, each supplement contains a greater percentage of the mineral, and you don't have to take as many pills to get the same amount of calcium. However, people who have decreased stomach acid—which can occur with age—absorb calcium citrate better. The carbonate form is absorbed best with food, but you can take the citrate form without food. Your doctor can help you choose the best type for your needs.

- Take no more than 500 milligrams of calcium at a time. When you take more at once, you absorb less.

- Calcium supplements can cause constipation, gas, and bloating. If this occurs, consider taking your calcium with meals, taking smaller doses throughout the day, or switching brands. See page 351 for Shopping Resources.

from your diet and also helps your kidneys hold on to calcium so it doesn't escape in urine. This vitamin is also special because your body produces it when sunlight hits your skin. Just a few minutes of sunlight exposure to your hands, face, and arms (without sunscreen) a few times a week produces ample vitamin D. The vitamin is also found in fortified dairy foods, fatty fish, and fortified nondairy "milks" like soy and rice milk.[4,1,15]

Experts recommend getting 400 to 800 IU of vitamin D each day. The North American Menopause Society recommends an amount at the higher end of that scale for women who don't get much sunlight because they are housebound or live in northern latitudes. Vitamin D is fat-soluble, meaning it is stored in the body. Taking high doses is toxic, so don't exceed

800 IU daily. Your health care provider can advise you on whether supplements would be helpful in your case.[3,4,15]

Practice weight-bearing exercise. Physical activity isn't just good for your muscles—it encourages healthy bones, too, says William Evans, PhD, a University of Arkansas expert on exercise's effects on aging bodies. It's important to incorporate a variety of physical activities—including weekly strength-training sessions—for good bone health.

When exercise puts stress on your bones, your body responds by increasing bone mass. In a 1994 study in which Dr. Evans was a researcher, 39 postmenopausal women were divided into two groups: One group did high-intensity strength training twice weekly for a year, while the other women maintained their usual exercise routines.[16] The strength trainers did five different exercises, lifting 80 percent of their maximum ability. (As you'll learn in the muscle section [page 195], you need to lift relatively heavy weights to reap muscle-building rewards.) Each session lasted 45 minutes.[16] At the end of the year, the women who lifted weights preserved their total bone mineral content . . . and the ones who didn't follow the routine lost some of theirs. In addition, the women who strength-trained increased their muscle mass and sense of balance while moving, which can reduce the risk of falling.[16]

Some forms of aerobic exercise are also helpful for strong bones. Activities with more impact, such as jogging, tennis, climbing stairs, tap dancing, or merely jumping up and down are thought to offer more bone-protecting potential. With weight-bearing exercise, the bone adapts to the stress and the impact by building more osteoblasts, thus becoming stronger.[18] Swimming and bicycling aren't especially useful for bone health, however, since your bones don't carry much load when you're in the water or on a bike saddle. Walking isn't extremely protective, either.

However, if you have osteoporosis or a history of fracture, certain activities can actually *hurt* you. Talk to your doctor before beginning any exercise program, and keep these tips in mind.[18,19]

- If you already have osteoporosis, skip high-impact activities such as jumping rope or jogging; activities that require you to twist or bend, like golf; and activities in which you may fall, like skiing, recommends the NIH.

- Use good posture when doing exercises. A qualified personal trainer can show you how to maintain good form.

- If you have to bend, do so from the hips and knees, not the waist. Skip the situps and toe-touches if you already have osteoporosis.

Put out the cigarettes. If you're still smoking, talk to your doctor about ways you can stop—particularly if menopause is approaching. Your bones need all the help they can get throughout your life, along with a minimal amount of harm to them. Stopping this habit as soon as possible will give your bones a little boost.[4]

Limit caffeine. Caffeine causes a brief rise in the amount of calcium that escapes your body. Moderate caffeine consumption may not play a major role over the long term in the amount of calcium in your body . . . but on the other hand, it might. If you're already consuming insufficient calcium in your diet, those regular little leaks of calcium out of your system may add up to a significant difference.[10] Studies have linked low bone mineral density or faster bone loss in postmenopausal women who drank 2 or more cups of coffee daily and didn't take in enough calcium.[10] This is yet another reason to keep your caffeine intake low, and if you're going to drink a caffeinated beverage, at least choose my favorite, which gives you an antioxidant boost. You know the one: green tea.

Know when to say when. Modest alcohol consumption has actually been linked to better bone density and lower bone loss in studies of big groups of people. Drinking more, though, puts the damper on bone formation and makes you more likely to fall down. Falls, of course, are a big source of broken bones.[10] Please don't *start* drinking for bone protection, and if you do drink alcohol, pour no more than one per day.[10]

Eat some soy. Okinawans have roughly half the risk of hip fractures that Americans do, according to Bradley Willcox, MD, and Craig Willcox, PhD, in their book *The Okinawa Program*. Natural estrogens in the soy foods they eat may play a role in their bone health. However, several studies from 2004 didn't find bone benefits from the isoflavones in soy. Still, these foods—such as tofu, miso, and edamame—are important elements of the *Positively Ageless* diet and can be a great source of calcium, too.

Prevent falls. Even if your bones are healthy, falling down can cause a painful injury. If your bones are weak, a fall could leave you with a lengthy recuperation. The NIH suggests the following strategies to stay upright.[20]

- Wear low-heeled shoes indoors and rubber-soled shoes with good traction outdoors.

- Be on the lookout for polished floors and slippery walkways.

- Keep your home free of clutter underfoot. Make sure power cords and phone cords are tucked away so you don't have to step over them.

- Ensure that stairwells are well lit and have handrails.

- Place a rubber bath mat in your tub.

- Keep a cordless phone with you when you're in your home so you don't have to rush to answer a ringing phone. Having phones strategically placed throughout your house is helpful, too.

chapter 15

MAINTAINING MUSCLE: MUCH MORE THAN AN EXERCISE IN VANITY

As we progress through our adult life, our muscles tend to become smaller and weaker. Some women just don't see this as a large concern, considering all the other myriad changes that we have to deal with as we get older. After all, shouldn't preserving muscle be more of a concern for men, who pump iron in an effort to maintain their days of football-playing, sleeveless-shirt-wearing, buffed-out youth?

And aren't dwindling muscles a given—a common fact of aging?

What do muscle mass and strength have to do with how well women age, anyway?

To answer those questions: No, no, and *a lot*.

After age 30, your muscle mass dwindles approximately 3 to 8 percent each decade. Once you hit 60, these losses accelerate even more quickly. The consequences are far more serious than an affront to your appearance. Declining muscle mass doesn't simply mean your shoulders are less toned or you can't achieve the same results in sports that you did as a teenager. These muscle changes have implications that are much bigger than your new pant size. The effects are serious and far-reaching. They determine how healthy and active you'll remain in your later years.

Decreased muscle mass means you'll burn fewer calories. If you take in the same amount that you did when you were younger, you'll start accumulating body fat. Your muscles require a lot of calories to maintain: Think of them like a bunch of high-strung, active family members visiting your home. They're always up, moving around. As a result, they're hungry and require a lot of food.

Imagine that these demanding visitors gradually leave, one by one, and the remaining folks start lying on the couch. This is like your muscles becoming smaller and weaker. These relaxed visitors don't need as much food, but you keep buying the same amount of groceries that you bought when you had a big group of active guests. This is like eating the same amount of calories you did when you had more muscle. Gradually, your cupboards and refrigerator overflow with unused food. This is like storing up fat from those unnecessary calories.

Even if your body weight stays the same, less of your weight is from muscle and more is from fat. That's because calories are stored (as fat) when there is less muscle to burn them. More fat equals less calorie-burning muscle. Internally, the extra fat increases your risk of diabetes, stroke, and some cancers. Externally, your body shape changes as muscle morphs to fat. This means bigger jeans and fewer fitted tops.

Also, the vigor of your muscles is related to the strength of your bones. Women are likely more focused on keeping their bones dense and strong than on maintaining their muscles, because the medical establishment, society, and the media have put more focus on preventing osteoporosis. However, when your muscles are weak, your bones are more likely to be weak. Exercise that helps your muscles helps your bones, too.

Declining muscle mass and strength also mean you'll be less likely to get around in your later years. Being able to move freely is a crucial component of healthy aging. Whether it's continuing your workout schedule at the gym, carrying groceries, cleaning your home, getting in and out of a chair, or stepping in and out of your shower, your ability to do these activities helps determine your independence.

Finally, shrinking muscles may grow less responsive to insulin. Your muscles are avid consumers of glucose, or blood sugar, but they need to use the hormone insulin so the blood sugar can enter their cells. When they become insulin resistant, the sugar can't enter. This puts you at greater risk for type 2 diabetes, which in turn raises your risk of heart disease, stroke, and perhaps Alzheimer's.

So maintaining your muscles isn't just an exercise in vanity. It's not about preserving a fleeting element of youthfulness that's best left to 20-somethings. It's about staying fit, vital, independent, and free of disease. Best of all, you have a lot of control over your muscle mass and strength—more than you realize. Experts have seen that declining muscle isn't just an unpreventable fact of aging. In large part it's due to lack of use. Even people in their nineties can show impressive strength gains with exercise.

Most women—whether young, boomers, or seniors—are in a prime position to prevent the serious consequences of muscle loss. Let's take a look at what happens in muscles that contributes to their changes as we get older, then we'll pursue the solutions.

Why Strength Fades Over the Years

As you age, a number of changes occur in your skeletal muscles, which are the ones that move your arms, your legs, and the rest of your body. You lose muscle mass—you simply have less of the stuff. Your nervous system becomes less efficient at prompting your muscles to move. Fat and connective tissue start developing within your muscles, leaving less muscle tissue to contract to move your body.

However, it's worth repeating: Although some muscle changes over the course of your life are caused by hormonal processes, shrinking muscle mass and decreasing strength aren't caused by age alone. Here are some of the factors that contribute to declining muscles as you venture into your later years.

Lack of use. Your body is designed to move, and lack of movement is a significant factor in muscle decline. Studies have shown that even young people's muscle mass and strength quickly deteriorate when they're confined to bed rest. And research has found that older men and women who are less active have less muscle mass and more disability. Conversely, training programs of just a few months in duration have been shown to significantly increase older people's strength. Even frail people who've already passed their 90th birthday can add muscle mass and strength. And if you can improve your muscles' capability deep into your nineties, there's no excuse for slacking off now whether you're 30-, 50-, or 70-something!

Insufficient protein. The current Recommended Daily Allowance for protein—the amount that people are supposed to get each day—is 0.8 grams per kilogram of body weight for adults. So if you weigh 130 pounds (59 kilograms), you need 47 grams of protein daily. On page 99, I recommend a guideline of 30 percent of your daily calories to be contributed by protein (with 45 percent from carbohydrate and 25 percent from fat). This is a little higher than the RDA, but you will be exercising and building muscle as a part of the *Positively Ageless* plan. Experts are discovering that many older people aren't getting enough protein in their diets . . . and that the 0.8 gram per kilogram recommendation may not be enough in the first place. Whether or not your goal is weight loss, if you're trying to build muscle (and burn fat), it's crucial that your protein needs are met. Individual protein recommendations vary per person, depending on weight and body composition. If you have any health conditions, such as kidney disease, that may affect your protein requirements, consult with your medical provider to determine your protein requirement.

Hormonal changes. If you're on hormone replacement therapy (HRT), you've probably learned firsthand that extra estrogen can cause a weight gain in fat, not muscle. Discuss the estrogen and progesterone balance of your HRT with your doctor, and be sure to stay on top of your exercise routine, even if that means consulting a personal trainer to get you started.

Biomarkers for Muscle Loss

Earlier you learned how to calculate your BMI to see if your weight is threatening your health. But it has a major drawback: It doesn't tell you how much of your weight is from unwanted fat and how much is from muscle. Thus, the following methods are helpful for telling you how much of you is fat and how much is lean body mass—those oh-so-important muscles, bones, and organs.

These different methods range from a guesstimate using a measuring tape to employing a highly sophisticated (and expensive) machine called a Bod Pod. Here are a few of the most commonly used methods, along with their pluses and minuses.

A tape measure. According to Rob Huizenga, MD, the sports doc behind NBC's *The Biggest Loser* program (and former team physician to the NFL Raiders), an ordinary tape measurement of your waist may be the most cost-effective way to follow your fat loss at home. Just ask a friend or family member to place a nonmetal tape measure around your waist, exactly parallel to the floor at belly-button level. After you let out a breath, have your helper take two waist circumference readings—do additional readings if these two are more than a half-inch different. This measurement, coupled with your baseline weight, can be an effective way to track your progress.

Body fat calipers. This handheld tool is popular in the fitness industry because it is inexpensive, portable, and relatively easy to use. However, its reliability is largely a function of the person using it—you want a pro who's familiar with the process to do it. Often, this is a personal trainer, dietitian, or gym instructor. For the test, the health professional gently pinches folds of skin at predetermined sites around your body, then measures the width of each fold with the calipers. The measurements are entered into formulas to quantify the amount of fat beneath your skin.

For accuracy, be sure to have the same person take your measurements each time. There is an art to using the tool as well as locating the various skin-fold sites. The most effective way for you to monitor progress with calipers is to record and date your skin-fold measurements and monitor their changes over time. Take measurements at the same time of day for each test, but not immediately after exercising. For optimal results, compare the results to those of a hydrostatic weighing test.

Hydrostatic weighing. Based on water displacement, this is a fairly accurate method of determining body fat and lean body mass. The downside is that the equipment is rather expensive and not as widely available as that for other methods. Hydrostatic weighing takes about 30 minutes to complete. First, your dry weight and lung volume are recorded. Next, dressed in minimal clothing or a swimsuit, you're seated on a chair that is suspended in shoulder-deep water from a scale above. You exhale completely, and then you're submerged briefly while your underwater weight is recorded. Several trials are performed and results recorded. Calculations determine your body density and estimate your body composition.

Bioelectrical impedance analysis. This method—BIA, for short—is a popular way to measure body fat because it's safe, quick, easy, and relatively inexpensive. To perform the test, you're first weighed. Your age, gender, height, and sometimes other characteristics such as physical activity level are entered into a small computer. Electrodes are attached to your hands and feet, and a very mild electrical current passes through your body. The machine measures the resistance—or *impedance*—to this electric signal as it travels through your muscle and body fat. Muscle contains water, and the greater the amount of water in a person's body, the easier it is for the current to go through it. Fat contains little water. The more body fat that is present, the more resistance to the current is measured.

The machine determines the amount of body fat based on your weight and the amount of lean tissue that is measured. The machine is used by fitness and health professionals and is considered reliable. However, its accuracy is dependent on the skill and knowledge of technicians as well as how well hydrated you are before testing.

Body fat scale. Many body fat scales look like typical bathroom scales, but they go beyond measuring weight. These scales estimate body fat, based on the principles of bioelectrical impedance. Unlike with the BIA device, your bare feet come into contact with electrodes when you step onto the metal plates on the scale, and impedance is measured through your legs and lower trunk. The most accurate and dependable models extrapolate a body fat percentage based on personal information including gender, age, height, and weight. For more information on body fat scales, see the Shopping Resources on page 351.

Bod Pod. This machine is a very useful tool to determine lean and fat mass ratios. While hydrostatic weighing uses water displacement, the Bod Pod displaces air to measure your mass and volume, then calculates your whole body density. It is extremely accurate and a very expensive piece of equipment. The machine is calibrated before every use to guarantee an accurate reading. The reading takes less than a minute and is performed twice for accuracy. The Bod Pod is capable of measuring people who weigh up to 500 pounds.

Now that you have your body fat measurements, what do they mean? If you weigh 150 pounds and have 10 percent fat, it means that your body has 15 pounds of fat and 135 pounds of lean body mass (like blood, bone, muscle, organ tissue, etc.). The following table, from the American Council on Exercise, puts body fat ranges into the following classifications.

CLASSIFICATION	% FAT (FOR WOMEN)
Essential fat (the minimum you need)	10–12
Athletes	14–20
Fitness	21–24
Acceptable	25–31
Obese	32–plus

The *Positively Ageless* Guide to Maintaining Your Muscles

Throughout this book, you've seen numerous references to exercising for 30 minutes most days of the week. Although aerobic exercise—things like running, bicycling, swimming, and dancing—are good workouts for your heart and lungs and help you lose weight, these aren't going to help you maintain your strength.

"The only type of exercise that prevents sarcopenia is resistance exercise," says William Evans, PhD, a professor of geriatrics, physiology, and nutrition at the University of Arkansas in Fayetteville who has studied how older people can address their muscle declines. (*Sarcopenia*, by the way, is the medical term for the muscle loss we've been talking about. It comes from the Greek for "poverty of the flesh.") Studies looking at athletes who have been running all their lives found that, though they're leaner and have lower risk of chronic diseases, their strength is similar to sedentary people of the same age.

You have to use resistance exercise to maintain and build your muscle. Some people refer to this type of activity as lifting weights, and pumping dumbbells and barbells certainly works. But you can also use strength-training machines at the gym or stretchy elastic bands. For some exercises, such as abdominal crunches, you simply lift your own body weight. But what all these activities have in common is that they require you to push your muscles against a form of resistance.

To appreciably increase your muscle size and strength, Dr. Evans says, you can't use weights that feel extremely light. Rather, you need to do exercises that incorporate at least 60 percent of the weight you can lift one time. In his studies, Dr. Evans typically has subjects lifting 80 percent of their maximum. Also, the weight you use should tire you out within eight to 12 repetitions. For example, if you can curl a 30-pound dumbbell once, you should aim for curling a 20-pound dumbbell up to 12 times. Curling a 10-pound dumbbell 20 times, by contrast, won't build your muscle strength. Likewise, if you can curl a 20-pound dumbbell once, you'll want to work on curling a 12-pound dumbbell up to 12 times.

If you're worried about building bulk—don't be. Few women actually gain significant muscle mass doing strength exercises, unless they're genetically predisposed to it. Do check with a trainer or someone at your gym if you're not certain of a safe starting weight.

Early in your resistance training, you'll notice quick improvements, Dr. Evans says. In even just 2 months, your strength may double. This isn't simply a matter of your muscles getting bigger—your brain learns how to use your muscles more efficiently, too.

But as you stick with it, your strength-training plan must be progressive. You have to add repetitions and use heavier weights (or thicker elastic bands). That's because your muscles get stronger, so they can adapt to lifting a certain weight. After you curl that 12-pound dumbbell 12 times for several sessions, it ceases to be a challenge, and you stop gaining strength. So once you can lift a weight 12 times, it's time to use a heavier weight and strive to lift it at least eight times.

Doing two sets of each exercise is a sufficient workout for your muscles, Dr. Evans says. That means you'd lift the weight—or stretch the band—a "set" of eight to 12 repetitions, then take a rest or do a different exercise, and then do another set.

Just two strength-training workouts a week, with exercises that work all your major muscle groups during each session, are adequate for building and maintaining your muscles. Your full-body workout would include exercises that focus on the fronts of your arms (biceps), backs of your arms (triceps), chest, shoulders, upper back, the fronts and backs of your thighs, your abdomen, and your lower back.

It's beyond the scope of the book to tell you everything you need to know about strength training. But here are some tips to keep in mind.

- Talk to your doctor before beginning any new type of exercise program. Lifting weights may not be appropriate for people with certain conditions, such as high blood pressure or joint problems.

- Strive for two strength-training workouts, each containing 10 or so exercises that give you a full-body workout. Do two sets of eight to 12 repetitions of each exercise.

- Consider working at least one session with a qualified fitness professional. A personal trainer can help you design a program, teach you how to do exercises, and observe your form to ensure it's correct.

■ Warm up for 5 to 10 minutes before a strength-training session and cool down afterward. Walking briskly and pumping your arms is a good warmup.

■ You have a lot of options for how to train. According to Dr. Evans, a simple and economical approach is to use elastic bands or tubes. You can do many exercises by standing on one end and tugging on the other, standing in the middle and pulling both ends, or holding each end and pulling them apart. Free weights, like dumbbells and barbells, also improve balance and coordination, but you need a spotter to help you with some exercises. Weight machines tend to be a little safer and easier to use, he says.

■ When you increase the amount of weight you lift or the difficulty of the elastic band you stretch, make the challenge only 5 to 10 percent harder. This will limit your risk of injury.

■ Don't do strength-training sessions for the same muscle groups on back-to-back days. Your muscles need more time to recover.

■ Work opposing muscles proportionally. That means working muscles on the fronts and backs of your upper arms, your upper back and chest, and your lower back and abdomen. Ignoring muscle groups throws your body out of balance.

■ Get plenty of protein. As you read earlier, the recommended daily allowance of protein for adults may not be enough to encourage sufficient muscle maintenance as you get older. Researchers haven't pinned down exactly how much you should strive to get. If you aim for getting 30 percent of your calories from protein, however, you should get enough to support muscle maintenance and growth. Get most of your protein from low-fat sources, Dr. Evans recommends. Protein will be much more efficient at building muscle when you eat it within 30 minutes after a workout, he says. Have a turkey sandwich, a low-fat cheese stick or yogurt, or nibble on some steamed edamame. Half a cup of these green immature soybeans contains a whopping 14 grams of protein.[23-28]

The *Positively Ageless* Program for Age-Proofing Your Bones and Muscles

At the end of each weekly section, you'll find an overview of specific tips to follow to incorporate the *Positively Ageless* diet into your lifestyle. These tips are broken down into stages. "Make One Change" is a list of easy-start changes. If you can only make one change per week, pick one from this list. "Quick Start" includes tips and strategies that are important but may take a bit longer to incorporate into your life. Suggestions you should follow for maximum antiaging benefit are listed in "Young for Life."

In addition, we've included a week's worth of meal plans that utilize the *Positively Ageless* ingredients. You'll find recipes for many of these menu items in the recipe section toward the back of the book.

Make One Change

If you can make only one change in your life, pick from this list. Research has shown these to be the most important strategies for slowing aging.

Check it out. Be sure to discuss your *Positively Ageless* plans with your doctor before beginning the exercise component of the program. He or she will want to evaluate your readiness for exercise, especially if it's been a long time since you were active.

Get your measurements. Measure your starting weight and take your body measurements (waist, hips, etc.) and blood pressure to establish your baseline. Measure yourself again later to track your improvements.

Check your meds. Discuss your bone density results with your doctor and determine whether any of your current medications may be interfering with your calcium absorption. Make changes accordingly.

Bone up on calcium. Based on bone density results, it may be time to begin supplementing your calcium intake. Ask your health care provider about your options. Your body's needs have increased, and it's time to really focus on keeping your bones strong. For more information, see Shopping Resources on page 351.

Do dairy. Be sure you're indulging in two daily servings of dairy (or calcium-fortified foods if you have lactose intolerance). Making a **Mango Mint Smoothie** (page 269) after your workout is a great start. If you haven't already tried kefir or fat-free ricotta with fruit, give it a whirl this week in your own smoothie concoction.

Rearrange it. Be sure your house isn't a hazard zone in terms of risks for falling. Unclutter your most traveled walkways, put a rubber mat in the tub, and be sure you have handrails on stairways.

Drink up. Stay on track with water and limit your caffeine intake. (If you haven't done so already, switch to green tea!) You're getting serious with exercise here, and your body needs the right type of fluids to elicit the best responses to your hard work. Water will keep your body hydrated and your body temperature well regulated, and it will escort nutrients to the muscles so they can grow and thrive. Too much caffeine can work against you.

Be decisive. Shop around for DVDs to guide your fitness program if you're planning to do part or all of it on your own at home. Design a fitness program tailored to your goals. Choose an instructor who exemplifies the style of workout and instruction you're most likely to enjoy.

Lift it. If you will be exercising at home, invest in basic equipment: dumbbells or resistance bands or tubing.

Keep on truckin'. This week it's time to increase your aerobic activity from 20 to 30 minutes a day. If you've been dividing your workout into two short periods per day during Weeks One and Two, try to combine them by this week's end to maintain 30 consecutive minutes of *Positively Ageless* aerobic activity.

Quick Start

These strategies are a little more involved, but the benefits will reflect the additional effort you're spending. They'll provide a jump-start for measurable results in a short period of time.

Measure it. For this more intense level of involvement, include as many baseline biomarkers as you can at your starting line. Ask your doctor or your trainer about options to have your body fat measured in addition to your starting weight. Whether it's with a Bod Pod, hydrostatic weighing, or calipers, it's always gratifying to track your improvements. The more baseline measurements you have, the more success you'll be able to measure. Remember that we're aiming to lose body fat here, not just pounds. Hopefully, you'll gain calorie-burning muscle while you rev up your metabolism.

Zone in on the bone. If you haven't already had DEXA, it may be time for your first bone density measurement. If your medical insurance doesn't cover it, see if your community health center has a mobile machine that frequents your area on a regular basis at a discounted rate.

Sound it. If DEXA is not an option for you, look for an ultrasound bone density testing to predict your bone mass based on testing of one area, such as your heel. Preserving and maintaining your bone mass is imperative for a long and healthy life. Don't neglect this pivotal step.

Work it out. Sign up for at least one session with a qualified fitness professional. A trainer will teach you how to actually do the exercises and observe your form to ensure it's correct.

Gear up. It pays to invest in a trained professional to help you choose the right equipment and design a program tailored to your weight, body, needs, and goals. Your muscles and bones are serious business, and they require a qualified professional to show you how to exercise them properly.

Warm it up. Before getting right down to it, start each workout with a warmup to relax your mind, get motivated, loosen up your muscles, and prevent injury. Five to 10 minutes should do it. This can be as basic as a brisk walk while pumping your arms or as extensive as a Pilates or yoga class.

Eat it! Sticking to a regular meal and snack schedule is important for your blood sugar and to keep your appetite harnessed, but adding a workout component makes it mandatory. Stick to your schedule of smaller frequent meals, and keep your metabolism supercharged.

Accessorize. At this level of commitment, you deserve a new outfit. Buy a gym bag to store your basics, and reward yourself with at least one workout ensemble that's comfortable and makes you feel as great as you're going to look.

Stay strong. Pay attention to any discomfort, injuries, or sprains while starting out. Address them before you move on. Staying hydrated and gradually building on your workouts will help you to avoid injury.

Catch some z's. Go to bed earlier. You're working out, possibly more than you've done in years. Be good to yourself, and give your muscles and bones a good rest. They may need time to catch up during the first few weeks.

Ring it. If you need to set the alarm for the first time in a while, do it. Finding a new routine to accommodate your *Positively Ageless* workouts may mean waking up earlier to exercise. A buff body payoff is priceless.

Take it to the burn. Focus on building all your major muscle groups during each of two *Positively Ageless* strength-training sessions per week. Include exercises for the fronts of your arms (biceps), backs of arms (triceps), chest, shoulders, upper back, front and back of thighs, abdomen, and lower back.

Lighten up. Start out with the minimal amount of weight and repetitions. This will minimize soreness as well as injury.

Cool off. End each workout with a cooldown to relax your muscles and your mind.

Inhale. Whether you're warming up, cooling down, or just taking a break to clear your head, breathing is key, especially when you're taxing your body to the limit with a new exercise regimen. Develop a mantra, such as "inhale confidence, exhale fear." You'll pull double duty, strengthening your fortitude while you strengthen your muscles and feed them with plenty of oxygen to do their best work.

Young for Life

This list of strategies is for those of you who are ready for a major lifestyle intervention. While you'll need to spend a bit more effort enacting these good habits, the payoff can be a dramatic, lasting impact on your health.

Change it. If there is a stretch or strength-training exercise that you flat-out don't like, experiment until you find one that works for you and that muscle group. Ask your trainer or a gym professional. We're in here for the long haul, and this needs to be enjoyable. There are many ways to work each muscle—find a move that you like.

Get extra activity. Whether or not it's your designated workout time, stay active and focus on working your muscles and elevating your metabolism. Standing up burns more calories than sitting down. Stand up to take phone calls (or to watch TV). Park your car at the far end of every lot when shopping or at work—as long as it's daylight and safe to do so. Look for situations to optimize calorie burning. Don't take the easy route—do everything the "hard" way!

Rest it. Take a day off to let your body and mind rest. You and your muscles deserve it.

chapter 16

EAT SMART, LIVE LONG MENUS

Positively Ageless Menus Week Three

The *Positively Ageless* menu plans are based on an average of 1,200 calories per day. If your calorie needs are a little higher (or lower), you can adjust accordingly. Adding a glass of 1 percent milk, 6 ounces of fat-free yogurt, one pear or a large apple, or a glass of red wine with dinner will each provide an additional 100 calories.

Positively Ageless **recipes** are listed in bold and designated as one serving size.

The two snacks can be scheduled between meals or one between meals and one after dinner.

DAY 1

1,218 calories; 27 grams fiber; 4,020 milligrams omega-3s

BREAKFAST

Baked Eggs in Savory Turkey Cups (page 266) (with pesto and Parmesan instead of salsa and Cheddar)

$^1/_2$ slice **Whole Grain Bread** (page 306)

$^3/_4$ cup diced watermelon

8 ounces iced green tea with lemon

MID-MORNING SNACK

$^1/_3$ cup fat-free vanilla yogurt sprinkled with 2 tablespoons sliced strawberries and 1 teaspoon ground flaxseed

LUNCH

Chicken Salad with $^1/_2$ cup cooked lentils, 3 ounces chopped grilled chicken breast, 1 cup diced tomatoes, 2 tablespoons chopped parsley, 2 tablespoons chopped fresh mint, and 1 teaspoon fresh lemon juice

Ruby Lemon Sorbet (page 343)

8 ounces green tea or ice water with orange slice

MID-AFTERNOON SNACK

Candied Pecans (page 291) and $^1/_4$ cup fat-free cottage cheese

DINNER

3 ounces grilled salmon fillet

2 cups wilted baby spinach with 1 teaspoon olive oil, 1 teaspoon balsamic vinegar, and 1 teaspoon grated Parmesan cheese

$^1/_2$ cup diced cantaloupe and $^1/_2$ cup fresh blackberries with 1 teaspoon fresh mint

8 ounces green tea with mint and ginger

DAY 2

1,216 calories; 29 grams fiber; 6,020 milligrams omega-3s

BREAKFAST

1/2 banana, sliced, and 1 teaspoon chopped mint

1/3 cup dry old-fashioned oatmeal cooked with 1 tablespoon ground flaxseed and 2/3 cup water, then sprinkled with cinnamon and 2 teaspoons chopped almonds

1/3 cup fat-free vanilla yogurt

1 serving (1 cup) mint tea or fat-free milk

MID-MORNING SNACK

1 fresh pear sliced and topped with 1/3 cup fat-free ricotta and drizzled with 1 teaspoon honey

LUNCH

Mediterranean turkey pita sandwich: 3 ounces thinly sliced lean turkey breast, 1/2 roasted red bell pepper, and 2 pieces romaine lettuce on a 4-inch whole wheat pita

Tahini Yogurt Sauce (page 284)

8 ounces iced green tea with lime

MID-AFTERNOON SNACK

1 low-fat cheese stick

1 medium tangerine

DINNER

3 ounces roast pork tenderloin

1 cup shredded red cabbage sautéed with 2 tablespoons minced onion and 1 teaspoon olive oil

Large tossed salad (2 cups mixed salad greens, 1/2 cup sliced cucumbers, and 1/4 cup sliced mushrooms) plus 1 tablespoon **Tomato Ginger Vinaigrette** (page 283)

4 ounces red wine

8 ounces green or white tea or sparkling water with lime wedge

DAY 3

1,172 calories; 28 grams fiber; 3,530 milligrams omega-3s

BREAKFAST

$\frac{1}{3}$ cup (2) scrambled egg whites with 1 teaspoon fresh herbs, $\frac{1}{4}$ cup chopped red onion, and $\frac{1}{4}$ cup sliced mushrooms

Old Fashioned Breakfast Sausage (page 259)

$\frac{1}{2}$ cup fresh raspberries with $\frac{1}{4}$ cup fat-free vanilla yogurt and 1 tablespoon ground flaxseed

8 ounces green tea with ginger or ice water

MID-MORNING SNACK

Whole Wheat Pita Chips (page 295) and **Zippy Hummus** (page 294)

LUNCH

Chicken Caesar salad with 3 ounces shredded roasted chicken breast, 1 cup chopped romaine lettuce, $\frac{1}{4}$ cup diced yellow bell pepper, $\frac{1}{2}$ cup halved cherry tomatoes, and 2 tablespoons low-fat Caesar dressing

Iced **Spicy Chai** (page 276)

MID-AFTERNOON SNACK

$\frac{1}{4}$ cup fat-free cottage cheese with $\frac{1}{2}$ cup tomato salsa

DINNER

Moroccan Fish Stew (page 328)

1 cup watercress salad with 1 tablespoon light balsamic vinaigrette

Gingerbread with Dried Cherries and Toasted Pecans (page 340)

Iced green tea

DAY 4

1,214 calories; 30 grams fiber; 3,340 milligrams omega-3s

BREAKFAST

½ cup chopped watermelon

Black Beans with Garlic (substitute black beans in **Black-Eyed Peas with Garlic**) (page 332)

1 omega-3 egg and 2 egg whites scrambled with 2 tablespoons chopped onion, 2 tablespoons chopped tomato, 1 tablespoon chopped cilantro, and 1 teaspoon olive oil

8 ounces iced green tea with fresh lemon

MID-MORNING SNACK

¼ cup fat-free yogurt with ½ sliced apple and 1 teaspoon chopped walnuts and 1 tablespoon ground flaxseed

LUNCH

Grilled chicken salad made with 3 ounces grilled chicken breast, 2 cups chopped romaine lettuce, ½ cup halved cherry tomatoes, ½ cup diced bell pepper, 2 tablespoons chopped green onion, 2 tablespoons chopped cilantro, 1 tablespoon grated low-fat Jack cheese, 1 tablespoon low-fat vinaigrette

1 whole grain Wasa Crispbread

1 medium nectarine

Iced green tea or water

MID-AFTERNOON SNACK

Hot Chocolate (hot or iced) (page 277)

DINNER

3 ounces medium shrimp sautéed with 1 teaspoon olive oil and 1 teaspoon chopped garlic

1 medium artichoke, steamed

⅓ cup whole wheat couscous with 2 tablespoons chopped onion, 2 tablespoons chickpeas, 1 teaspoon chopped fresh cilantro, and 1 tablespoon low-fat Dijon vinaigrette

8 ounces green tea or water

DAY 5

1,224 calories; 33 grams fiber; 4,390 milligrams omega-3s

BREAKFAST

Creamy Almond Kasha (page 261) with 1 tablespoon ground flaxseed

1 wedge honeydew melon

1 cup fat-free milk

8 ounces green tea

MID-MORNING SNACK

Asparagus Spears with Smoked Salmon and Tangy Mustard Dressing (page 293)

LUNCH

Roast-beef wrap: 3 ounces thinly sliced lean roast beef (or chicken or turkey or pork), $1/2$ cup shredded romaine lettuce, 2 medium tomato slices, 1 teaspoon horseradish, and 1 teaspoon Dijon mustard in a 6-inch whole wheat tortilla

$1/2$ cup cooked lentils with 1 teaspoon chopped basil and 1 tablespoon light Caesar vinaigrette

Iced green tea with lemon or water

MID-AFTERNOON SNACK

$1/3$ cup warm unsweetened applesauce with $1/3$ cup fat-free vanilla yogurt, 1 tablespoon chopped almonds, and a dash of ground cinnamon

DINNER

3 ounces grilled salmon or halibut fillet

$1/2$ cup sliced mushrooms sautéed with 1 teaspoon olive oil, $1/4$ cup chopped red onion, $1/4$ cup sliced yellow bell pepper, and 1 tablespoon chopped parsley

1 cup arugula salad with $1/4$ cup halved cherry tomatoes and 1 tablespoon miso dressing

4 ounces red wine

8 ounces green tea or water

DAY 6

1,199 calories; 28 grams fiber; 1,920 milligrams omega-3s

BREAKFAST

Breakfast burrito made with 1 medium whole wheat tortilla,
3 scrambled egg whites, 2 tablespoons fat-free refried black beans,
2 tablespoons salsa, 1 tablespoon grated low-fat Cheddar, and
1 teaspoon fresh cilantro

1 cup diced watermelon

1 cup fat-free milk

8 ounces green tea or water

MID-MORNING SNACK

Sparkling Melon Agua Fresca (page 272)

LUNCH

Savory Beet Stew (page 298)

Spinach salad made with 2 ounces smoked salmon, 2 cups baby
spinach leaves, 1/2 cup halved cherry tomatoes, 1 tablespoon light
vinaigrette, and 1 teaspoon grated Parmesan cheese

8 ounces green tea or ice water with orange slice

MID-AFTERNOON SNACK

1 low-fat cheese stick

1/4 cup red grapes

DINNER

3 ounces poached salmon or halibut

Gingered Edamame with Fire-Roasted Tomatoes (page 331)

Chocolate Almond Pudding (page 338)

8 ounces green tea or fat-free milk

DAY 7

1,198 calories; 35 grams fiber; 2,110 milligrams omega-3s

BREAKFAST

Breakfast frittata with ½ cup (3 large) egg whites, 2 tablespoons chopped bell peppers, 2 tablespoons chopped spinach, 1 tablespoon shredded part-skim mozzarella, and 1 teaspoon pesto

½ slice **Whole Grain Bread** (page 306)

1 cup fresh raspberries

8 ounces green tea, ice water, or fat-free milk

MID-MORNING SNACK

½ cup fat-free vanilla yogurt with 2 teaspoons ground flaxseed and ¼ cup chopped peach or pear

LUNCH

Spanish Meatball Soup (page 303)

Tomato cucumber salad with 3 slices fresh tomato, ¼ cup sliced cucumber, 1 teaspoon fresh chopped thyme, 1 tablespoon crumbled low-fat feta cheese, and 1 tablespoon low-fat vinaigrette

1 medium orange

Iced green tea with lemon

MID-AFTERNOON SNACK

Smoothie made with ½ cup fat-free milk, ½ banana, 3 tablespoons fat-free yogurt, 1 tablespoon natural peanut butter, and 2 tablespoons sliced strawberries

DINNER

3 ounces red snapper baked with 1 teaspoon olive oil, 1 teaspoon lemon juice, and ½ teaspoon fresh thyme

½ cup spaghetti squash with 1 teaspoon olive oil and 1 teaspoon grated Parmesan cheese

1 cup steamed green beans sprinkled with 1 teaspoon slivered almonds

8 ounces green tea or water with lemon

YOUR OUTSIDE PARTS

Though they don't sustain your longevity like your brain, heart, and other vital organs do, your outside parts play a crucial role in how well you age. The youthfulness of your skin, hair, and teeth influences how you feel about your own vitality and how you project it to others. And your eyes allow you to take in the beauty surrounding you as you travel on life's journey. These parts also provide visible evidence that your efforts to age gracefully are paying off!

chapter 17

PROTECT THE SKIN YOU'RE IN

Let's face it—changes in our skin are often the first signs of aging that we notice. A wrinkle here or a brown spot there serves as a small but brutal warning that time is marching forward in our body. For many of us, our cosmetic "issues" are the most dreaded of any aging concerns. After all, our faces are the one part of our anatomy that everyone sees, so it's not always easy to conceal some of our new and not-so-desirable features.

Sure, successful aging is about how you *feel*. You want energy to enjoy your life and your activities with vigor. You want freedom from pain. You want to be strong so you can move freely, without excess fat weighing you down. And you want to be free of major diseases that can taint your quality of life or end your days too early.

Feeling good is vital to staying young, but successful aging also applies to how we *look*. Wanting to stay youthful looking isn't a pursuit in vanity—it's a legitimate concern as we get older. If you feel exuberant and vital on the inside, it makes sense to want the world to see that in your external appearance. And when you know that your youthful appearance comes from making smart lifestyle choices, your fleeting glimpses in the mirror remind you that your savvy decisions are keeping you young on the *inside*, too.

Of course, you can't expect to always have the supple skin and radiant face that you had in your twenties . . . and there's nothing wrong with having a few wrinkles to flaunt the wisdom you've accumulated over the years. However, you can do a lot to prevent the extreme skin changes that make people look far older than their years.

The Anatomy of Aging Skin

Thinking of your skin as simply an outer wrapper does this fascinating part of your body a disservice—and even puts it at risk. "Skin is an organ,

THE DERMATOLOGIST'S PANTRY

Antiaging author and dermatologist Nicholas Perricone, MD, has no trouble listing the top foods that will help protect your skin as the years pass by. Be sure to keep your kitchen stocked with his favorite picks.

1. Cold-water fish. Wild salmon, mackerel, albacore and bluefish tuna, herring, anchovies, and sardines are great sources of omega-3 fatty acids. They're a healthy protein source, too. And certain fish contain a powerful antioxidant called DMAE, which protects you from free radical damage and preserves your skin tone, he says.

2. Green leafy vegetables. These give you a rich dose of antioxidants and other nutrients for healthy skin.

3. Kefir and yogurt. These dairy foods are a source of protein, calcium, and probiotics.

4. Fresh fruits, especially berries. These are great sources of antioxidants and fiber.

5. Good fats. The low-fat craze that swept the country years ago brought with it a wave of bad skin. Having an ample amount of good fats in your diet, by contrast, helps keep your skin supple and healthy. Make room in your diet for olive oil, avocados, flaxseed, nuts, and, of course, omega-3-rich fish.

and it's not just a simple organ; it's a very dynamic organ," says Nicholas Perricone, MD, a dermatologist, author, and guru of skin self-care.[1]

Your skin is composed of layers and contains oil glands, blood vessels, immune cells, and components that give it structure and elasticity. Obviously, a lot of factors in the environment—especially sunlight—can damage your skin. After all, your skin is constantly exposed to these external elements. But your skin is also exposed to many factors on the inside of your body, such as the foods you eat, that can change its appearance over the years.[2,1]

Until recently, the public—and even many dermatologists—didn't give proper credit to the role that food plays in your skin's health, Dr. Perricone says. "I heard a *tremendous* amount of ridicule and skepticism over changing the way you look through your diet. But the books I've written have convinced enough people that there's been a tipping point."[1]

Intrinsic aging is dictated by our genes and includes the events that naturally happen as we accumulate the years. These factors include:

- A slower turnover of cells in the outer layer of the skin—the epidermis. In young people, this turnaround process takes about 28 days; in the elderly, it takes 40 to 60 days. This makes the skin thinner and more translucent, so structures beneath become more apparent (think of the veins and bones in your hands).[4,5]

- More difficulty for nutrients to pass from the deeper layer of the skin—the dermis—to the outer layer.[4]

- Less activity in the pigment-producing cells in the epidermis and fewer of them. This leads to mottled coloring and makes you more likely to get sunburned.[2]

- A decrease in a kind of immune-system cell that resides in the skin. The loss of these cells and the pigment-producing cells raises your risk of skin cancer.[2]

- Less *collagen*, which provides support for the skin, and *elastin*, which provides elasticity. This contributes to sagging and wrinkles.[3,4]

- Reduced blood supply and fewer oil glands. Your skin becomes thinner and drier.[4]

Taken together, that sounds like an awful lot of changes going on in your skin for everyone to see. But these issues vary in severity from person to person, and, according to the medical literature, intrinsic aging doesn't cause major visible effects.[4] It's more the *extrinsic* aging processes you need to worry about. These have major effects on your appearance—and they're issues you can control. These include:[4]

- Sunlight. This is the main cause of changes in your skin as you age. Experts refer to sun damage as *photoaging*. The sun's ultraviolet waves cause deep wrinkles, rough patches, sagging, discolorations, age spots, and skin cancer. The ultraviolet light called UVA causes most of the photoaging, and it generally does it by triggering free radicals in the skin that damage DNA, proteins, and other substances. Photoaging accumulates over the years, a few minutes of sun exposure at a time. The collagen and elastin that kept your skin firm and smooth in your youth become damaged, blood vessels become more visible in your face and other sun-exposed places, and your appearance slowly changes.[4,2]

■ Smoking. This habit also speeds up aging changes in the skin, causing deep wrinkles, yellowing, and a leathery texture.[3]

These are factors that you can control. Another problem that can cause signs of aging that you can affect is advanced glycation end products (AGEs). Remember those? They're the troublemakers that form when glucose attaches to proteins in your body, and they're related to all sorts of internal diseases.[6,1] AGEs accumulate on collagen, making cross-links. These extra connections within the collagen make your skin stiffer and prone to developing deep wrinkles and grooves.[6,1]

In addition, skin changes can be a consequence of menopause. Estrogen influences skin functions, and once your levels of the hormone decline, the change can contribute to wrinkles, thinning, sagging, and dryness of the skin. Unfortunately, studies on hormone replacement therapy's benefits on skin have had mixed results—and hormone therapy carries risks that may outweigh any benefit you'd get for your skin. Not much is known about the usefulness of plant estrogens—like in soy—for skin aging, either.[7]

So there you have it. Some of the changes in your skin are factors you can't do anything about. They're simply souvenirs to show for your time on Earth. But much of the most significant damage that can leave marks on your skin *is* avoidable. If you take action now, you can ensure that your appearance in the mirror matches the vibrant image that you see when you picture yourself in your mind.

Biomarkers for Skin Aging

Simply looking at your skin to observe wrinkles and discolorations, along with feeling it for changes in texture, will tell you a lot about its health, says Dr. Perricone. For example, pinch the skin on the back of your hand. If it stays "tented up" instead of falling back in place, it's a sign that the collagen underneath has undergone age-related changes.[1]

SIMPLE PROCEDURE BRINGS OUT A FRESHER FACE

As we get older, our skin doesn't regenerate as quickly as it used to, and as our estrogen supply dwindles, our skin becomes thinner, too. We lose that fresh, dewy look found in glowing, vital, younger skin.

Microdermabrasion is an exfoliating procedure that "sandblasts" the skin with very fine crystals of aluminum oxide or other compounds to remove the top layer of dead skin cells. This reveals a newer layer of fresh cells just below. There are a variety of materials and technologies used for microdermabrasion, including kits and creams for doing mild exfoliation at home. Stronger and more vigorous treatments can be done in a physician's office.

Prices range from about $20 for a home kit to more than $200 for professional treatments. Microdermabrasion is usually performed on the face and décolleté (upper chest), but it can be done on the hands or back as well.

In addition, you may find a device at health fairs or a dermatologist's office that shines a special light on your face as you look in a mirror, which makes the hidden signs of sun damage become visible. Since photoaging accumulates gradually and shows itself slowly over the years, this can be a good way to remind yourself to protect your skin now.

The *Positively Ageless* Guide to Healthy Skin

Stay out of the sun! One of the most important ways to slow down your skin's aging process is to stop casting your shadow outdoors so much. Remember, sun exposure really puts the process on a fast track. Though you can't totally prevent sunlight from hitting you—nor should you for at least one important reason—you can minimize its harmfulness.

- Be particularly careful to limit your sun exposure between 10:00 a.m. and 4:00 p.m., when you'll get the strongest dose of UV rays.[8,3]

KEEP YOUR LIPS FULL AND YOUTHFUL

The fullness of your lips can melt away as your estrogen supply wanes . . . but collagen injections are not the only answer! To optimize the fullness of your lips and maintain your va-va-voom:

- Protect your lips from sun and wind damage like you do the rest of your skin. Wear a moisturizer or lip balm with an SPF of 15 or higher.

- When exfoliating your face, don't forget your lips! Buf-Pufs work well; an everyday washcloth also works wonders. Moisturized, exfoliated lips become a protective layer for lip color, which will now look smoother and cleaner.

- Lip liner is a lifesaver for thin lips. If you have thinning lips, outline your natural lip shape slightly *beyond* the edge of your lip to regain any lost territory! Not only can this resolve a lip size problem, you can also use the liner to correct any shape imperfections. Lining your lips will also help keep your lipstick in place and avoid that dreaded seeping of color into the skin around your mouth. Be sure the liner is not visible once your lipstick is applied.

- Get glossy. A little gloss will brighten up your face, even if you're not wearing color under it.

- Your lip color sends a message and can age you if you choose the wrong color. Be careful with brown shades. They can make you look older and your teeth appear yellow.

- Use a sunscreen with an SPF (sun protection factor) of 15 or higher, suggests the National Institutes of Health (NIH). This number, which goes from 2 to more than 30, is a measure of how long it protects you. You should also use a type that says it's "broad spectrum" on its label so it'll protect you from both UVA and UVB rays. Apply it 20 minutes before you go outside. It should also be water resistant, but be sure to reapply it after you've been in the water or perspiring. Sunscreens may not offer 100 percent protection, though, so they don't give you a license to bask in the blazing sun all day.[5,3,8]

- Wear protective clothing outdoors. This includes a wide-brimmed hat that shades your face, neck, and ears; sunglasses that offer at least 99 percent protection from UV rays; and long-sleeved shirts and pants or a long skirt made of lightweight fabric.[3,5]

- Avoid tanning booths and sunlamps.[5]

- If you really crave that bronzed look, there are plenty of self-tanners available. It takes minutes to rub the cream in, then a couple hours for the color to set in, which will last several days.

Having said all this, *do* expose your face, arms, and hands to 5 to 10 minutes of sunlight on most days, Dr. Perricone suggests. Your skin produces vitamin D upon sun exposure, which is vital for keeping your bones strong. "I'll take the fine line or wrinkle over osteoporosis any day of the week," he says. However, a few minutes are all you need—more exposure isn't better.

Drink lots of water. Staying well hydrated keeps your skin's cells plump and firm. When you don't take in enough water, the deficiency encourages dry, wrinkled skin.

Think of a bunch of grapes—firm and smooth and fresh. Leave them in a hot, dry environment so they lose their fluid, and what do you get? Raisins . . . soft, deeply wrinkled raisins. This image probably oversimplifies what happens to your skin's cells when you don't drink enough water, but the point is that your body is filled with fluid, and you need to be constantly replacing it. It washes toxins out of your body, helps bring nutrients to your cells, and keeps all your processes working properly—on the inside *and* the outside of your body.

Eat foods rich in antioxidants. Your skin has a natural antioxidant system to neutralize free radicals and protect cells from damage. However, as you get older, your antioxidant protection drops, particularly in sun-damaged skin. Eating a diet rich in antioxidants can help protect your skin. According to a paper in a 2006 issue of the *Journal of Investigative Dermatology*, researchers around the world are searching for ways to prevent the skin damage—particularly skin cancer—resulting from free radicals. Laboratory work indicates that antioxidants such as green and black tea, resveratrol (found in grapes), the spice curcumin (also known as turmeric), and vitamin C may prove to be helpful in protecting your skin.[4,9]

(continued on page 228)

NEED REJUVENATION? TRY THESE TOPICAL RECIPES FOR YOUR SKIN

The following topical recipes are loaded with antioxidant-rich, revitalizing ingredients. These inventive (and edible!) potions are for cleansing, exfoliating, peeling, toning, moisturizing, and overall refreshing. Most were developed by Kyle O'Hara, a former surgical nurse who has developed a line of natural antiaging skin care products for her Napa, California–based business, Maintain Youth.

Carrot Coconut Scrub
(good for sensitive skin)

½ young coconut, freshly grated

¼ cup fresh carrot juice milk

¼ teaspoon ground turmeric

1 teaspoon almond oil

2–3 tablespoons rice flour

Mix everything in a ceramic bowl, adding just enough rice flour to make a paste. Moisten your skin with warm water, then massage this mixture into your skin with an upward/outward motion, leaving it on at least 5 minutes before rinsing with warm water. This is also great for the entire body.

Sesame Mint Scrub

Sesame seeds are also mildly abrasive, and their oil is a great emollient. I like the black sesame seeds when I can get them, since they seem firmer than white ones. The honey is also very exfoliating, and the dried herbs are invigorating.

½ cup raw honey (to thin it, add a little warm water)

¼ cup whole sesame seeds

1 teaspoon sesame oil (optional)

½ teaspoon dried lavender leaf

½ teaspoon dried mint

Mix everything in a ceramic bowl. Moisten your skin with warm water, then massage this mixture into your skin with an upward/outward motion, leaving it on at least 5 minutes before rinsing with warm water. This is also great for the entire body.

Cornmeal Yogurt Scrub

Cornmeal acts as a mild abrasive. In this recipe, it's combined with a normal skin-nourishing formula of yogurt and olive oil.

¼ cup stone-ground cornmeal

¼ cup plain yogurt

1 teaspoon extra-virgin olive oil

Mix everything in a ceramic bowl. Moisten your skin with warm water, then massage this mixture into your skin with an upward/outward motion, leaving it on the skin at least 5 minutes before rinsing with warm water.

Oatmeal Exfoliating Scrub
(for face, neck, and décolleté)

Oatmeal is a naturally abrasive, bulking, and absorbing agent in skin care preparations. Oats also contain a colloid that has soothing properties and provides a whole natural vegetable protein that leaves the skin soft, reduces redness and irritation (from sunburn and chemical irritation), and absorbs excess oil. It also has considerable cleansing properties and soothes sensitive skin.

¼ cup dry rolled oats (coarsely ground in blender or food processor)

2 teaspoons sea salt (medium to coarse grind)

¼ cup raw honey

¼ cup plain natural yogurt

1 teaspoon almond, grape seed, or sesame oil

Mix all the ingredients in a ceramic bowl immediately before use. Moisten your skin with warm water, then massage this mixture gently into your skin with an upward/outward motion, paying particular attention to areas that tend to get congested—the nose, forehead, and chin. Also, gently cleanse your neck and your chest area right above the breast line. Overall treatment should take about 5 minutes. Rinse the scrub with warm water and follow with a mask or moisturizer. Your skin should be glowing afterward.

(continued)

MASK RECIPES

Kyle likes to follow her scrubs with a special mask because the treated skin is especially able to take in nourishment and retain moisture. Both the avocado and egg mask recipes are for mature skin and are basically rich moisturizing masks, but yogurt added to any mask will balance it for normal skin types. Avocado is rich in vitamin E, and egg yolk is rich in vitamin A and zinc.

Avocado Banana Mask

1 large ripe avocado

1 ripe banana

1 teaspoon raw honey

1 teaspoon extra-virgin olive oil

Mash the avocado and banana in a ceramic bowl. Mix in the honey and oil to make a smooth paste. Apply to your face, neck, and décolleté and leave on for at least 20 minutes. Rinse with warm water.

Omega-3 Egg Mask

1 omega-3 egg yolk

1 teaspoon raw honey thinned with a little warm milk

1 teaspoon almond, grape seed, or sesame oil

You're already eating foods rich in antioxidants, such as vitamins C and E and the mineral selenium—and getting more antioxidants from all those cups of green tea—to help keep your heart healthy and the rest of your body cancer free. Remind yourself that those daily *Positively Ageless* habits help your skin, too. It's easy to forget about protecting the health of your insides because you can't see them. Let your skin be a constant reminder to make healthy choices to reduce signs of aging.[4,8]

In addition to its antioxidant protection, vitamin C plays an important role in the production of collagen, a protein that provides structure and softness to your skin. Selenium is a component of your body's antioxidant enzymes, and it's been shown to help protect skin from damage from UV

Beat the yolk thoroughly, then blend together with the honey and oil. Apply in a thin layer all over your face, neck, and décolleté and leave on for at least 20 minutes. Rinse with warm water.

Cheryl's Sea Salt Body Scrub

My friend John loves to indulge himself in pampering spa treatments and salt scrubs. After hearing about the latter, I experimented to make my own concoction. I couldn't believe how easy (and effective) this is. This exfoliating scrub will leave your skin baby soft. If you have sensitive skin, try a test run on a small area before applying to your entire body.

1 cup olive oil

1½ cups sea salt or kosher salt

1½ teaspoons scented essential oil (optional)

Place the salt in a wide-mouthed jar, pour the oil over it, and stir well. The mixture can be stored in the refrigerator for about a month.

To use body scrub: Dampen yourself in a shower. Apply the scrub with your hands or a bath mitt and gently massage it into your skin, using a circular motion. Rinse with warm water. Note: Be careful not to apply salt scrub to any cuts, scratches, or freshly shaven legs. Also, be sure you have a bath mat in place, since the scrub can make the tub very slippery.

rays.[10] That's a great reason to occasionally pop Brazil nuts, an exceptionally good source of the mineral, into your mouth.

In addition to the antioxidants you eat, topical treatments containing the antioxidant vitamins C and E, which you rub into your skin, can help protect you from sun damage.[1]

Cut out the sugar. A burst of sugar in your bloodstream encourages inflammation and skin-stiffening AGEs in your body, according to Dr. Perricone. Follow the rules established earlier for keeping your blood sugar on an even keel: Eat small portions often during the day, stick with complex carbs, and steer clear of foods made of white sugar and flour.[1]

Eat plenty of protein. "The days you don't eat protein are the days you age," Dr. Perricone says—and women typically don't get enough protein. When you eat protein, your body breaks it down into amino acids that are then used to repair cells in your skin, cartilage, muscles, and other structures. According to Dr. Perricone, a long-term deficiency of protein in the diet can contribute to sagging skin, so be sure to include a source of high-quality protein with each meal and snack. His favorite source: fish (see the box on page 220). As you've read throughout this book, certain types are high in omega-3 fatty acids. In addition to all the internal health improvements they provide, these can make your skin softer and probably reduce the appearance of wrinkles, too!

Go for vitamin A. When you're ladling hefty portions of veggies onto your plate, regularly make room for the ones that are rich in vitamin A. This nutrient helps maintain the integrity of your skin and works as an antioxidant, helping to protect your skin from UV rays. A 1997 study followed more than 2,000 people with a history of sun damage, such as actinic keratoses (precancerous changes) or skin cancers called carcinomas. For the next 5 years, some of them took daily vitamin A and some took a placebo (an inactive substance). Those taking the vitamin A had a "significantly lower" chance of developing a new case of one type of carcinoma than did the people who took the placebo.[11] Many foods that are appropriate for the *Positively Ageless* diet, such as carrots, spinach, cantaloupe, and mangoes,[12] are rich in carotenoids that can be converted into vitamin A in your body,

Get enough vitamin B$_6$. Vitamin B$_6$ is crucial for optimal function of many body tissues, including muscles, the nervous system, and the skin. A range of skin disorders can occur if this vital nutrient is deficient.

Ditch the smokes. It's been said that if smoking caused the same damage on the outside of the body as on the inside, then people wouldn't want to smoke. The truth is that smoking causes plenty of visible damage—it just takes a while to accumulate. Why spend your hard-earned money on a habit that makes your skin leathery, yellow, and creased . . . if it doesn't kill you first? Instead, invest those dollars wisely in a few quality products that *protect your skin*, not poison it.

chapter 18

HAIR: THERE'S PLENTY YOU CAN DO TO PROTECT YOUR MANE

Not all the changes that happen to our maturing bodies threaten our health. Take our hair, for instance. It's virtually a given that our natural color will change as years go by. Our hair will first be invaded and then overcome by an increasing number of renegade gray hairs. Our tresses may also lose some of the luster, thickness, and volume they used to have. But even though these hair changes don't harm our health, and we know that at least some of this change is inevitable, gray or thinning hair can be a source of genuine emotional distress.

Compared to the other topics in this book, you don't have as much control over what happens to your hair; self-care steps won't necessarily protect it from the aging process. However, some factors that you can alter may play a role in some conditions that affect your hair. You may be able to improve your hair thickness—and hair color is probably the easiest and least expensive problem to remedy.

Portrait of an Aging Scalp

The story of how your hair goes gray is pretty simple. The hair follicles in your scalp contain cells called melanocytes, which produce pigment that gives your hair its familiar color. As you get older, melanocytes drop in number, and those that remain become less active. Eventually, the hairs turn white. This may have already started happening to you in young adulthood, or you may not have even seen your first white hair yet.[13]

What causes hair loss is a little more complicated. Although this is thought of as more of a "guy problem," perhaps because it tends to be more noticeable in men, women's hair grows thin, too. In fact, more than one-third of women show some signs of hair loss after menopause.[14] A common cause is androgenetic alopecia. (*Alopecia* simply means "hair loss.") In men, this process is called male pattern baldness and results in the familiar strip of remaining hair over the ears and the back of the head. Women's hair tends to grow thinner on top rather than receding from the front. This is caused by a hormone called DHT, which is converted from testosterone in your body. (Yes, women have testosterone, too).[15,16]

In people who are genetically susceptible, DHT affects hair follicles so that they don't produce hairs like they previously did. Normally, the hair on your head goes through a years-long cycle of growing, resting, and falling out, then the follicle grows a new hair in the vacated spot. DHT causes follicles to wither. Some die altogether, and some become capable of only growing hairs that are shorter and thinner.[15,17]

Other conditions may also cause hair loss. A problem called alopecia areata, thought to be an autoimmune disorder, causes bare patches to develop relatively quickly. Also, a number of factors can temporarily cause your hair to shed more rapidly than normal, resulting in noticeable hair loss. These include hormonal changes, such as childbirth or menopause; deficiencies of certain nutrients, such as iron or protein; certain medications; and stress.[315]

Biomarkers for Hair Loss

A variety of tests are used to determine particular causes of hair loss. These include evaluating hormone levels, checking thyroid function, and measuring iron levels.[14,15]

The *Positively Ageless* Guide to Age-Related Hair Changes

See your doctor. If you're concerned about hair loss, visit your doctor. A wide variety of issues can cause you to shed hair, and some are treatable. Your doctor can run a number of tests to look for underlying problems and recommend medications to treat androgenetic alopecia or alopecia areata. In addition, certain medications, including birth control pills, can *cause* hair loss, so bring a list of all the medications you're taking and discuss with your doctor whether they may be playing a role.[14,15]

Eat a balanced diet. Since a lack of protein or iron has been associated with hair loss, make sure you eat protein throughout the day from high-quality sources such as fish, poultry, dairy, and eggs. Iron-rich foods include clams and whole grain cereals. Also, ask your doctor to check your iron levels to ensure that you have enough of the mineral in your body.[14,15]

Other nutrients, such as omega-3 fatty acids and zinc, are also associated with healthy hair. Be sure to get a wide variety of all the nutrients that the *Positively Ageless* diet is intended to provide. Aim to meet your nutritional needs with your diet, and use caution with nutrient supplements—excessive amounts of particular nutrients, such as vitamin A, may influence hair loss.[18]

In addition, if you need to lose weight, do it slowly and gradually. Crash dieting is another cause for hair loss.[3]

Meet with a great hairstylist. A hairdresser can work wonders to make your hair look more youthful. You can cover up gray with color, of course, but a talented pro can also give you an age-appropriate style that flatters your face and helps make thinning areas less noticeable. Simple changes such as side-swept bangs or a hair length just below the chin may trim away years.

Get a fashion makeover. Certain clothing colors and jewelry styles complement gray hair. If you decide to flaunt your natural colors, consult a fashion advisor who can help you make wardrobe choices that flatter your hair and maximize its beauty.

Careful with your eyebrows. Like the hair on your head, the growth of your body hair changes as you age. This includes your eyebrows! Don't overpluck them. The regrowth will not be as responsive as it once was, and they'll be less apt to grow back if you pluck too much.

chapter 19

BITE INTO GOOD HEALTH

A gorgeous smile can be your greatest physical attribute. It's easy to take it for granted if you're blessed with great teeth, but even the brightest pearly whites are subject to unanticipated changes as we age.

We all know that a healthy mouth is better than one that's filled with cavities, sore gums, and missing teeth. The signs of poor oral health don't look or feel good. But did you know that an ailing mouth can influence your overall health and even your longevity?

It's no surprise that people who are missing teeth have difficulty chewing many foods. Unfortunately, it's often the most nutritious foods—like fresh fruits and vegetables and nuts—that become the biggest obstacles. And when people are reluctant to eat in front of others, they miss out even further. They lose the protective effects of self-confidence and being social, which keep you active, healthy, and vital.[19]

But the perils of an unhealthy mouth go far beyond that. Research has linked gum disease with an increased risk of heart disease and stroke. Gum disease may contribute to these problems by allowing bacteria from your mouth to enter your bloodstream, where they create inflammation that encourages plaque to develop in your arteries.[20,21]

Older adults tend to have more dental problems than younger people, which makes sense because these changes are cumulative. According to the American Academy of Periodontology, more than half of people over age 55 have periodontitis (inflammation and infection of the supportive tissues around the teeth). And nearly one-quarter of people age 65 and older have lost all their teeth, though that situation is much less common than it used to be.[22] Issues that may be age-related that affect the mouth include:[19,23]

- Normal wear and tear on the teeth and shrinkage of the gums, exposing the roots of the teeth, which become susceptible to decay (cavities)

- Hormonal changes of menopause, which may put women at increased risk of periodontal disease and tooth loss

- Diabetes, which is more common in older adults and is linked to an increased risk of cavities and periodontal disease

So as you're taking the smart steps to keep your heart, brain, and other Very Important Parts well maintained for a healthy life, spend some time on your teeth and gums, too. They face special risks as you get older . . . but preserving their strength will keep you healthy and smiling for longer.

Biomarkers for Periodontal Disease

To diagnose periodontal disease, your dentist will check for redness, swelling, and other signs of inflammation, as well as loose teeth, and will ask whether your gums bleed when you brush them. Dentists also use a thin probe to check for any pockets that have formed between your teeth and gums and measure their depth.[24,25]

Your dentist may diagnose a cavity through a visual inspection, while prodding your teeth with a special instrument, or by finding a hidden spot of decay on an x-ray.[26]

The *Positively Ageless* Guide to Dental Health

Eat a balanced diet. Your gums, your tongue, and the lining of your mouth are easily affected by nutrient deficiencies. For example, a classic sign of scurvy—an extreme vitamin C deficiency that affected sailors hundreds of years ago—was inflamed and bleeding gums. Eating a diet rich in fruits, vegetables, whole grains, and lean sources of protein will help ensure that you get adequate levels of the vitamins and minerals that play a role in keeping your mouth healthy: vitamins A, B complex, C, D, E, and K and the minerals calcium, copper, magnesium, and zinc.[23]

See your dentist regularly. Visit your dentist for regular checkups—he or she can tell you how often that should be for you. Be sure to mention any symptoms of problems such as pain, bleeding gums, tooth sensitivity, changes in tooth color, persistent bad breath, or changes in your bite. Let your dentist know if you have diabetes or if you smoke. They both affect oral health and may be a cause for more frequent checkups. In addition, your dentist is in a good position to spot lumps and other suspicious changes that may indicate oral cancer.

Brush and floss! The American Dental Association (ADA) recommends that you brush twice a day with fluoride toothpaste and clean between your teeth daily with floss or an interdental cleaner. This removes plaque, a sticky film of bacteria that covers your teeth and contributes to cavities and gum problems. Replace your toothbrush every 3 months, since a worn-down brush doesn't clean your teeth as well and also harbors bacteria.[27,28]

It's a good idea to brush your tongue or use a tongue scraper—available at pharmacies and department stores—to remove bacterial buildup there, too. Take a peek at your tongue the next time you brush. It should look nice and pink. If it has a white or off-color coating, you're not finished cleaning. If you've never brushed your tongue before, you're in for a surprise. You'll love how much cleaner it makes your mouth look and feel.

If you have gingivitis, a mild form of gum disease marked by swelling and bleeding that can lead to periodontitis, ask your doctor to recommend an antibacterial mouth rinse.

Steer clear of sweet snacks. According to the ADA, each time you eat a food containing sugar or starch, bacteria on your teeth create acid after coming in contact with it. This acid stays on your teeth for at least 20 minutes and can lead to tooth decay. Sodas, whether sugary or diet, also contain acids that can cause damage over time. That's why it's a good idea to limit eating to regularly scheduled healthy meals and snacks, rather than munching on sugary treats throughout the day. Be especially wary of sugary foods that stick to your teeth. When you do indulge in a sweet treat, brush your teeth afterward.

Don't smoke. Smoking damages far-flung regions all over your body, so it shouldn't come as a surprise that it harms the part of your body where the smoke enters. According to the Centers for Disease Control and Prevention (CDC), smokers have seven times more risk of gum disease than nonsmokers.

Treat reflux. If you have acid reflux—acid rising out of your stomach and up into your esophagus—the harsh fluid may damage your teeth and the tissues in your mouth. Take the steps listed on page 74 to reduce the acidic attack.[13]

Keep your teeth away from damaging objects. Avoid chewing ice or using your teeth as tools to open packages or tear materials. These habits can damage your teeth.[13]

Watch your blood sugar. If you have diabetes, strive to keep your blood sugar in check (see the diabetes section starting on page 127 for a reminder of how to do that), and be especially diligent about keeping your teeth clean. Excess blood glucose encourages bacteria to grow in your mouth, setting the stage for gum disease and possible tooth loss.[29]

Ask about medications. Some medications reduce the flow of saliva in your mouth. Saliva contains components that protect your teeth and minimize bacterial growth in your mouth. When you don't have enough, you're at risk of infections and cavities. If your mouth has become dry, ask your doctor whether any medications could be contributing to the problem and, if so, what you can do to address the issue.[19,30] Also tell your dentist if you have dry mouth—you may need an added level of care and advice to keep your teeth and gums healthy.

Prevent tooth grinding with a mouth guard. Some people clench their jaws and grind their teeth during sleep, which can crack and wear down the teeth. This obviously doesn't bode well for the future of your chompers. If you suspect that you grind your teeth at night—symptoms include jaw soreness and headaches—discuss with your doctor whether you should wear a protective mouth guard while you sleep. Some people don't even realize they have a problem until their dentist makes the connection between lost fillings and nocturnal grinding.

Go for the sparkle! Dentists now have amazing techniques to work wonders on teeth that are discolored or unsightly. If your smile could use a makeover and your resources allow it, consider having your teeth whitened or other cosmetic dental work done. It won't necessarily improve your physical health, but it's hard not to smile when your teeth are dazzling!

chapter 20

KEEP YOUR EYES
ON THE PRIZE

Once you have a few decades of living behind you—okay, maybe more than a few decades—you've seen a lot of wonderful things. And when you practice the *Positively Ageless* lifestyle, you improve your chances of seeing a lot more during your life: new additions to your family, reunions with old friends, travels to exotic locales, and an unending parade of enriching experiences that you'll experience when you have optimal health.

It's important to make sure you protect your eyesight to fully enjoy all that's still ahead. That's because our bones and joints aren't the only things that stiffen as we age. The lenses of our eyes get stiff, too, making it more difficult to focus at different distances. So it's natural to lose some of our visual acuity with age, most noticeably in our forties or fifties. Luckily, this can easily be remedied with prescription or OTC reading glasses. The choices for new eyewear frames are so seductive, I choose to look at this as my opportunity for a new fashion accessory rather than an age-related "handicap."

A number of more serious conditions can also develop during adulthood and rob you of your vision. Several of these are at least partially preventable by your lifestyle.

Age-related macular degeneration (AMD). Your macula is the part of your retina responsible for seeing details in your central vision—or the things you see right in front of you.[31,32] It comes in two forms, "dry" and "wet." The dry form involves damage to cells in the macula, causing your central vision to gradually become blurry. The wet form is caused by leaky new blood vessels growing underneath the macula. It typically causes straight lines to appear crooked, and it may cause a blurry blind spot in your field of vision.[31,32]

People over the age of 60 have the highest risk of AMD. According to the National Eye Institute (NEI), smoking may increase the risk of the condition, and obesity may make early stages more likely to develop to advanced AMD.[31,32] High blood pressure, a deficiency of antioxidant nutrients in your diet, and cardiovascular disease may also increase your risk.[32]

Cataracts. Light entering your eye travels through the lens, a clear disc at the front of your eye that focuses the incoming light on your retina. Proteins within the lens can gather together, making a cloudy spot. This is a cataract. The cataract causes fuzziness in your field of vision, and the size of the blurry spot depends upon the size of the cloudy area on your lens.

Age is a factor in cataracts—most people with vision problems from cataracts are over 60. Experts also think that oxidative damage to the proteins within the lens plays a role in cataract development. Diabetes, smoking, and excessive sunlight exposure also raise your risk, according to the eye institute.

Diabetic retinopathy. This is a common cause of blindness among adults. It affects the retina—the thin layer of tissue lining the back wall of the eyeball. This condition causes blood vessels in the retina to swell and leak fluid or to grow new blood vessels, causing blurriness and blacked-out areas in your field of vision.[33,34] The longer you have diabetes, the higher your risk of developing these problems. Out-of-control blood sugar levels and high blood pressure also increase your risk.[33,34]

Biomarkers for Vision Changes

An eye specialist can perform a variety of tests to look for age-related conditions.

The *Positively Ageless* Guide to Preventing Age-Related Eye Problems

Get an eye exam. The NEI recommends that people age 60 and over have a comprehensive dilated eye exam at least once every 2 years. The doctor uses special eyedrops to make your pupils widen and allow a better look at your retinas and optic nerves.[35] Heed your doctor's advice if he or she recommends "readers"—and don't self-prescribe by picking your own at the drugstore without a proper exam first. Using glasses that are too strong can reduce the ability of your eyes to focus normally. And many of us don't have the same vision in both eyes. A prescription will adjust for that.

Use your glasses faithfully. I keep extra pairs in my car and purse so there's no excuse to strain my eyes any further. I figure I have many more decades of reading before me.

If you have early stage AMD, get a comprehensive eye exam every year. If you have diabetes, get a thorough eye exam *at least* once every year.[33,31] In addition, if you notice any of the following problems, make an appointment to discuss them with your doctor.

- Having to hold books closer
- Needing more light to see
- Dry eyes
- Eye fatigue
- Poor vision at night
- Blurry or double vision
- Headaches after reading

Keep your blood sugar in check. Research has found that people with diabetes who strive to keep their blood sugar near normal levels have later development and slower progression of diabetic retinopathy.[34] But even if you don't have diabetes, it's a good idea to keep your blood sugar restrained. AGEs—those familiar combinations of sugar and proteins—may play a role in the development of cataracts. So be sure to eat small meals containing fiber and protein throughout the day, and limit your consumption of sweets and other foods that quickly raise your blood sugar.[36]

Wear shades. Whether or not they're prescriptive, sunglasses protect your eyes from those wicked UV rays. Wraparound styles block out the most damaging light. Shading your eyes with sunglasses and a hat with a brim (another fashion accessory!) may help protect you from cataracts.[35]

Eat foods rich in nutrients for eye health. Antioxidants may reduce your risk of cataracts, and a diet rich in green leafy vegetables may lower your risk of AMD. Two carotenoids called lutein and zeaxanthin, found in leafy greens, may be particularly helpful for reducing the risk of AMD and cataracts.[37] So load your plate with a variety of green leafy vegetables and other deeply colored fruits and vegetables. Also make use of healthy oils and lean sources of protein. All together, these will give you the vitamins C, E, and A and the mineral zinc that may help keep your eyes healthy.[31,35,38]

In addition, the NEI has found that a high-dose formula of vitamins C and E, beta-carotene, zinc, and copper reduces the risk of advanced AMD. If you're at high risk, ask your doctor if you'd benefit from taking these supplements, since it's hard to get the high levels of these nutrients that were used in the research just from your diet.[31]

Stop smoking. If you're still smoking, keep in mind that the habit may leave you in the dark someday. There's no better time to stop than right now!

The *Positively Ageless* Program for Age-Proofing Your Outside Parts

At the end of each weekly section, you'll find an overview of specific tips to follow to incorporate the *Positively Ageless* diet into your lifestyle. These tips are broken down into stages. "Make One Change" is a list of easy-start changes. If you can only make one change per week, pick one from this list. "Quick Start" includes tips and strategies that are important but may take a bit longer to incorporate into your life. Suggestions you should follow for maximum antiaging benefit are listed in "Young for Life."

In addition, we've included a week's worth of meal plans that utilize the *Positively Ageless* ingredients. You'll find recipes for many of these menu items in the recipe section toward the back of the book.

Make One Change

If you feel able to make only one change in your life, pick it from this list. Research has shown these to be the most important strategies for slowing the aging clock.

Scope it out. If you're under 40, have a dermatologist give you a top-to-bottom skin exam every few years, starting at your scalp and ending at the soles of your feet. If you're over 40, schedule one annually. If you've spent a lot of time in the sun, or have lots of moles, freckles, or pigment changes or a family history of skin cancer, you should be examined even more frequently.

Polish your pearls. Be sure to see the dentist at least once a year for an exam and a cleaning. The powerful colors of all of the antioxidant-rich (and pigment-rich) foods like blueberries, tea, and red wine in your *Positively Ageless* diet may leave unsightly marks on your teeth while they put their beneficial mark on your health. Keep an extra brush and floss in your purse and in your car so there's never a reason not to have a dazzling smile.

Block it. The best prevention for skin cancer or sun damage is a simple tube of sunscreen (or avoiding the sun altogether). Be sure your moisturizers and foundation have SPF protection, too. You never know when you may unexpectedly find yourself being drenched in sunlight—so be prepared.

Say bye-bye to tanning booths. They're just as damaging as the real thing. If you simply have to have a bronzed glow, buy a great self-tanning product. They're inexpensive and offer a priceless sheen, compared with exposure from damaging UV rays.

Feed it. Wonderful topical products provide antioxidant protection for your skin. Invest in a cleanser, moisturizer, eye cream, and sunscreen for daily use. A weekly exfoliating scrub will restore that radiant glow while improving skin texture. Be sure to choose products suited to your skin's sensitivity and moisture level (dry to oily). And feed your skin from the inside out with the *Positively Ageless* diet: rich in antioxidants, anti-inflammatories, lean dairy, and omega-3-rich proteins. And don't forget lots of water.

Scrub it. As we get older, our skin cells regenerate much more slowly. Give them a helping hand by removing the dead outer layer once a week to let the dewy skin below shine through. If microdermabrasion is out of your budget, buy a home kit.

Pass the salt, please. Try an allover exfoliation with Cheryl's Sea Salt Body Scrub (page 229). This invigorating indulgence will leave your body smooth, soft, and radiant.

Load up on lutein. Lutein and zeaxanthin are the plant forms of vitamin A that concentrate in your macula. Make a special place on your plate each day for leafy greens, broccoli, squash, or avocados.

Zero in on 3s. Omega-3-rich proteins such as fish and flaxseed will provide the healthy fats that nourish hair and skin. Since omega-3s promote soft skin, this can help minimize the appearance of wrinkles. From flaxseed in your yogurt to salmon in your snacks, find ways to sneak in omega-3s throughout the day.

Pass the protein, please. Your body's working hard to stay lean and healthy. Don't forget the pivotal role of protein. It should be included with every snack and meal.

Quick Start

These strategies are a little more involved, but the benefits will reflect the additional effort you're spending. They'll provide a jump-start for measurable results in a short period of time.

Love your lips. Unlike the rest of your body, your lips don't have a thick protective outer layer of skin, oil glands to keep them moist, or protective melanin. They're vulnerable to dryness and sun damage, so keep them moisturized (or glossed), and don't forget that they like exfoliation, too.

Slather it. The delicate skin around your eyes is even thinner now and sometimes is the first place to wrinkle. Treat yourself to a rich eye cream to delay and minimize the appearance of fine lines. Ask your dermatologist about retinoid creams to keep fine lines from becoming wrinkles.

Bank it. You only pass this way once, and you only have one chance to protect your skin. Make a budget to pamper your skin and have a facial each month. If that's beyond your means, invest in a good scrub or peel and moisturizers. Once the wrinkles set in, there's no going back (unless "nip and tuck" is music to your ears).

Sleep it off. Getting enough sleep is underrated—it's a top antiager. Be disciplined and treat yourself to this luxury, whether it's napping during the day or going to bed earlier. Lack of sleep taxes your body from head to toe—and it shows.

High five for hands. It's easy to abuse our hands, and sometimes they're the first parts to show our age: They have few oil glands and thinner skin, and they get more sun exposure than any other part of the body. Treat them with the same care you give your face. Wear moisturizer (with SPF) and keep hand cream everywhere—the car, your desk, and near every sink. Once a week, give your hands a nighttime pampering with a rich moisturizer and a pair of cotton gloves to provide an intensive treatment while you sleep.

Now see this. If you've never had an eye exam, you should schedule one at age 40, even if you don't yet have a vision problem, and have an eye exam every other year after that. Follow your doctor's advice. If he or she recommends glasses, wear them. There's a lot of beautiful scenery on the road ahead. Keep your eyes healthy so you can savor it all.

Young for Life

This list of strategies is for those of you who are ready for a major lifestyle intervention. While you'll need to spend a bit more effort enacting these good habits, the payoff can be a dramatic, lasting impact on your health.

Experience exfoliation. Whether it's a professional treatment or do-at-home enzyme peels or microdermabrasion creams, keep your face dewy fresh and rub away that lifeless layer of outer skin.

Big on brows. If you haven't had a professional shaping before, treat yourself. You may be amazed at how the correct brow shape can change your appearance. It can open your eyes and even make you look happier. Remember not to overtweeze, as these hairs won't grow back as fast as they used to.

Sparkle, shimmer, and shine. If you haven't tried whitening your teeth, you're in for a real surprise. Whether you have this professionally done or use whitening strips at home, you will be dazzled at what tooth whitening can do. A brighter smile means more of them—and soaring self-confidence, too.

Pick up a tongue scraper (or just use your toothbrush). It's quick and easy to clear away bacteria and debris that settle on your tongue. If you've been battling bad breath, this may be the cure you've been seeking.

Get plenty of pairs. Be sure to keep extra readers on hand, especially if your vision is the same in both eyes (enabling you to buy inexpensive OTC glasses). Keep them in the car, your desk, and by your bedside. Treat your eyes well, and give them a little assistance now and then.

Don't forget to wear your shades. Keep them everywhere. Squinting doesn't only strain your eyes—it crinkles the thin skin around them. Don't add to the wrinkle momentum. Wraparound glasses provide the best protection for your eyes as well as the delicate skin.

Work it. It's time to bump up the exercise routine you've been working on the past few weeks. If you really want to push your workout to the limit, try adding a second mini-workout each day until you achieve the results you desire. Tack on an additional 20 to 30 minutes of aerobic exercise in the evening, 5 days per week. You may want to do this before dinner as a late-afternoon or evening workout (although some people find this impedes sleep). Mix it up with a different activity than you do in the mornings. For example, if you cycle in the morning, run in the evening.

Intensify it. By adding intense "intervals" in your aerobic sessions, you can really burn fat and rev up your metabolism. For example, jog for 4 minutes, run fast for the fifth minute, then go back to jogging, and repeat over and over. Your body will work harder and burn more fat. When you fall into a comfortable exercise routine, your metabolism slacks off, so keep it interesting and supercharged.

Accessorize. Sun hats are a must, so be sure to choose a style that you'll love wearing. Keep a hat or baseball cap in the car in case you suddenly find yourself exposed to the sun.

Love your locks. If you have any issues with hair loss, be sure to check with your doctor right away to determine the cause. The *Positively Ageless* diet will provide the nutrients and vitamins required to promote healthy hair.

Style it. Your tight body, glowing skin, and dazzling teeth will shine with an age-appropriate hairstyle. If you've been sporting the same do since college, it may be time for a new cut (and color).

Top it off. If your closet looks like a fashion flashback, it's time for a wardrobe makeover, starting from the inside out. Toss those granny bloomers and find some sexy lingerie to hug your curves. Many of us tend to choose the wrong clothing colors as well as the wrong styles for flattering our figures. This is a new chapter in your life, and it's time for some head-turning fashion changes. Now's the time to see an image consultant (or a fashion-savvy friend) to bring your attire out of the Dark Ages.

chapter 21

EAT SMART, LIVE LONG MENUS

Positively Ageless Menus Week Four

The *Positively Ageless* menu plans are based on an average of 1,200 calories per day. If your calorie needs are a little higher (or lower), you can adjust accordingly. Adding a glass of 1 percent milk, 6 ounces of fat-free yogurt, one pear or a large apple, or a glass of red wine with dinner will each provide an additional 100 calories.

Positively Ageless **recipes** are listed in bold and designated as one serving size.

The two snacks can be scheduled between meals or one between meals and one after dinner.

DAY 1

1,170 calories; 33 grams fiber; 6,660 milligrams omega-3s

BREAKFAST

Breakfast wrap: 1 small whole wheat tortilla with 1 omega-3 egg, 2 egg whites, **Zippy Hummus** (page 294), 2 tomato slices, and 1 slice avocado

1 nectarine

8 ounces iced green tea with lemon

MID-MORNING SNACK

Smoothie with 1/3 cup kefir, 1/3 cup fat-free milk, 2 tablespoons sliced strawberries, and 1 teaspoon ground flaxseed

LUNCH

Tuna salad with 3 ounces water-packed tuna, 1/2 cup cooked lentils, 1 cup chopped tomatoes, 2 tablespoons chopped parsley, and 1 tablespoon **Tomato Ginger Vinaigrette** (page 283)

1 medium orange

8 ounces green tea or ice water with orange slice

MID-AFTERNOON SNACK

Zinger Green Tea (page 271)

1 Wasa Crispbread with 1 ounce sliced turkey and 1 tablespoon **Watercress Sauce** (page 289) **or Tahini Yogurt Sauce** (page 284)

DINNER

3 ounces grilled salmon fillet

Lima Beans with Parsley and Red Cabbage (page 335)

1/2 cup wild or brown rice

1/2 cup diced watermelon and 1/2 cup fresh blueberries with 1 teaspoon fresh mint

8 ounces green tea with ginger

DAY 2

1,235 calories; 28 grams fiber; 2,700 milligrams omega-3s

BREAKFAST

Positively Ageless Flax Cereal (page 260)

⅓ cup fat-free vanilla yogurt

½ medium banana, sliced, and ⅓ cup fresh raspberries

1 serving (1 cup) green tea or fat-free milk

MID-MORNING SNACK

⅓ cup fat-free cottage cheese with ½ sliced pear and 1 teaspoon chopped pecans

LUNCH

3 ounces poached salmon served with

Sliced Avocados and Oranges with Tahini Yogurt Sauce (page 316)

1 cup watercress with ½ tablespoon low-fat vinaigrette

8 ounces iced green tea with lime

MID-AFTERNOON SNACK

1 low-fat cheese stick

1 Granny Smith apple

DINNER

Roast Pork Tenderloin with Citrus, Green Tea, and Spices (page 329)

1 cup wilted green cabbage sautéed with 2 tablespoons finely chopped onion and 1 teaspoon olive oil

½ cup stone-ground polenta sprinkled with 1 teaspoon grated Parmesan cheese

4 ounces red wine

8 ounces green or white tea or sparking water with orange wedge

DAY 3

1,215 calories; 38 grams fiber; 2,320 milligrams omega-3s

BREAKFAST

Morning smoothie blend: $^2/_3$ cup fat-free milk or soy milk, $^1/_4$ cup fat-free vanilla yogurt or 4 ounces soft tofu, and $^3/_4$ cup mixed chopped fruit (berries, banana, melon, or mango)

Bran Yogurt Muffin (page 264)

8 ounces green tea with ginger or ice water

MID-MORNING SNACK

$^1/_2$ ounces roasted soy nuts

1 tangerine

LUNCH

Southwest Salmon Burger (page 324)

Chopped salad: 1 cup chopped romaine lettuce, $^1/_2$ cup watercress, $^1/_2$ cup halved cherry tomatoes, 1 tablespoon low-fat Caesar dressing, and 1 tablespoon chopped cilantro

Sweet Pumpkin Polenta (page 339)

1 cup iced green tea with lime wedge

MID-AFTERNOON SNACK

2 tablespoons fat-free refried beans and $^1/_4$ cup salsa

Whole Wheat Pita Chips (page 295)

DINNER

Sesame Turkey Stir-Fry with Cabbage and Green Beans (page 326) (made with chicken instead of turkey)

$1^1/_2$ cups mixed baby greens with 1 teaspoon extra-virgin olive oil, 1 teaspoon balsamic vinegar, and $^1/_2$ teaspoon chopped thyme

1 poached pear

Iced green tea or ice water

DAY 4

1,209 calories; 26 grams fiber; 3,390 milligrams omega-3s

BREAKFAST

Breakfast yogurt parfait: alternating layers of **Positively Ageless Flax Cereal** (page 260); ⅓ cup fat-free vanilla yogurt; 2 tablespoons blueberries; 2 tablespoons raspberries; and ½ medium apple, diced

8 ounces iced green tea with fresh lemon

MID-MORNING SNACK

Quesadilla: 1 small corn tortilla, 2 tablespoons low-fat Cheddar, and 1 tablespoon salsa

LUNCH

Green Tea Miso Soup (page 297)

3 ounces poached salmon or sea bass

⅓ cup diced mango with ⅓ cup fresh blueberries

Iced green tea or water

MID-AFTERNOON SNACK

Almond Berry Bar (page 346)

Green tea with lemon

DINNER

3 ounces chicken breast grilled with **Barbecue Sauce** (page 285)

Rainbow Radicchio Slaw (page 315)

½ medium artichoke, steamed

⅔ cup diced honeydew with 1 tablespoon fat-free vanilla yogurt and 1 teaspoon chopped pecans

8 ounces green tea or water

DAY 5

1,222 calories; 27 grams fiber; 1,910 milligrams omega-3s

BREAKFAST

½ seven-grain English muffin

1 poached omega-3 egg

½ cup fresh strawberry slices

1 cup steamed fat-free or soy milk sprinkled with cinnamon and nutmeg

8 ounces green tea

MID-MORNING SNACK

1 whole grain Wasa Crispbread spread with ½ tablespoon cashew or almond butter and **Easy Blueberry Jam** (page 288)

LUNCH

Chicken salad: 3 ounces grilled skinless chicken (or turkey) breast, chopped, served over 1 cup baby lettuce leaves with ½ cup diced pear and 1 tablespoon dried cranberries and dressed with 1 tablespoon balsamic vinegar

Wild Rice with Radicchio and Dried Cherries (page 309)

Iced green tea with lemon or water

MID-AFTERNOON SNACK

Asparagus Spears with Smoked Salmon and Tangy Mustard Dressing (page 293)

DINNER

3 ounces grilled halibut fillet with **Miso Marinade** (page 287)

Gingered Edamame with Fire-Roasted Tomatoes (page 331)

1 cup wilted Swiss chard sautéed with 1 teaspoon olive oil and 1 teaspoon chopped garlic

4 ounces red wine

8 ounces green tea or water

DAY 6

1,213 calories; 28 grams fiber; 2,540 milligrams omega-3s

BREAKFAST

Nutty breakfast smoothie: 1 cup fat-free or soy milk, 2 ounces silken tofu (or $\frac{1}{2}$ cup fat-free yogurt), 1 tablespoon natural peanut butter, 1 medium frozen banana, and $1\frac{1}{2}$ tablespoons natural cocoa powder

8 ounces green tea or water

MID-MORNING SNACK

Spicy Chai (page 276)

Bran Yogurt Muffin (page 264)

LUNCH

Spanish Meatball Soup (page 303)

2 cups mixed baby greens with $\frac{1}{2}$ cup halved cherry tomatoes, 2 tablespoons chopped yellow bell pepper, 2 tablespoons chopped cucumber with peel, 1 tablespoon crumbled low-fat feta cheese, and 1 tablespoon light vinaigrette

8 ounces green tea or ice water with orange slice

MID-AFTERNOON SNACK

Sparkling Melon Agua Fresca (page 272)

4 almonds

DINNER

3 ounces grilled salmon or halibut

1 cup sautéed baby spinach

Sweet Potatoes with Onion Confit (page 333)

Ruby Lemon Sorbet (page 343)

8 ounces green tea or fat-free milk

DAY 7

1,234 calories; 35 grams fiber; 2,410 milligrams omega-3s

BREAKFAST

Cheesy Vegetable Frittata (page 262)

½ slice **Whole Grain Bread** (page 306)

½ cup fresh raspberries

8 ounces green tea, ice water, or fat-free milk

MID-MORNING SNACK

½ small whole wheat pita stuffed with **Zippy Hummus** (page 294), 2 slices tomato, and 4 slices cucumber

LUNCH

Baby Spinach Salad (page 314; recipe prepared with chicken instead of turkey)

1 small peach

Iced green tea with lemon

MID-AFTERNOON SNACK

½ cup fat-free cottage cheese with ½ medium apple, chopped; 1 tablespoon ground flaxseed; and 2 tablespoons chopped celery

DINNER

Lebanese Kebabs (page 322)

Cumin-Spiced Bulgur and Lentils (page 308)

1 cup steamed Swiss chard

½ cup halved red cherry tomatoes

Rich Cocoa Sorbet (page 342)

4 ounces red wine

8 ounces green tea or water with lemon

POSITIVELY AGELESS RECIPES

WHAT'S HIGH IN ANTIOXIDANTS?

Nutritional values for *Positively Ageless* recipes have been calculated using data from the USDA National Nutrient Database for Standard Reference, Release 18, and the Food Processor software program, ESHA Research, Inc., in Salem, Oregon. Analyses include:

- Calories

- Protein

- Carbohydrates (carbs)

- Total fat

- Saturated fat (sat fat)

- Monounsaturated fat (mono fat)

- Omega-3s*

- Fiber

- Sugar

- Sodium

*The available nutritional databases do not provide omega-3 values for all foods; therefore, actual omega-3 values may be higher than what is stated. Additionally, the data provided do not distinguish between the types of omega-3s; e.g., ALA, DHA, EPA. The milligrams of omega-3s per serving are provided as a learning tool to reflect the types of foods that are rich in either type of omega-3s, whether derived from plant or animal sources.

ABOUT THE ORAC CHARTS

The ORAC (oxygen radical absorbency capacity) measurement quantifies a food's ability to neutralize cell-damaging free radicals. We don't yet know how this translates to its performance in our bodies. The science is still emerging in terms of how much of a food's antioxidants we actually absorb. We do know enough, however, to warrant making them a focal point in our diets. The charts in this section identify highest-ranking foods in each category in terms of their average antioxidant capacity in lab measurements. If you don't see a particular food listed, that does not mean that it doesn't contain a measurable amount of antioxidants. It may mean that either the food hasn't been studied yet or those measurements were not available for us to include. For recommended daily amounts of ORAC, see the Introduction (page 1).

Breakfast

Old-Fashioned Breakfast Sausage

Positively Ageless Flax Cereal

Creamy Almond Kasha

Cheesy Vegetable Frittata

Bran Yogurt Muffins

Baked Eggs in Savory Turkey Cups

Breakfast Polenta with Berries and Vanilla

Old-Fashioned Breakfast Sausage

MAKES 8 SERVINGS (2 LINKS EACH)

Toast or fruit is not enough for breakfast. Protein plays an important part of every meal, including breakfast. Pork tenderloin is sometimes overlooked as a lean protein choice, although ground turkey can be substituted in this recipe for an equally delicious result.

> 1 pound pork tenderloin (or very lean ground pork)
> 3 tablespoons finely grated onion
> 1 teaspoon dried sage
> $\frac{1}{2}$ teaspoon dried thyme
> 2 cloves garlic, chopped
> 1 teaspoon agave nectar
> $\frac{3}{4}$ teaspoon salt
> $\frac{1}{4}$ teaspoon ground black pepper
> 1 tablespoon olive oil

Remove all visible fat from the pork. Cut the pork into $\frac{1}{2}$" pieces.

Place the pork, onion, sage, thyme, garlic, agave, salt, and pepper in the bowl of a food processor. Pulse just until the mixture is well combined and cohesive. Transfer to a bowl, cover with plastic, and refrigerate for at least an hour (or overnight) to allow flavors to marry. There will be about 2 cups of mixture.

Using approximately 2 tablespoons of the mixture per sausage, quickly shape into 16 patties about $2\frac{1}{2}$" in diameter (or links about 3" long and 1" in diameter).

Heat the oil in a large nonstick sauté pan. Add the sausages, cover, and cook over medium heat for about 3 minutes. Remove the cover, turn the sausages, reduce the heat to medium-low, cover the pan, and cook until the sausages are crisp and cooked through, about 2 minutes longer. (You may have to do this in two batches, depending on size of the pan.) Drain on paper towels. Serve immediately. Overcooked sausage will be dry.

✱ **PORK TENDERLOIN FACTOID:** It's lean. A 3-ounce serving of broiled pork tenderloin actually contains less total fat than the same weight of skinless broiled chicken breast.

NUTRIENT ANALYSIS PER SERVING
85 calories, 11 g protein, 1 g carbohydrates, 4 g total fat, 1 g saturated fat, 2 g monounsaturated fat, 20 mg omega-3s, < 1 g fiber, < 1 g sugar, 245 mg sodium

Positively Ageless Flax Cereal

MAKES 24 SERVINGS (½ CUP EACH)

It's easy and inexpensive to make your own high-fiber, high-protein breakfast cereal. For even more antiaging fiber and antioxidants, serve with fresh berries.

4 cups old-fashioned rolled oats

1½ cups oat or wheat bran

1 cup low-fat soy flour

1 cup raw wheat germ

1 cup nonfat dry milk

½ cup chopped pecans or slivered almonds (optional)

⅔ cup agave nectar

½ cup water

2 tablespoons pure vanilla extract

¾ cup ground flaxseed

Preheat the oven to 250°F.

In a large mixing bowl, combine the oats, bran, soy flour, wheat germ, milk, and nuts (if using).

In a small bowl, combine the agave, water, and vanilla extract. Stir well to combine.

Pour the agave mixture over the dry ingredients and combine well. Divide the mixture between 2 ungreased 15" × 10" baking sheets and spread evenly. Bake for 1 hour, stirring every 15 minutes to ensure even browning. Cool completely. Sprinkle with the flaxseed. Store in the refrigerator in airtight containers.

Note: It is important that the wheat germ is purchased raw and not already toasted; otherwise, it will burn during the slow toasting process. Raw wheat germ is available at health food stores.

❋ **FLAX FACTOID:** Although some of the ALA omega-3s found in flax are converted to the EPA or DHA form found in fish, the conversion rate and amount depend on your gender and the composition of the rest of your diet. Conversion rate is greater in women, possibly due to the effects of estrogen.

NUTRIENT ANALYSIS PER SERVING

173 calories, 28 g carbohydrates, 9 g protein, 4 g total fat, 0 g saturated fat, 1 g monounsaturated fat, 1,040 mg omega-3s, 6 g fiber, 10 g sugar, 39 mg sodium

Creamy Almond Kasha

MAKES 8 SERVINGS ($\frac{1}{2}$ CUP EACH)

Toasted buckwheat is called kasha. Toasting separates the grains and adds a nutty flavor, and slow cooking in extra liquid softens them—as in this recipe, which takes minutes to put together before placing in the oven to bake. This dish can also be prepared the night before, then reheated in an oven at low heat or the microwave.

2 cups hot fat-free milk or soy milk

$\frac{1}{4}$ cup agave nectar or sorghum syrup

$\frac{1}{2}$ cup kasha (toasted buckwheat)

$\frac{1}{2}$ cup chopped almonds or walnuts

2 tablespoons ground flaxseed

$\frac{1}{2}$ cup dried berries (optional)

Preheat the oven to 350°F.

Pour the hot milk into a $1\frac{1}{2}$-quart soufflé or casserole dish. (Or heat the milk in the soufflé dish using the microwave for about 3 minutes.)

Stir in the sweetener, kasha, nuts, flaxseed, and berries (if using). Bake uncovered for 35 minutes. The kasha should be bubbling and just starting to brown. (It will continue to absorb liquid as it cools.) Serve with fresh fruit, if desired.

Note: To pare back calories and fat, omit the nuts. That brings the calories down to 113, and the fat grams drop to 2 per serving.

❊ **BUCKWHEAT FACTOID:** Buckwheat is a grainlike seed. Porous and absorbent, it is quick and easy to prepare. Buckwheat has a bundle of plant chemicals called rutin. Studies have shown that this compound helps lower cholesterol, maintain bloodflow, and protect against heart disease. Buckwheat also contains magnesium, which relaxes blood vessels while lowering blood pressure.

NUTRIENT ANALYSIS PER SERVING
152 calories, 24 g carbohydrates, 6 g protein, 6 g total fat, 0 g saturated fat, 3 g monounsaturated fat, 510 mg omega-3s, 5 g fiber, 12 g sugar, 29 mg sodium

Cheesy Vegetable Frittata

MAKES 6 SERVINGS

Like most of the recipes in this book, it's easy to make this one your own by substituting ingredients and flavorings. If you don't like mushrooms, substitute a cup of sliced artichoke hearts. If you prefer oregano to basil, plug that in—or use both. Any way you slice it, this frittata is a delicious way to sneak antioxidant-rich herbs and vegetables into your breakfast routine.

6 egg whites

2 whole omega-3 eggs

3 teaspoons olive oil

1 cup chopped onion

1 cup chopped bell pepper

1 cup sliced mushrooms

1 cup chopped tomato

1 tablespoon chopped garlic

1 cup fat-free ricotta cheese

2 tablespoons fresh basil, chopped

$\frac{1}{2}$ teaspoon salt

$\frac{1}{4}$ teaspoon cracked black pepper

2 tablespoons grated Parmesan cheese, for garnish

Fresh basil sprigs, for garnish

Lightly coat an 8" × 8" square baking pan with cooking oil spray. Preheat the oven to 400°F.

In a large mixing bowl, combine whole eggs and egg whites. Set aside.

Heat 1 teaspoon of the oil in large nonstick sauté pan over medium-high heat. Add the onion and bell pepper and cook for 5 minutes, until the vegetables are soft. Transfer to a baking sheet to cool.

Add another teaspoon of the olive oil to the same pan. Add the mushrooms and sauté for a few minutes until the mushrooms are cooked. Transfer to the baking sheet to cool. Add the remaining 1 teaspoon oil to the pan. Add the tomato and garlic and cook for 3 to 4 minutes, or until the tomatoes are cooked and most of the juices have evaporated. Transfer to the baking sheet to cool.

Whisk the reserved eggs. Add the ricotta and whisk again until smooth. Stir in the basil, salt, pepper, and cooled vegetables. Pour the frittata mixture into the prepared pan. Bake for 25 minutes, or just until set. Serve immediately, garnished with the cheese and basil sprigs.

✳ **BELL PEPPER FACTOID:** Bell peppers are an excellent source of vitamins A, C, and B$_6$. Bell peppers have a recessive gene for capsaicin, the plant chemical responsible for the heat in other peppers. This is the reason they aren't hot like the others.

NUTRIENT ANALYSIS PER SERVING
133 calories, 1 g carbohydratess, 11 g protein, 4 g total fat, 1 g saturated fat, 2 g monounsaturated fat, 160 mg omega-3s, 2 g fiber, 5 g sugar, 151 mg sodium

Bran Yogurt Muffins

MAKES 12 MUFFINS

These moist, fiber-loaded bran muffins are a staple in my kitchen. I usually make a double batch and keep some in the freezer. Try using flavored yogurt, or stir in your favorite fresh berries or nuts if you want even more flavor or texture.

1¾ cups wheat bran or oat bran

1 cup stone-ground whole wheat flour, or ¾ cup whole wheat flour + ¼ cup sorghum flour

¼ cup ground flaxseed (see note)

1 teaspoon ground cinnamon

1 teaspoon baking soda

¼ teaspoon salt

1 cup fat-free plain yogurt

¾ cup soy or low-fat milk

½ cup agave nectar or sorghum syrup

2 tablespoons olive oil

1 large omega-3 egg

1 teaspoon pure vanilla extract

Position a rack in the center of the oven and preheat the oven to 400°F.

Lightly coat 12 (2¼" × 1½") nonstick muffin cups with olive oil cooking spray.

In a medium bowl, combine the bran, flour, flaxseed, cinnamon, baking soda, and salt. Set aside.

In another medium bowl or in a blender, combine the yogurt, milk, agave or syrup, oil, egg, and vanilla extract and stir until smooth.

Make a well in the center of the dry ingredients and pour in the liquid mixture. Using a spoon, stir just until combined. Do not overmix.

Spoon about ¼ cup of batter into each prepared muffin cup. Bake for 14 minutes, or until the tops spring back when pressed gently in the centers. Do not overbake. Cool in the pan on a wire rack for 10 minutes before removing from the cups. Serve warm or cool completely on the rack.

Note: Grind whole flaxseeds in a clean spice grinder to the consistency of cornmeal.

❄ **YOGURT FACTOID:** Probiotics are healthy bacteria that discourage the growth of harmful bacteria. Some manufacturers add "live" healthy bacteria cultures to their dairy or soy products during processing to enhance the health-promoting potential. These cultures may include *Lactobacillus acidophilus*. The probiotic bacteria pass through the stomach to the gastrointestinal (GI) tract, where they help maintain a good balance between the many kinds of bacteria that live there while promoting GI health. There is some scientific evidence that fermented foods containing probiotics may help to prevent some forms of cancer, too.

NUTRIENT ANALYSIS PER MUFFIN
153 calories, 6 g protein, 26 g carbohydrates, 5 g total fat, 1 g saturated fat, 2 g monounsaturated fat, 740 mg omega-3s, 7 g fiber, 10 g sugar, 142 mg sodium

Baked Eggs in Savory Turkey Cups

MAKES 6 SERVINGS

Fresh egg whites deliver the best flavor, but egg substitute can be used for convenience. You can also use whole omega-3 eggs if you haven't exceeded your weekly cholesterol allotment.

6 ounces very thinly sliced deli turkey

12 tablespoons (1½ cups) salsa or chopped grilled veggies

9 large egg whites or 1 cup + 2 tablespoons liquid egg white or egg substitute (see note)

2 tablespoons chopped fresh cilantro

2 tablespoons grated low-fat Cheddar cheese

Preheat the oven to 400°F. Lightly coat each cup of a standard-size nonstick muffin pan with olive oil cooking spray.

Line each muffin cup with ½ ounce of the turkey. There will probably be a little excess extending from the top of each cup. Spoon 1 tablespoon of the salsa or veggies into each cup.

Measure 3 tablespoons of the egg whites or egg substitute (or a whole omega-3 egg, if using) into each muffin cup. (After the first "muffin," you can pour the whites from the liquid measuring cup to the same level as the first muffin cup, rather than measuring 3 tablespoons each time.)

Place the muffin pan in the oven and bake for 10 to 12 minutes, or until the eggs are puffed and the center is set. Carefully remove the baked eggs from the pan and place two muffins on each serving plate. Garnish with the cilantro and cheese.

Note: If using fresh eggs, separate 9 whites into a medium mixing bowl. Add ½ teaspoon salt and whisk lightly. Transfer to a liquid measuring cup. Let stand while you prepare the rest of the ingredients.

✱ **EGG WHITE FACTOID:** A large egg white measures about 2 tablespoons. Adding salt will thin the whites slightly and make them easier to measure by the tablespoon.

NUTRIENT ANALYSIS PER SERVING
68 calories, 3 g carbohydrates, 11 g protein, 1 g total fat, 0 g saturated fat, 0 g monounsaturated fat, 20 mg omega-3s, 1 g fiber, 1 g sugar, 220 mg sodium

Breakfast Polenta
with Berries and Vanilla

MAKES 4 SERVINGS

This delicious twist on a savory grain results in a satisfying breakfast dish that is high in fiber and flavor. If you're counting calories, cook the cereal with water instead of soy milk and omit the sweetener. Result = 100-calorie version.

⅓ cup stone-ground cornmeal or polenta

2 cups low-fat or fat-free milk

2 tablespoons ground flaxseed

2 tablespoons oat bran

¼ teaspoon ground cinnamon (optional)

Pinch of salt

1 tablespoon agave nectar

½ teaspoon pure vanilla extract

1 cup fresh blueberries, raspberries, or sliced strawberries

Pour the cornmeal or polenta into a 1-quart saucepan over medium heat. Stir for 2 to 3 minutes until very lightly toasted.

Carefully pour in the milk. Bring to a boil, stirring to avoid lumps. When the mixture just starts to boil, reduce the heat to simmer and stir in the flaxseed, oat bran, cinnamon (if using), and salt. Simmer for 1 minute, stirring. Turn off the heat. Cover and let stand for 5 minutes. Stir in the agave and vanilla extract. Divide the cereal between 4 bowls. Top each with ¼ cup blueberries. Serve hot.

✳ **CORNMEAL FACTOID:** Unlike most commercial brands, stone-ground cornmeal has a chewy texture and includes the nutritious germ.

NUTRIENT ANALYSIS PER SERVING
176 calories, 8 g protein, 30 g carbohydrates, 4 g total fat, 0 g saturated fat, 1 g monounsaturated fat, 130 mg omega-3s, 5 g fiber, 7 g sugar, 73 mg sodium

Beverages

Mango Mint Smoothie

Nutty Chocolate Shake

Zinger Green Tea

Sparkling Melon Agua Fresca

Pinolillo (Spanish Chocolate Shake)

Spicy Chai

Hot Chocolate

Grapefruit Lassi

Mango Mint Smoothie

MAKES 2 SERVINGS (1 CUP EACH)

This is a great pre- or postworkout drink, as it has a nice blast of protein from the tofu. Be sure the mango is very ripe. You can add a splash of agave nectar for extra sweetness.

$^3/_4$ cup very ripe mango, roughly chopped

$^3/_4$ cup silken tofu

$^1/_2$ cup almond milk*

1 tablespoon finely chopped fresh mint leaves

$^1/_8$ teaspoon ground nutmeg

1 cup crushed ice or ice cubes

Agave nectar (optional)

Combine all the ingredients in the jar of a blender or bowl of a food processor. Blend or process until smooth.

*Choose a brand that is either unsweetened or sweetened with brown rice syrup, such as Pacific's Almond Non-Dairy Beverage.

✳ **MANGO FACTOID:** Originally cultivated in India, the tropical mango tree is a member of the cashew family.

NUTRIENT ANALYSIS PER SERVING

199 calories, 6 g protein, 18 g carbohydrates, 3 g total fat, 0 g saturated fat, 2 g monounsaturated fat, 30 mg omega-3s, 4 g fiber, 11 g sugar, 75 mg sodium

Nutty Chocolate Shake

MAKES 2 SERVINGS (1¼ CUPS EACH)

There are a variety of ready-to-drink nut milks on the market, which are made by soaking nuts or seeds in water, then blending and straining the liquid. Try to find an unsweetened brand or use soy milk or fat-free milk. This creamy shake is thickened and sweetened with frozen banana.

> 1 cup almond, fat-free milk, or soy milk
>
> ⅓ cup soft silken tofu
>
> 1 very ripe banana, peeled and frozen
>
> 1½ tablespoons natural cocoa powder
>
> 1 teaspoon agave nectar (optional)
>
> ½ teaspoon vanilla extract
>
> 4 ice cubes

Combine all of the ingredients in the jar of a blender or bowl of a food processor. Blend or process until smooth. Pour into a glass and serve immediately.

Note: Pour leftover smoothie into a small plastic bag and store in the freezer. When ready to serve, thaw slightly and remix in the blender.

✳ **TOFU FACTOID:** Silken or Japanese-style tofu is made from soy milk that is strained before adding a coagulant. The coagulating protein is not hardened into curds, nor is the whey drained off. This makes a smooth and creamy texture, whether it's soft, firm, or extra-firm. That's why silken tofu is a good choice for making desserts or smoothies.

NUTRIENT ANALYSIS PER SERVING
126 calories, 7 g protein, 23 g carbohydrates, 1 g total fat, < 1 g saturated fat, < 1 g monounsaturated fat, 20 mg omega-3s, 3 g fiber, 13 g sugar, 62 mg sodium

Zinger Green Tea

MAKES 6 SERVINGS OR 1½ QUARTS

Packed with antioxidants, this tea is bursting with flavor, too. Fresh lime juice gives it a tangy zing and a wallop of vitamin C.

6 cups water

1 cup firmly packed fresh mint leaves

3 green tea bags

⅓ cup agave nectar

⅓ cup fresh lime juice

6 lime slices, for garnish

Bring the water to boil in a 3-quart saucepan. Add the mint and tea bags, remove from the heat, and let steep for 5 minutes. Strain. Stir in the agave and lime juice. Serve hot or iced, garnished with the lime slices.

❄ **MINT FACTOID:** The mint family includes basil, marjoram, oregano, thyme, and rosemary, among others. All are excellent sources of antioxidants. Their leaves have glands containing essential oils, which provide their distinctive flavors.

NUTRIENT ANALYSIS PER SERVING

43 calories, 0 g protein, 12 g carbohydrates, 0 g total fat, 0 g saturated fat, 0 g monounsaturated fat, 30 mg omega-3s, 2 g fiber, 1 g sugar, 13 mg sodium

Sparkling Melon Agua Fresca

MAKES 6 SERVINGS OR 1½ QUARTS

Agua fresca translates from Spanish to "fresh water." Try this with different melons or juices to find your own flavor favorites. If you don't like carbonated water, you can omit it and enjoy the undiluted version.

4 cups chopped cantaloupe (about 3½ pounds)

¼ cup fresh lime juice

Ice cubes

8 ounces sparkling water

4 tablespoons Pomegranate Syrup (page 282)

Fresh lime wedges, for garnish

Place the cantaloupe and lime juice in the jar of a blender or bowl of a food processor. Blend or puree until smooth. There will be about 2½ cups of puree. Divide among four 8-ounce glasses.

Add a few cubes of ice to each glass. Add 2 ounces of the sparkling water to each glass, and carefully spoon 1 tablespoon of the Pomegranate Syrup onto top of each glass. Garnish with the fresh lime wedges.

Note: Melon puree can be stored and refrigerated for 1 day.

❉ **MELON FACTOID:** Cantaloupe is also called muskmelon, and it provides more beta-carotene than other members of the melon family.

NUTRIENT ANALYSIS PER SERVING

66 calories, 1 g protein, 17 g carbohydrates, 0 g total fat, 0 g saturated fat, 0 g monounsaturated fat, 40 mg omega-3s, 1 g fiber, 15 g sugar, 26 mg sodium

Pinolillo (Spanish Chocolate Shake)

MAKES 1 SERVING

Pinolillo is a distinctively flavored Spanish drink that contains toasted corn and the classic ingredients of a mole—cocoa, spices, and chili flakes. This rendition has a simplified preparation but the same complex flavors.

1 tablespoon toasted stone-ground cornmeal (see note)

1 tablespoon natural cocoa powder

1 tablespoon agave nectar

Pinch of ground cinnamon

Pinch of ground cloves

Pinch of chili flakes (optional)

2 drops pure vanilla extract

1 cup very cold light soy, almond, or fat-free milk

5 ice cubes

Combine all of the ingredients in the jar of a blender. Blend until smooth. Serve immediately.

Note: Toast cornmeal in a small dry skillet over low heat, stirring constantly until golden and fragrant.

❋ **CORNMEAL FACTOID:** Stone-ground cornmeal contains the nutritious and flavorful germ. Yellow cornmeal has more carotene and antioxidants than its white counterpart.

NUTRIENT ANALYSIS PER SERVING
150 calories, 9 g protein, 25 g carbohydrates, 2 g total fat, 0 g saturated fat, 1 g monounsaturated fat, 20 mg omega-3s, 2 g fiber, 16 g sugar, 205 mg sodium

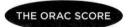

HERBS AND SPICES: FLAVOR YOUR WAY TO A YOUNGER YOU

Spices and herbs are powerful allies in the *Positively Ageless* pantry. Not only do they provide complex layers of flavor to replace what salt and fat deliver, but many of them are loaded with antioxidants and beneficial phytochemicals. Cinnamon contains a compound called MHCP (methylhydroxy chalcone polymer) that makes insulin more

SPICES	ORAC PER 1/2 TSP
Cloves, ground	3,144
Cinnamon, ground	2,675
Turmeric	1,593
Oregano leaf, dried	1,334
Curry powder	485
Black pepper, whole peppercorns	451
Mustard seed, ground	440
Chili powder	354
Basil leaf, dried	338
Ginger, ground	288
Black pepper, ground	251
Paprika	179
Parsley, dried	124
Garlic powder	101
Onion powder	57
Poppy seed	8

sensitive. Turmeric contains a potent antioxidant with anticarcinogenic properties, and oregano has loads of antioxidants and antibiotic benefits. Here are a few well-endowed seasonings whose antioxidant capacities have been measured.

HERBS	ORAC PER ½ TSP
Tarragon	933
Oregano	838
Thyme	658
Marjoram	655
Sage	641
Basil	127
Peppermint	87
Parsley	49
Dill	25
Rosemary	6
Chives	3

Spicy Chai

MAKES 6 SERVINGS

Chai is traditionally prepared by steeping tea and spices in hot water and adding milk and sweetener. Though black tea is more often used, you can use green tea as well.

5 cups water

1 cup low-fat milk or soy milk

1 teaspoon natural cocoa powder

1 teaspoon ground ginger

$\frac{1}{2}$ teaspoon ground cardamom

$\frac{1}{4}$ teaspoon ground cinnamon

$\frac{1}{8}$ teaspoon ground cloves

4 black tea bags

2 tablespoons chopped mint

2 tablespoons agave nectar (optional)

Combine the water, milk, cocoa, ginger, cardamom, cinnamon, and cloves in a 2-quart saucepan over medium heat. Bring to a boil, then reduce the heat. Add the tea bags and mint and simmer for 4 minutes. Remove from the heat and strain. Sweeten with the agave, if desired. Chai may be enjoyed hot or chilled. Store for 2 to 3 days in the refrigerator.

✳ **TEA FACTOID:** Doubling tea's infusion time from 3 to 6 minutes may double the caffeine content, but, depending on the tea, it may become too astringent if steeped any longer. Tea bags contain broken leaves of smaller size and greater surface area. They will produce an infusion with more caffeine than loose tea does.

NUTRIENT ANALYSIS PER SERVING

20 calories, 1 g protein, 2 g carbohydrates, < 1 g total fat, 0 g saturated fat, 0 g monounsaturated fat, 10 mg omega-3s, 0 g fiber, 2 g sugar, 22 mg sodium

Hot Chocolate

MAKES 6 SERVINGS (6 OUNCES EACH)

Delicious hot or cold, this takes just minutes to make. Store leftovers in the fridge for up to 2 days. Leftover Hot Chocolate is a great base for a postworkout smoothie. Just add a frozen banana and a dollop of vanilla yogurt for a thick and frosty treat.

⅓ cup unsweetened natural cocoa powder

4 cups fat-free milk or soy milk

½ cup water

¼ cup agave nectar

1 teaspoon pure vanilla extract

Place the cocoa in a 2-quart saucepan. Add about ½ cup of the milk to make a smooth paste. Stir well to remove all lumps. Gradually whisk in the water, agave, and the remaining milk. Place over medium-high heat and bring just to a simmer; do not boil. Stir in the vanilla extract.

✳ **COCOA FACTOID:** Unsweetened cocoa powder's high starch content makes it difficult to dissolve in liquid. To prevent lumps from forming, use cold liquid, which can help separate the starch particles.

✳ **OMEGA-3 FACTOID:** Preliminary British studies show that organic milk contains more omega-3s, likely due to the diet of the organic cows. Though the nutrition database for analyzing this recipe does not reveal the omega-3 milligrams for milk, choosing organic is optimal.

NUTRIENT ANALYSIS PER SERVING

101 calories, 6 g protein, 19 g carbohydrates, 1 g total fat, 0 g saturated fat, 0 g monounsaturated fat, 0 mg omega-3s, 0 g fiber, 16 g sugar, 77 mg sodium

Grapefruit Lassi

MAKES 2 SERVINGS

Lassi (or lhassi) is an Indian yogurt drink. A savory lassi may be flavored with spices such as cumin, and may even contain salt. This sweet lassi is made with antioxidant-rich pink grapefruit juice. Creamy Greek-style yogurt is high in protein, making this frosty treat a perfect on-the-go breakfast or a welcome refresher after a great workout.

8 ounces 100% pink grapefruit juice

1 cup nonfat Greek-style yogurt

1 tablespoon chopped fresh mint (optional)

$\frac{1}{2}$ teaspoon pure vanilla extract

8 ice cubes

1 tablespoon agave nectar, honey, or sweetener

Fresh mint sprig for garnish, if desired

Combine all ingredients in blender jar. Blend until smooth. Add sweetener, if desired.

Garnish with fresh mint sprig.

✱ **GRAPEFRUIT JUICE FACTOID:** A recent study at the University of Florida revealed that pink grapefruit juice had more nutrients per calorie than the commonly consumed 100 percent fruit juices This means that comparatively, grapefruit juice was lower in calories and higher in essential nutrients, such as vitamin C, potassium, and folate. Orange juice ranked second, and white grapefruit juice ranked third.

NUTRIENT ANALYSIS FOR ONE SERVING
130 calories, 11 g protein, 20 g carbohydrates, 0 g total fat, 0 g saturated fat, 0 g monounsaturated fat, 10 mg omega-3s, 0 g fiber, 8 g sugar, 45 mg sodium

Condiments

Curried Tomato Dipping Sauce

Tangy Mustard Dressing

Pomegranate Syrup

Tomato Ginger Vinaigrette

Tahini Yogurt Sauce

Barbecue Sauce

Mango Butter

Miso Marinade

Easy Blueberry Jam

Watercress Sauce

Curried Tomato Dipping Sauce

MAKES 12 SERVINGS ($\frac{1}{4}$ CUP EACH) OR 3 CUPS

This flavorful sauce is a delicious dipper for grilled shrimp or a great condiment for your favorite sandwich. If you can't find the fire-roasted tomatoes, canned tomatoes or fresh tomatoes work well.

1 tablespoon olive oil

$\frac{1}{4}$ cup finely chopped onion

1 teaspoon ground cumin

1 teaspoon ground coriander

1 teaspoon curry powder

$\frac{1}{2}$ teaspoon ground ginger

$\frac{1}{8}$ teaspoon ground cloves

$\frac{1}{8}$ teaspoon ground mace

2 tablespoons agave nectar or sorghum syrup

$1\frac{3}{4}$ cups (14.5-ounce can) fire-roasted tomatoes (Muir Glen brand)

6 ounces tomato paste

$1\frac{1}{2}$ cups water

Salt

Heat the oil in a 3-quart saucepan over medium heat. Add the onion and sauté for about 5 minutes, until lightly browned. Add the cumin, coriander, curry powder, ginger, cloves, and mace and cook for 1 minute longer, until fragrant.

Carefully add the syrup or agave, tomatoes, tomato paste, and water and bring to a boil. Reduce the heat and simmer for 3 minutes. Remove from the heat and cool slightly. Carefully transfer the sauce to the jar of a blender or bowl of a food processor. Blend or process until smooth. Add salt to taste.

✳ **TOMATO FACTOID:** Store tomatoes at room temperature until ripe so they develop their full flavors. Refrigeration can cause them to lose more than 30 percent of their flavor, and direct sunlight can cause them to ripen unevenly.

NUTRIENT ANALYSIS PER $\frac{1}{4}$ CUP

42 calories, 1 g protein, 7 g carbohydrates, 1 g total fat, 0 g saturated fat, < 1 g monounsaturated fat, 10 mg omega-3s, 1 g fiber, 3 g sugar, 92 mg sodium

Tangy Mustard Dressing

MAKES 1¼ CUPS

This addictive dressing goes together in a flash. The best surprise is that there is no added oil. It's great on salad or as a condiment for grilled salmon or chicken.

¾ cup silken tofu

¼ cup white miso

¼ cup unseasoned rice wine vinegar

¼ cup Dijon mustard

¼ cup fresh lemon juice

1 tablespoon brown rice syrup

2 cloves garlic

½ teaspoon Worcestershire sauce (with no added salt or sugar; available at health food stores)

¼ teaspoon ground black pepper

Combine all of the ingredients in the jar of a blender or bowl of a food processor. Blend or process until smooth.

✳ **MUSTARD FACTOID:** Mustard seeds and mustard greens contain potent antioxidants that fight free-radical damage. They also contain sulfur compounds with antibacterial, antiviral, anticancer, and antifungal properties.

NUTRIENT ANALYSIS PER 2 TABLESPOONS

39 calories, 2 g protein, 6 g carbohydrates, 1 g total fat, 0 g saturated fat, 0 mg monounsaturated fat, 0 mg omega-3s, 1 g fiber, 3 g sugar, 373 mg sodium

Pomegranate Syrup

MAKES 2½ CUPS

Although you can buy premade pomegranate syrup, it's usually sweetened with sugar. This antioxidant-rich version is easy to make and keeps about 2 months, refrigerated. Add a splash to tea, yogurt, or a smoothie for an antioxidant boost.

4 cups refrigerated pomegranate juice
1 cup agave nectar

In a medium saucepan, combine the juice and agave. Bring to a boil. Reduce the heat to medium and simmer 20 minutes, or until reduced by almost half. Syrup will thicken as it cools. Cool completely, pour into a jar, seal tightly, and refrigerate.

✱ **POMEGRANATE FACTOID:** Although the levels of polyphenol antioxidants are not affected, most (although not all) of the vitamin C in pomegranate juice is, unfortunately, eliminated during the pasteurization process.

NUTRIENT ANALYSIS PER TABLESPOON

27 calories, 0 g protein, 7 g carbohydrates, 0 g total fat, 0 g saturated fat, 0 g monounsaturated fat, 0 mg omega-3s, 0 g fiber, 7 g sugar, 7 mg sodium

Tomato Ginger Vinaigrette

MAKES 16 SERVINGS (1 TABLESPOON EACH) OR ¾ CUP

Packed with omega-3s, this zippy dressing will wake up your salad or add a kick to your sandwich or grilled chicken. Be sure to store it in the refrigerator so the oil stays fresh.

2 tablespoons balsamic vinegar

2 tablespoons rice wine vinegar

2 tablespoons finely chopped sun-dried tomatoes

2 tablespoons water

1 tablespoon Dijon mustard

2 teaspoons finely chopped fresh ginger

½ cup flaxseed oil

Salt and ground black pepper

1 tablespoon chopped fresh cilantro

In the jar of a blender or bowl of a food processor, combine the vinegars, tomatoes, water, mustard, and ginger. Blend or process until very smooth. It may take a few minutes. Continue blending and slowly add the oil in a steady, continuous stream. Season to taste with the salt and pepper and stir in the cilantro.

✴ **FLAXSEED FACTOID:** Flaxseed is a preeminent plant source of the essential omega-3 ALA, aka alpha-linolenic acid. ALA does convert to the EPA/DHA forms of omega-3s in the body, but the process is long and inefficient, so the resulting amount of EPA/DHA is much less than the amount of ALA consumed.

NUTRIENT ANALYSIS PER TABLESPOON

64 calories, < 1 g protein, 1 g carbohydrates, 7 g total fat, 1 g saturated fat, 0 g monounsaturated fat, 3,620 mg omega-3s, < 1 g fiber, 0 g sugar, 33 mg sodium

Tahini Yogurt Sauce

MAKES 1 CUP

This is a fabulous condiment for grilled chicken or fish or on sandwiches, and it's delicious with Lebanese Kebabs *(page 322).*

³⁄₄ cup fat-free plain yogurt (preferably Greek-style)

¹⁄₄ cup tahini (sesame paste)

¹⁄₄ cup Dijon mustard

2 tablespoons water

2 tablespoons chopped fresh cilantro

1 teaspoon lemon juice

¹⁄₂ teaspoon ground cumin

Combine all of the ingredients in the bowl of a food processor or jar of a blender. Process or blend until smooth. Sauce should be the consistency of thick cream.

✳ **SESAME FACTOID:** A prized ingredient in Middle Eastern and Asian cuisines, sesame seeds are rich in vitamins B and E, calcium, iron, and zinc.

NUTRIENT ANALYSIS PER TABLESPOON
27 calories, 1 g protein, 2 g carbohydrates, 2 g total fat, 0 g saturated fat, 1 g monounsaturated fat, 20 mg omega-3s, < 1 g fiber, 1 g sugar, 57 mg sodium

Barbecue Sauce

MAKES 16 SERVINGS (2 TABLESPOONS EACH) OR 1 QUART

Slather it on chicken or turkey breast or use it as a condiment—this flavorful sauce is a snap to make and keeps well in the fridge. If you can't find fire-roasted tomatoes, canned or fresh tomatoes work well. They just won't have the smoky tang.

2 tablespoons olive oil

1 cup finely chopped onion

1 tablespoon minced garlic

3 cups (28 ounces) finely chopped fire-roasted tomatoes

½ cup fresh lime juice

½ cup balsamic vinegar

½ cup agave nectar

2 tablespoons chili powder

Heat the oil in a 2-quart saucepan over medium heat. Add the onion and cook, stirring occasionally, for 3 minutes, or until soft and translucent. Stir in the garlic and cook, stirring occasionally, until softened; do not brown. Add the tomatoes, lime juice, vinegar, agave, and chili powder and simmer for 20 minutes. Cool.

Transfer to the jar of a blender or bowl of a food processor and blend or process until smooth. Transfer to a glass jar and refrigerate.

✳ **CHILI FACTOID:** Compounds found in chili powder have antioxidant effects and may be helpful for diabetics in controlling blood sugar.

NUTRIENT ANALYSIS PER SERVING

69 calories, 1 g protein, 14 g carbohydrates, 2 g total fat, 0 g saturated fat, 1 g monounsaturated fat, 10 mg omega-3s, 1 g fiber, 10 g sugar, 49 mg sodium

Mango Butter

MAKES 16 SERVINGS (1 TABLESPOON EACH) OR 1 CUP

There is no butter or added fat in this recipe. The name comes from its smooth, buttery texture. This creamy spread is great on toast or stirred into yogurt or hot cereal.

3 mangoes
½ cup water
2 tablespoons lime or lemon juice
¼ cup agave nectar
½ teaspoon ground ginger (optional)
½ teaspoon ground cinnamon (optional)

Clean, cut, and finely chop the mangoes. Place in the bowl of a food processor and pulse until the mixture is just smooth. There will be about 1½ cups of mango puree.

Place the puree in a 2- to 3-quart saucepan. Add the water, juice, and nectar. Simmer, stirring occasionally for the first 10 minutes. Stir more and more frequently after that, as the juices reduce, or the mango will stick and burn. After about 30 minutes total, the juices will have reduced and the puree will thicken to the consistency of applesauce. Remove from the heat. Cool. Stir in the ginger and cinnamon, if desired. Transfer to a jar and refrigerate. Mango butter will keep for about 2 weeks.

✱ **MANGO FACTOID:** Though mango pulp is sweet and delicious, beware of its outer skin. The sap sometimes found on a mango tree contains an oil called urushiol, the same toxin found in poison ivy. Contact may result in a skin rash that can be painful and prolonged. Be sure to wash your hands immediately after handling the fruit.

NUTRIENT ANALYSIS PER SERVING

37 calories, < 1 g protein, 10 g carbohydrates, 0 g total fat, 0 g saturated fat, 0 g monounsaturated fat, 10 mg omega-3s, 1 g fiber, 9 g sugar, 4 mg sodium

Miso Marinade

MAKES 1 CUP

This tasty marinade works well with chicken, fish, vegetables, or tofu. A tablespoon is all that's needed to flavor one chicken breast or piece of fish.

½ cup white or yellow miso
½ cup mirin (see factoid) or sake
2 tablespoons water
1 tablespoon soy sauce
2 teaspoons minced garlic
1 teaspoon finely chopped fresh ginger

Combine all of the ingredients in a blender or food processor. Blend or process until smooth. Transfer to a glass jar and store in the refrigerator.

To use the marinade: Place chicken or fish in a shallow baking dish. Pour the marinade over and turn the fish or chicken to coat both sides. Marinate for 2 to 4 hours. Bake or grill.

✻ **MISO FACTOID:** This thick paste is made from combining sea salt; a Japanese mold called *koji;* soybeans; and, sometimes, a grain such as rice or barley.

✻ **MIRIN FACTOID:** Mirin is a Japanese cooking wine. Light gold in color, it is sweet in flavor and made from rice.

NUTRIENT ANALYSIS PER TABLESPOON

35 calories, 1 g protein, 5 g carbohydrates, 1 g total fat, 0 g saturated fat, 0 g monounsaturated fat, 40 mg omega-3s, 0 g fiber, 3 g sugar, 354 mg sodium

Easy Blueberry Jam

MAKES 12 SERVINGS (2 TABLESPOONS EACH) OR 1½ CUPS

Now that you know the incredible benefits that blueberries provide, here's another way to cook them. This is as great on whole grain toast as it is stirred into plain yogurt.

3 cups fresh blueberries or 12 ounces frozen blueberries, unsweetened

⅓ cup agave nectar or sorghum syrup

2 tablespoons fresh lemon juice

¼ teaspoon pure vanilla extract

1 tablespoon grated lemon peel

¼ teaspoon ground cinnamon

Place the blueberries in the bowl of a food processor and pulse until roughly chopped but not pureed. Transfer to a 2-quart saucepan. Add the sweetener and lemon juice. Bring to a boil over medium-high heat. When the mixture boils, reduce the heat to low. Simmer for about 3 minutes (slightly longer if using frozen berries), stirring occasionally, or until the juices have reduced slightly and mixture has thickened. Remove from the heat and cool. Stir in the vanilla extract, lemon peel, and cinnamon. Keeps refrigerated for about 2 weeks.

✳ **BLUEBERRY FACTOID:** The rich, vibrant color of this berry is a beacon to the powerhouse that lies within. The plethora of antioxidants helps reduce the risk of diseases such as cancer, heart disease, and Alzheimer's.

NUTRIENT ANALYSIS PER SERVING
34 calories, < 1 g protein, 9 g carbohydrates, 0 g total fat, 0 g saturated fat, 0 g monounsaturated fat, 0 mg omega-3s, < 1 g fiber, 5 g sugar, 5 mg sodium

Watercress Sauce

This sauce is an adaptation of the original served at Cindy Pawlcyn's famous Napa Valley restaurant, Mustards Grill. The real thing has a little mayo and sour cream—I substituted yogurt. The rest of the antiaging ingredients are the same. It's delicious on salmon, turkey, or chicken and great as a dip or sandwich spread.

³⁄₄ cup low-fat or fat-free plain yogurt (preferably Greek-style)

2 tablespoons chopped shallot

2 teaspoons minced garlic

½ bunch watercress, coarse stems removed

1½ teaspoons Dijon mustard

1 teaspoon fresh lemon juice

Pinch of salt

Pinch of ground black pepper

Combine all of the ingredients in the jar of a blender or bowl of a food processor. Blend or process by pulsing until ingredients are well combined but not completely pureed. There should still be flecks of green from the watercress, rather than one homogeneous color.

✳ **WATERCRESS FACTOID:** Watercress is an excellent source of ALA, the essential omega-3 fatty acid that the body does not produce.

NUTRIENT ANALYSIS PER SERVING

33 calories, 3 g protein, 4 g carbohydrates, 1 g total fat, 0 g saturated fat, 0 g monounsaturated fat, 40 mg omega-3s, < 1 g fiber, 3 g sugar, 53 mg sodium

Snacks

Candied Pecans

Indian Olives with Citrus and Panch Puran

Asparagus Spears with Smoked Salmon and
Tangy Mustard Dressing

Zippy Hummus

Whole Wheat Pita Chips

Candied Pecans

MAKES 8 SERVINGS (2 TABLESPOONS EACH) OR 1 CUP

These crunchy nuggets are great sprinkled on a salad or stirred into your favorite whole grain dish. Try using walnuts or almonds or your own favorite seasoning combinations.

2 tablespoons sorghum syrup, agave nectar, or brown rice syrup

$\frac{1}{2}$ teaspoon Italian seasoning (dried chopped basil, thyme, oregano, and rosemary)

$\frac{1}{4}$ teaspoon salt

1 cup roughly chopped pecans (about 4$\frac{1}{4}$ ounces)

Preheat the oven to 325°F. Use a nonstick baking sheet or coat a baking sheet with cooking oil spray.

In a small bowl, combine the sweetener, seasonings, and salt and stir to combine. Add the pecans and toss to coat. Spread on the prepared baking sheet in a single layer (some nuts may clump together). Bake for 12 minutes, or until the pecans are golden and sugary mixture is bubbling. Stir once during baking time to break up clumps. Watch carefully so they don't burn. Cool completely on the baking sheet. Store in airtight container for up to 3 days.

Note: It's not a good idea to make these in humid weather. The added moisture in the air doesn't allow them to stay crispy for long.

✷**PECAN FACTOID:** Pecans contain healthy fats plus beta-sitosterol, a plant sterol that competes with the absorption of cholesterol in the body and may help lower blood cholesterol.

NUTRIENT ANALYSIS PER SERVING

116 calories , 1 g protein, 5 g carbohydrates, 11 g total fat, 1 g saturated fat, 6 g monounsaturated fat, 15 mg omega-3s, 1 g fiber, 1 g sugar, 79 mg sodium

Indian Olives with Citrus and Panch Puran

MAKES 16 SERVINGS (1 OUNCE EACH, OR ABOUT 3 OLIVES)

Panch puran is an East Indian spice blend of fennel, cumin, black cumin, fenugreek, and mustard seeds. This spice variation combines with citrus to infuse extraordinary flavor into ordinary olives. These delicious nibbles take minutes to make and are a perfect snack to keep on hand for surprise guests.

1 pound brine-packed olives

1/4 cup olive oil

2 teaspoons whole fennel seeds

1/2 teaspoon white sesame seed

1/2 teaspoon whole yellow mustard seed

1/4 teaspoon whole coriander seeds

1/4 teaspoons cumin seeds

Zest of 1 lemon

Zest of 1 lime

Rinse the olives under cool water, drain, and transfer to mixing bowl.

Heat the oil in a small pan until nearly hot but not smoking. Remove from the heat. Carefully add spices. Cool.

Pour the cooled seasoned oil over olives. Add the lemon and lime zest and toss well to coat. Allow to marinate for an hour at room temperature. Transfer to a quart-size jar and refrigerate.

Note: When the olives are gone, the flavorful oil is delicious for sautéing chicken, fish, or vegetables or for making vinaigrette.

✳**OLIVE FACTOID:** The flavor of olives (and olive oils) varies widely; some are mild, others are nutty in flavor. Colors range from yellow to green, depending on the time of harvest. Olives can be stored for a year unopened. After opening, olives in brine can be refrigerated for several weeks in a clean nonmetal jar.

NUTRIENT ANALYSIS PER SERVING

51 calories, 1 g protein, 1 g carbohydrates, 5 g total fat, 0 g saturated fat, 3 g monounsaturated fat, 7 mg omega-3s, 1 g fiber, 0 g sugar, 448 mg sodium

Asparagus Spears with Smoked Salmon and Tangy Mustard Dressing

MAKES 4 SERVINGS (4 SPEARS EACH)

This is a great last-minute appetizer idea. Thicker asparagus spears are easier to handle for wrapping.

1 pound asparagus, tough ends snapped (about 16 spears)

2 teaspoons extra-virgin olive oil

Sea salt and freshly ground pepper

4 thin slices smoked salmon (about 4 ounces), each cut in 4 lengthwise strips

2 tablespoons Tangy Mustard Dressing (page 281)

Cilantro sprigs or toasted sesame seed, for garnish

Preheat the grill to medium-high heat.

Lightly coat the asparagus with the oil. Season with salt and pepper to taste.

Grill for 2 to 3 minutes, or until al dente but not soft. Remove from the grill. The asparagus will continue to cook as they cool. Do not overcook or the spears will be too soft and difficult to handle. When cool enough to handle, wrap each spear with a slice of the salmon. Arrange on a serving platter and drizzle with the dressing. Garnish with the cilantro or sesame seed and serve immediately, or chill to serve later.

This recipe also works well with grilled asparagus spears.

✳**SALMON FACTOID:** Chinook salmon is found in Pacific waters from Alaska to Southern California. A 4-ounce piece (raw) has about 200 calories and a whopping 2,300 milligrams of omega-3s.

NUTRIENT ANALYSIS PER SERVING
92 calories, 8 g protein, 7 g carbohydrates, 4 g total fat, 1 g saturated fat, 2 g monounsaturated fat, 150 mg omega-3s, 3 g fiber, 3 g sugar, 661 mg sodium

Zippy Hummus

MAKES 16 SERVINGS (2 TABLESPOONS EACH) OR 2 CUPS

This tasty spread takes minutes to prepare and will keep for several days, refrigerated. It's the perfect accompaniment for Whole Wheat Pita Chips (opposite), or serve it in a sandwich on a warm pita with sliced tomatoes and shredded lettuce. Lime juice and mint add a zippy twist, but you can substitute lemon juice and cilantro if you prefer a traditional flavor.

1½ cups cooked garbanzo beans, white beans, or mature (white) soybeans or 1 can (15 ounces), rinsed and drained

⅓ cup tahini (sesame paste)

⅓ fresh lime juice

2 tablespoons water

1 teaspoon minced garlic

1 teaspoon ground cumin

1 teaspoon salt

1 tablespoon chopped fresh mint, without stems

Place the beans, tahini, lime juice, water and garlic in the bowl of a food processor or blender. Process or blend until very smooth, about 4 minutes. Transfer to a bowl. Stir in the cumin and salt. Sprinkle with mint before serving.

✳**GARBANZO BEAN FACTOID:** Also known as chickpeas, garbanzos are an excellent source of fiber and manganese. One of the key antioxidant enzymes in the body (superoxide dismutase) requires manganese as a cofactor to neutralize free radicals.

NUTRIENT ANALYSIS PER SERVING

57 calories, 2 g protein, 6 g carbohydrates, 3 g total fat, < 1g saturated fat, 1 g monounsaturated fat, 30 mg omega-3s, 2 g fiber, 1 g sugar, 151 mg sodium

Whole Wheat Pita Chips

MAKES 16 SERVINGS (6 CHIPS EACH)

I always keep whole wheat pitas in the freezer and garbanzos in the cupboard for a quick-to-fix hors d'oeuvres. My friends eat a lot of hummus and pita chips when they drop in unannounced.

6 (6") whole wheat pitas
Olive oil cooking spray

Preheat the oven to 375°F.

With a sharp knife, cut each pita in half, then each half into 4 triangles. Separate each triangle into 2 pieces. There should be 16 chips (triangles) per pita. Arrange in a single layer on two baking sheets. Lightly coat the triangles with cooking spray.

Bake for 7 minutes. Remove from the oven and, using a metal spatula, gently turn the triangles over and continue to bake until crisp and golden brown, about 7 minutes longer. Chips will continue to crisp as they cool. Store in airtight containers or self-sealing plastic bags.

✻OLIVE OIL FACTOID: Olive oil is made by crushing and then pressing freshly picked olives. Extra-virgin oil is from the first pressing and has a more assertive flavor, richer color, and higher concentration of antioxidants.

NUTRIENT ANALYSIS PER 6-CHIP SERVING

64 calories, 2 g protein, 13 g carbohydrates, 1 g total fat, < 1g saturated fat, 1 g monounsaturated fat, 10 mg omega-3s, 2 g fiber, < 1 g sugar, 128 mg sodium

Soups and Stews

Green Tea Miso Soup

Savory Beet Stew

Red Bean Mole Soup

Italian Vegetable Soup

Spanish Meatball Soup

Green Tea Miso Soup

MAKES 4 SERVINGS

Green tea lends a subtle flavor to this Japanese classic. If you don't like mushrooms, toss in a cup of edamame instead.

4 cups fat-free, low-sodium chicken or vegetable broth

2 green tea bags

1 tablespoon olive oil

1 cup finely chopped yellow onions

1 tablespoon finely chopped, peeled fresh ginger

2 tablespoons sweet white miso (see factoid)

4 ounces firm tofu, drained and cut into 1/4" pieces

1 cup fresh spinach leaves, cut in fine ribbons

1 cup thinly sliced mushrooms

1/2 cup finely chopped fresh tomato

1 green onion (white and green parts), very thinly sliced, for garnish

Heat 1 cup of the broth to boiling. Remove from the heat. Add the tea bags and steep for 3 minutes. Remove the tea bags and discard. Set aside the tea-broth mixture.

Heat the oil in a 2-quart saucepan over medium heat. Add the onion and cook, stirring frequently, for 8 minutes, or until just starting to brown. Add the ginger and cook, stirring frequently, for 1 minute. Add the remaining 3 cups broth and bring to a boil.

Whisk in miso until dissolved. Add the tofu, spinach, mushrooms, tomato, and the reserved tea-broth mixture and simmer for 1 minute. Serve warm, garnished with the green onions.

✳MISO FACTOID: Nonpasteurized miso not only contains beneficial bacteria and their enzymes (probiotics), it also contains richer flavors and aromas that are otherwise lost in the process of pasteurization.

NUTRIENT ANALYSIS PER SERVING

108 calories, 7 g protein, 11 g carbohydrates, 5 g total fat, 1 g saturated fat, 4 g monounsaturated fat, 50 mg omega-3s, 3 g fiber, 5 g sugar, 313 mg sodium

Savory Beet Stew

MAKES 6 LARGE SERVINGS

Most of us have tried the classic cold version of beet soup, also known as borscht. This hot version is loaded with flavor. And don't toss the greens—they're just as loaded with antioxidants as the bottom half.

4 medium beets with greens attached (see note)

¼ cup + 2 tablespoons balsamic or red wine vinegar, divided

2 tablespoons olive oil

2 cups finely chopped yellow onions

1 cup finely chopped tomato

1 teaspoon chopped fresh dill (or ½ teaspoon dried)

4 cups fat-free chicken or vegetable broth

2 cups water

Salt

Trim the tops off the beets, leaving about 1" of stems attached. Clean the tops and set aside the greens. Scrub and rinse the beets well.

In a 4-quart pan, combine the beets, enough water to cover, and 2 tablespoons of the vinegar. Bring to a boil. Reduce the heat, cover, and simmer until the beets are tender when pierced, about 30 minutes. With a slotted spoon, lift the beets out of the pan and let cool. Discard the liquid. Clean the pan.

Heat the oil in the pan over medium-high heat. Add the onions and sauté for 8 to 9 minutes, or until the onions are very soft and just starting to brown. Add the remaining ¼ cup vinegar, stir well, and cook for a few minutes longer, until the juices have evaporated. Add the tomato and dill and cook for three minutes, or until the tomato is soft.

Add the broth and water and bring to a boil. Meanwhile, slip off the beet skins and cut into ½" pieces. Set aside. Chop the beet greens into ½" pieces.

Add the beets and greens to the soup. Bring to a boil, reduce the heat, and simmer for 5 minutes longer, or until the greens are soft. Add salt to taste.

Note: If your beets didn't come with greens attached, or the greens are not in good shape, you can substitute 3 cups of chopped raw spinach, Swiss chard, or another leafy green.

✳ **BEET FACTOID:** Cooking with beets provides double antiaging nutrition because the roots contain powerful anthocyanin antioxidants. The leaves contain both chlorophyll and carotenoids.

NUTRIENT ANALYSIS PER SERVING
105 calories, 2 g protein, 14 g carbohydrates, 5 g total fat, 1 g saturated fat, 2 g monounsaturated fat, 40 mg omega-3s, 3 g fiber, 10 g sugar, 278 mg sodium

Red Bean Mole Soup

MAKES 8 SERVINGS

Mole (pronounced moh-LAY) is a classic and complex Spanish blend of spices, chili, and cocoa powder. If you like things extra spicy, add a little chipotle chile.

2 small (6") stone-ground corn tortillas, torn or crumbled

1/2 cup almonds, toasted

2 tablespoons sesame seeds, toasted

2 tablespoons unsweetened natural cocoa powder

2 tablespoons minced garlic

1 teaspoon coriander seeds

1 teaspoon ground cinnamon

1/2 teaspoon red chili flakes (optional)

1/4 teaspoon ground cloves

1/4 teaspoon fennel seeds

6 cups nonfat no-salt-added chicken broth (or vegetable broth)

2 tablespoons olive oil

1 large yellow onion, finely chopped

1 cup dry red beans soaked overnight, rinsed, and drained

1/2 teaspoon salt

2 tablespoons fresh chopped cilantro, without stems, for garnish

In the bowl of a food processor, combine the tortillas, almonds, sesame seeds, cocoa, garlic, coriander, cinnamon, chili flakes (if using), cloves, fennel seeds, 1 cup of the broth, and 1 tablespoon of the oil. Process to a smooth paste. This will take several minutes.

Heat the remaining 1 tablespoon oil in a 3-quart saucepan over medium-high heat. Add the onion and cook for 5 minutes, or until lightly golden. Add the spice paste to the pan. Cook about 5 minutes, or until bubbly and fragrant, stirring constantly. If the paste is too thick, add ¼ cup water. Add the remaining 5 cups broth to the pan and bring to a boil. Add the beans. Reduce the heat to low and cover. Simmer for 1 hour, or until the beans are tender, stirring occasionally. Season with the salt. Garnish with the cilantro and serve immediately.

✳ **RED BEAN FACTOID:** Researchers found dry red beans to have more antioxidants than highly ranked blueberries. It is uncertain, however, how much of the antioxidant content is lost during cooking and how much is actually absorbed by the body.

NUTRIENT ANALYSIS PER SERVING
179 calories, 8 g protein, 21 g carbohydrates, 8 g total fat, 0 g saturated fat, 5 g monounsaturated fat, 130 mg omega-3s, 7 g fiber, 2 g sugar, 174 mg sodium

Italian Vegetable Soup

MAKES 12 LARGE SERVINGS

Loaded with fiber, this recipe makes a large batch of soup, which freezes well, too. For more protein, add shredded roast chicken or turkey or 1 cup cooked and crumbled Old-Fashioned Breakfast Sausage (page 259).

2 tablespoons olive oil

1 cup finely chopped onions

1 cup finely chopped carrots

½ cup thinly sliced celery

2 tablespoons minced garlic

1 pound tomatoes, finely chopped, or 1 can (14.5 ounces) chopped tomatoes

8 cups fat-free chicken or vegetable broth

1 tablespoon chopped fresh oregano (or 1 teaspoon dried)

1 tablespoon chopped fresh basil (or 1 teaspoon dried)

1 tablespoon chopped fresh thyme (or 1 teaspoon dried)

1 cup dry bulgur

2 cups finely shredded cabbage

1½ cups cooked white beans, such as cannellini or Great Northern

1½ cups cooked red or black beans

Salt (see note)

¼ cup chopped Italian parsley, for garnish

Heat the oil in a 3- to 4-quart soup pot over medium-high heat. Add the onion, carrots, and celery and cook for 5 minutes, or until the vegetables are soft, stirring occasionally. Add the garlic and cook for 1 minute longer. Do not brown.

Add the tomatoes, broth, oregano, basil, and thyme and bring to a boil. Add the bulgur and cabbage and reduce the heat to a simmer. Cook for 20 to 30 minutes longer, or until the bulgur is tender. Stir in the beans and simmer for 5 minutes longer. Season with salt if desired. Garnish with the parsley and serve hot.

Note: If using unsalted or homemade stock, you may wish to add a little salt to taste. The nutrient analysis includes a purchased stock containing salt.

✷ **OREGANO FACTOID:** Recent studies revealed that oregano's antioxidant activity is as much as 20 times higher than that of other herbs.

NUTRIENT ANALYSIS PER SERVING

145 calories, 7 g protein, 25 g carbohydrates, 3 g total fat, 0 g saturated fat, 2 g monounsaturated fat, 80 mg omega-3s, 8 g fiber, 3 g sugar, 347 mg sodium

Spanish Meatball Soup

MAKES 8 SERVINGS (1 CUP EACH) OR 2 QUARTS

The ingredient list looks daunting, but this flavorful soup takes only minutes to make. Add a cup or two of your favorite beans or lentils to kick up the fiber.

1 tablespoon olive oil

1 cup finely chopped onions

1 tablespoon + 1 teaspoon minced garlic

1 bay leaf

4 cups fat-free chicken broth

1 cup fresh tomato sauce

¼ cup chopped fresh cilantro

¾ pound lean ground turkey

¼ cup stone-ground yellow cornmeal

1 omega-3 egg

2 teaspoons chopped fresh oregano (or ¾ teaspoon dried)

½ teaspoon salt

½ teaspoon ground black pepper

½ teaspoon ground cumin

1 cup cooked brown or wild rice

2 cups sliced zucchini

Heat the oil in a heavy, large pot over medium-high heat. Add ¾ cup of the onions. Sauté for 5 minutes, or until very soft. Add 1 tablespoon of the garlic and the bay leaf and sauté 1 minute longer. Add the broth, tomato sauce, and cilantro and bring to a boil. Reduce the heat and simmer for 5 minutes.

Meanwhile, combine the turkey, cornmeal, egg, oregano, salt, pepper, cumin, and the remaining ¼ cup onions and 1 teaspoon garlic. Mix well. Shape by tablespoonfuls into about 32 balls. Add the meatballs to the simmering broth. Cover and simmer for 5 minutes, or until the meatballs are tender, stirring occasionally. The meatballs will float when done. Remove the bay leaf. Add the rice and zucchini. Simmer a few minutes longer until heated through. Ladle into bowls and serve.

✱ **BAY LEAF FACTOID:** It doesn't have the same antioxidant bang as oregano, but bay leaf possesses antioxidants, too, and has shown antibacterial properties in a variety of studies.

NUTRIENT ANALYSIS PER SERVING

150 calories, 11 g protein, 14 g carbohydrates, 3 g total fat, 1 g saturated fat, 2 g monounsaturated fat, 80 mg omega-3s, 2 g fiber, 1 g sugar, 201 mg sodium

Grains

Barley Risotto with Wilted Greens

Whole Grain Bread (or Buns)

Cumin-Spiced Bulgur and Lentils

Wild Rice with Radicchio and Dried Cherries

Barley Risotto with Wilted Greens

MAKES 6 SERVINGS

I used to make barley risotto when I worked at Postrio, a Wolfgang Puck restaurant in San Francisco. This is a lighter version, though you can turn it into a main course by stirring in roasted chicken or turkey at the end. Do not use pearl barley, which is more refined and cooks very quickly.

1 tablespoon olive oil

1 cup finely chopped yellow onion

1/2 cup finely chopped carrot

1/4 cup finely chopped celery

1 tablespoon chopped garlic

1/4 cup white wine

1 cup hulled barley

3 1/2 cups fat-free chicken or vegetable broth

2 teaspoons chopped fresh thyme (or 1 teaspoon dried)

4 cups baby spinach leaves or torn leafy greens, such as Swiss chard

2 tablespoons freshly grated Romano cheese (optional)

Salt and ground black pepper

Heat the oil in a shallow 3-quart saucepan over medium-high heat. Add the onion, carrot, celery, and garlic. Cook, stirring occasionally, for 5 minutes, or until the vegetables are soft. Pour in the wine and cook, stirring constantly, until the liquid is completely absorbed. Add the barley and stir well.

Carefully pour in 2 cups of the broth and bring to a boil. Reduce the heat to medium-low and simmer until the liquid is absorbed, stirring frequently. This will take about 10 minutes. Add the thyme and the remaining 1 1/2 cups broth. Turn up heat until the broth comes to a boil, then reduce the heat to low. Simmer for 10 minutes, stirring occasionally, until the barley is tender but still al dente. Stir in the greens.

Remove from the heat and let sit for a minute or two until the greens wilt. For a brothier risotto, add extra broth or hot water. Add the cheese, if desired. Season with salt and pepper to taste. Serve immediately.

✻ **BARLEY FACTOID:** Hulled barley, also known as barley groats, is the least processed form of the grain. Only the outermost hull is removed, unlike pearl barley, which is stripped of both the hull and the nutritious bran layer. Hulled barley takes slightly longer to cook but has more texture, fiber, and antioxidants.

NUTRIENT ANALYSIS PER SERVING

179 calories, 32 g protein, 6 g carbohydrates, 3 g total fat, 0 g saturated fat, 2 g monounsaturated fat, 70 mg omega-3s, 7 g fiber, 4 g sugar, 356 mg sodium

Whole Grain Bread (or Buns)

MAKES 1 LOAF (16 SLICES) OR 8 SANDWICH BUNS

It's getting easier to find delicious high-fiber whole grain baked goods, but nothing beats the taste (or smell) of freshly baked bread. If you can't find flax-seed meal, you can purchase whole flaxseed and grind it in a clean coffee grinder.

1½ cups warm water

¼ cup olive oil

2 tablespoons agave nectar, sorghum syrup, or dark honey

2 packages active dry yeast

3½ cups whole wheat flour

¼ cup sorghum flour or whole wheat flour

¼ cup ground flaxseed

¼ cup oat bran

¼ cup untoasted wheat germ

1 teaspoon salt

2 teaspoons stone-ground cornmeal

In a large bowl, combine the water, oil, sweetener, and yeast. Allow to rest for 5 minutes to activate yeast.

Add 3 cups of the whole wheat flour, the sorghum or whole wheat flour, flax-seed, bran, wheat germ, and salt. Turn out on a lightly floured board and knead for 5 minutes. Place in a lightly oiled bowl, cover, and let rise 1 hour.

Uncover the bowl and punch the dough down. Preheat the oven to 350°F.

Turn the dough out onto a lightly floured surface and knead gently. Shape into a loaf and place in a lightly oiled 8" × 4" bread pan.

Cover and let rise until doubled, about 30 minutes.

Bake the bread for about 35 minutes or until loaf is golden and sounds hollow when thumped on the bottom.

Alternatively, the dough can be shaped into buns for sandwiches. With a sharp knife, divide the dough into 8 pieces. Lightly oil a 15" × 10" baking sheet and sprinkle with the cornmeal.

Preheat the oven to 400°F.

Roll pieces of dough into balls and flatten into disks approximately 3½" across. Place on the prepared baking sheet. Cover and let rise for 20 minutes, or until almost doubled. Bake for 12 to 15 minutes, or until golden brown. Remove from the oven and cool on racks. When ready to use, split the buns in half horizontally.

✳ **SORGHUM FLOUR FACTOID:** There are several types of sorghum plants, including sorghum cane, which is used for making syrup. The grain is used to make an antioxidant-rich, gluten-free flour.

NUTRIENT ANALYSIS PER SLICE

144 calories, 5 g protein, 23 g carbohydrates, 5 g total fat, 1 g saturated fat, 3 g monounsaturated fat, 40 mg omega-3s, 4 g fiber, 2 g sugar, 152 mg sodium

Cumin-Spiced Bulgur and Lentils

MAKES 10 SERVINGS

Grains and legumes team up to make a side dish that's loaded with protein and fiber. Toss in shredded chicken and you have a meal.

3 cups fat-free vegetable broth (or chicken broth), divided

1 cup coarse bulgur

1 tablespoon olive oil

½ cup finely chopped yellow onion

1 tablespoon minced garlic

1 teaspoon chopped fresh thyme (or ½ teaspoon dried)

¾ teaspoon ground cumin

½ teaspoon ground mustard seed

½ teaspoon salt

1 cup brown lentils, rinsed

GARNISH

¼ cup chopped sun-dried tomatoes

¼ cup chopped green onion

¼ cup chopped fresh cilantro or parsley leaves

2 tablespoons chopped green olives

Heat 1 cup of the broth. Place the bulgur in a small mixing bowl. Pour the warm broth over the bulgur, cover, and allow to soak for 30 minutes.

Heat the oil in a saucepan over medium heat. Add the onion and sauté for 5 minutes, or until tender. Add the garlic, thyme, cumin, mustard, and salt and cook, stirring frequently, for 1 minute longer, but do not brown the garlic. Add the remaining 2 cups broth and bring to a boil. Add the lentils, reduce the heat to low, and simmer for 15 minutes. Add the bulgur and simmer for 10 minutes longer. Remove from the heat. Cover and let stand for 10 minutes.

Garnish by stirring in the tomatoes, onion, cilantro, and olives. Serve hot or warm.

✳ **BULGUR FACTOID:** This form of whole wheat has been cleaned, ground, and sifted into different sizes from fine to coarse. Unlike cracked wheat, bulgur has been pre-cooked.

NUTRIENT ANALYSIS PER SERVING

134 calories, 7 g protein, 25 g carbohydrates, 1 g total fat, 0 g saturated fat, 0 g monounsaturated fat, 30 mg omega-3s, 7 g fiber, 2 g sugar, 386 mg sodium

Wild Rice with Radicchio and Dried Cherries

MAKES 10 SERVINGS

My friend Robin loves to use fruit in savory dishes to create distinctive flavors and rich textures. This is her recipe for a great side dish that doubles as a salad or grain dish.

½ cup dried cherries or dried cranberries

½ cup dry red wine

1 head radicchio (12 ounces), cored and finely chopped

3 green onions, chopped, with some green tops

2 cups cooked wild rice

¾ cup chopped parsley

3 tablespoons balsamic vinegar

1 tablespoon Dijon mustard

¼ cup olive oil

½ teaspoon salt

¼ teaspoon ground black pepper

2 tablespoons slivered almonds, lightly toasted

Parmesan cheese (optional)

In a small bowl, cover the cherries or cranberries with the wine and let soak for about 2 hours or overnight. Drain, discarding the wine or reserving for another use.

In a large bowl, toss the radicchio, onions, rice, parsley and drained cherries.

In a small bowl, whisk together the vinegar, mustard, oil, salt, and black pepper. Pour over the radicchio mixture and toss gently. Serve at room temperature, sprinkled with the almonds. Add shavings of Parmesan, if desired.

✳ **RED WINE FACTOID:** Though a 4-ounce glass of Cabernet Sauvignon or Chardonnay has roughly the same number of calories (about 90), the Cabernet has nearly six times the antioxidant bang. That's because most antioxidants are found in the pigment component of whole foods. Unlike white wines, red wines are left in contact with their deeply pigmented skins during the fermentation process.

NUTRIENT ANALYSIS PER SERVING

147 calories, 3 g protein, 17 g carbohydrates, 7 g total fat, 1 g saturated fat, 2 g monounsaturated fat, 630 mg omega-3s, 3 g fiber, 5 g sugar, 152 mg sodium

Salads

Arthur's Tomato Salad

Baby Spinach Salad

Rainbow Radicchio Slaw

Sliced Avocados and Oranges
with Tahini Yogurt Sauce

Broccoli Salad with Caramelized Onions
and Toasted Almonds

Arthur's Tomato Salad

MAKES 4 SERVINGS

My dear friend Arthur enjoyed this dish growing up in Hawaii. His father always made it for him, and one day, Arthur shared their prized recipe with me.

1 pound fresh tomatoes

1 tablespoon finely chopped fresh ginger

1 tablespoon low-sodium soy sauce

1 tablespoon rice wine vinegar, seasoned

1 tablespoon chopped fresh cilantro, for garnish

Slice the tomatoes about ¼" thick and layer them in a spiral fashion on a dinner-size plate. Sprinkle with the ginger and drizzle evenly with the soy sauce and vinegar. Garnish evenly with the cilantro. Try to prepare about ½ hour before serving to allow the flavors to marry at room temperature. The tomatoes are delicious the next day as well.

✱ **TOMATO FACTOID:** Raw or cooked—which is better? Fat-soluble nutrients such as lycopene become more concentrated when tomatoes are cooked. Vitamin C, on the other hand, is more abundant in raw tomatoes. Enjoy this antiaging "fruit" both ways for optimal benefits.

NUTRIENT ANALYSIS PER SERVING
22 calories, 1 g protein, 5 g carbohydrates, 0 g total fat, 0 g saturated fat, 0 g monounsaturated fat, 0 mg omega-3s, 1 g fiber, 3 g sugar, 139 mg sodium

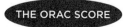

POSITIVELY AGELESS VEGETABLES

As far as veggies go, they're *all* antiagers. But which is better—raw or cooked? Some vitamins, such as B and C, are water-soluble, meaning they're lost through cooking. Other fat-soluble vitamins, such as the carotenoids, become more concentrated when cooked.

- Beta-carotene is one of many forms of carotenoids in foods that convert to the fat-soluble vitamin A in the body. It is usually found in red and orange vegetables (and fruits) and in some dark green ones, such as beet greens, where the other colors are masked by chlorophyll in the plant.

- Lycopene, another carotenoid found in tomatoes and watermelon, is one of the most powerful antioxidants and appears to protect against many diseases, including cancers. Because the carotenoid is fat-soluble, lycopene becomes more concentrated when tomatoes are cooked.

- Lutein, another type of carotenoid, may decrease risk of developing macular degeneration. Foods rich in lutein include avocados, broccoli, Brussels sprouts, kale, and spinach.

- Vitamin C plays an important role in fighting infections, keeping the walls of blood vessels firm, and promoting healthy gums. Unlike the carotenoids, vitamin C is water-soluble and not retained in the body, so try to replenish it throughout the day.

VEGETABLE	SERVING SIZE	ORAC
Artichoke hearts	½ cup	3,952
Broccoli rabe, raw	½ bunch	2,621
Red cabbage, cooked	½ cup	2,359
Asparagus, raw	½ cup	2,021
Yellow bell peppers, raw	1 medium	1,905
Beets, raw	½ cup	1,896
Orange bell peppers, raw	1 medium	1,830
Asparagus, cooked	½ cup	1,480
Radicchio, shredded	1 cup	1,415

VEGETABLE	SERVING SIZE	ORAC
Broccoli rabe, cooked	½ bunch	1,322
Yellow onion, cooked	½ cup	1,281
Red leaf lettuce, raw	4 outer leaves	1,213
Sweet potato, cooked	1	1,195
Radishes, sliced	1 cup	1,107
Red bell peppers, raw	1 medium	1,072
Spinach, raw	4 leaves	1,058
Eggplant, raw	½ cup	1,039
Broccoli, cooked	½ cup	982
Red cabbage, raw	½ cup	788
Carrot, raw	1 medium	741
Broccoli, raw	½ cup	700
Green bell peppers, raw	1 medium	664
Green leaf lettuce, raw	4 leaves	620
Red bell peppers, chopped, cooked	½ cup	576
Tomato, cooked	½ cup	552
Sweet onion, raw	½ cup	492
Green peas, frozen	½ cup	480
Cabbage, raw	½ cup	476
Corn, cooked	½ cup	434
Butterhead lettuce	4 leaves	427
Green bell peppers, chopped, cooked	½ cup	418
Tomato, raw	1 medium	415
Romaine lettuce, raw	4 inner leaves	396
Celery, raw, chopped	½ cup	344
Green peas, cooked	½ cup	326
Cauliflower, raw	½ cup	324
Lima beans, cooked	½ cup	301
Baby carrots, raw	6 medium	262
Snap beans, cooked	½ cup	197
Carrots, cooked	1 medium	171
Snap beans, raw	½ cup	147
Iceberg lettuce, raw	4 leaves	144
Cucumber, peeled, sliced	½ cup	74
Cucumber with peel, sliced	½ cup	60

Baby Spinach Salad

MAKES 4 APPETIZER OR 2 MAIN-COURSE SERVINGS

This gorgeous salad is flecked with chewy bits of cranberries and an explosion of flavors and textures in every bite.

2 cups baby spinach leaves

1 cup watercress

8 ounces shredded or chopped roast turkey breast

3 tablespoons chopped dried cranberries

2 tablespoons chopped fresh mint

1 large navel orange

2 tablespoons apple cider vinegar

1 tablespoon Dijon mustard

1 teaspoon agave nectar

1 teaspoon horseradish

$\frac{1}{4}$ teaspoon salt

$\frac{1}{4}$ teaspoon ground black pepper

$\frac{1}{4}$ cup olive oil or canola oil

Salt and ground black pepper

2 tablespoons sliced almonds, toasted, for garnish

In a large mixing bowl, place the spinach, watercress, turkey, cranberries, and mint.

Scrub the orange lightly with an abrasive sponge to remove any surface impurities. Rinse thoroughly and dry well. Remove the peel from the orange with a zester or citrus grater. Peel the orange. Cut the orange in half vertically, then slice the halves horizontally into $\frac{1}{4}$"-thick pieces. Set aside in small bowl to catch any juices.

In a small bowl, whisk together the vinegar, mustard, agave, horseradish, salt, pepper, and oil. Add 3 tablespoons of dressing to the salad and toss well.

To assemble: Arrange the reserved orange slices around the outer edge of chilled plates. Mound the salad in the center. Garnish with the almonds. Pass the remaining vinaigrette.

✳ **ORANGE FACTOID:** One medium orange has a full day's requirement of vitamin C, a water-soluble antioxidant that is not stored by the body and must be replenished throughout the day for optimal antiaging protection.

NUTRIENT ANALYSIS PER APPETIZER SALAD

189 calories, 12 g protein, 15 g carbohydrates, 9 g total fat, 1 g saturated fat, 6 g monounsaturated fat, 70 mg omega-3s, 3 g fiber, 9 g sugar, 201 mg sodium

Rainbow Radicchio Slaw

MAKES 8 SERVINGS

My friend Robin loves to bring this dish when we have picnics together. The confetti of bright colors makes a beautiful salad that's as rich in flavor as it is in antioxidants.

1 head (12 ounces) radicchio, cored and shredded
1 cup peeled and shredded jicama
1 green bell pepper, seeded and cut into thin strips
¾ cup shredded carrot
½ cup chopped parsley
½ sweet onion, peeled and thinly sliced
⅓ cup cider vinegar
¼ cup olive oil
¼ cup fruit-sweetened ketchup
2 tablespoons Dijon mustard
2 tablespoons agave nectar
¾ teaspoon salt + more to taste
½ teaspoon ground black pepper + more to taste

In a large bowl, toss the radicchio, jicama, bell pepper, carrot, parsley, and onion. In a small bowl, whisk together the vinegar, oil, ketchup, mustard, agave, salt, and pepper. Pour dressing over slaw and toss; season to taste with more salt and pepper.

* **RADICCHIO FACTOID:** The three most popular types of radicchio are named after the Italian towns where they are thought to have originated: Chioggia, Treviso, and Castelfranco.

NUTRIENT ANALYSIS PER SERVING

107 calories, 1 g protein, 11 g carbohydrates, 7 g total fat, 1 g saturated fat, 5 g monounsaturated fat, 60 mg omega-3s, 2 g fiber, 5 g sugar, 338 mg sodium

Sliced Avocados and Oranges with Tahini Yogurt Sauce

MAKES 4 SERVINGS

This salad is an interesting marriage of sweet and savory flavors and creamy and juicy textures. Sweet grapefruit makes an equally delicious substitution for the oranges. For a heftier appetizer, top with a few grilled prawns.

1 medium avocado, peeled and sliced

2 medium seedless navel oranges, peeled and segmented

4 tablespoons Tahini Yogurt Sauce (page 284)

1 tablespoon chopped parsley or fresh cilantro, for garnish

1 teaspoon lightly toasted sesame seeds, for garnish

Arrange the avocado slices alternately with orange segments on 4 salad plates. Drizzle 1 tablespoon Tahini Yogurt Sauce over each salad. Garnish with the parsley or cilantro and sesame seeds and serve immediately.

Note: If the sauce is too thick to drizzle, you may need to add a teaspoon or two of water.

✻ **AVOCADO FACTOID:** Found primarily in nuts and seeds, two phytosterols—beta-sitosterol and campesterol—are also found in avocados. Their cholesterol-cloning property enables them to simulate cholesterol's presence in the body, thus decreasing the amount of cholesterol the body produces and absorbs, subsequently promoting cardiovascular health.

NUTRIENT ANALYSIS PER SERVING

125 calories, 3 g protein, 12 g carbohydrates, 10 g total fat, 1 g saturated fat, 7 g monounsaturated fat, 20 mg omega-3s, 3 g fiber, 7 g sugar, 57 mg sodium

Broccoli Salad with Caramelized Onions and Toasted Almonds

MAKES 4 SERVINGS

⅔ cup finely chopped yellow onion
¼ cup balsamic vinegar
⅔ cup water
1 teaspoon agave nectar
4 cups broccoli florets (about 12 ounces)
1 tablespoon top-quality extra-virgin olive oil
½ teaspoon salt
¼ teaspoon freshly ground black pepper
2 tablespoons lightly toasted almonds
1 tablespoon fresh lemon peel, grated

In a small saucepan, place the onion, vinegar, water, and agave. Bring to a boil and simmer over low heat for 30 minutes, or until the liquids have nearly evaporated. Watch carefully, stirring occasionally so the mixture doesn't burn. Let cool.

Bring a medium saucepan of salted water to a boil. Blanch the broccoli 3 minutes, or until just al dente. Immediately transfer to a bowl of ice water. Drain well and transfer to a mixing bowl.

Drizzle the oil over the broccoli and toss lightly. Add the onions and toss again. Season to taste with the salt and pepper. Divide among four plates. Sprinkle with the almonds and lemon peel.

✱ **BROCCOLI FACTOID:** This veggie is an excellent source of vitamins A, B, and C as well as iron and potassium. Its powerful antioxidants (beta-carotene, indoles, and isothiocyanates) help prevent carcinogens from forming.

NUTRIENT ANALYSIS PER SERVING
100 calories, 4 g protein, 14 g carbohydrates, 4 g total fat, < 1 g saturated fat, 3 g monounsaturated fat, 130 mg omega-3s, 3 g fiber, 7 g sugar, 323 mg sodium

Entrées

Asian-Style Fish

Grilled Salmon with Almond Pomegranate Sauce

Lebanese Kebabs

Southwest Salmon Burgers

Sesame Turkey Stir-Fry
with Cabbage and Green Beans

Moroccan Fish Stew

Roast Pork Tenderloin
with Citrus, Green Tea, and Spices

Asian-Style Fish

MAKES 4 SERVINGS

This recipe is delicious with any kind of fish—chicken breast would work, too. The poaching broth turns into a sumptuous sauce. Serve with brown or wild rice.

½ tablespoon olive oil

½ cup finely chopped yellow onion

½ cup thinly sliced mushrooms

1 tablespoon finely chopped fresh ginger

1 pound fresh plum tomatoes, cored and finely chopped

½ cup brewed green tea

4 fillets (4 ounces each) halibut or salmon, preferably 1" thick

9 ounces raw baby spinach leaves (6 cups)

1 tablespoon mirin (Japanese cooking wine)

1 teaspoon soy sauce

2 tablespoons chopped green onion or fresh cilantro

Heat the oil in a deep sauté pan over medium-high heat. Add the yellow onions and cook, stirring frequently, for 5 minutes, or until soft and just starting to brown. Add the mushrooms and ginger and cook for 2 minutes longer, stirring frequently. Add the tomatoes and simmer for 3 minutes, or until the juices are released but the tomatoes still hold their shape. Add the tea. When the mixture boils, reduce the heat to a simmer.

Carefully add the fish to the pan. When the mixture returns to a boil, cover and cook for 3 minutes. Add the spinach, cover again, and cook for 3 minutes longer, or until the fish flakes easily. Thicker fish will take slightly longer to cook. If the fillets are thin, they will take only a few minutes.

Carefully mound the cooked spinach in the middle of each of four dinner plates. Place the fish on top of the spinach and keep warm.

Add the mirin, soy sauce, and green onion or cilantro to the pan. Increase the heat and cook the poaching liquid at a steady, high simmer for 1 to 2 minutes, or until the juices are slightly reduced and the mixture is saucy. Ladle sauce over the fish fillets. Serve immediately.

❋ **CILANTRO FACTOID:** Also known as Chinese parsley or Mexican parsley, cilantro is an herb. The seed of the plant is called coriander and has been studied for its antibacterial properties.

NUTRIENT ANALYSIS PER SERVING

234 calories, 33 g protein, 14 g carbohydrates, 5 g total fat, 1 g saturated fat, 2 g monounsaturated fat, 640 mg omega-3s, 4 g fiber, 4 g sugar, 235 mg sodium

Grilled Salmon
with Almond Pomegranate Sauce

MAKES 4 SERVINGS

This complex sauce is inspired by a Middle Eastern stew called fesenjan. *Ground almonds add richness to a spice-infused sauce made tangy with homemade Pomegranate Syrup.*

SAUCE

1 teaspoon olive oil

$\frac{1}{2}$ medium yellow onion, chopped

$\frac{1}{2}$ teaspoon ground turmeric

$\frac{1}{8}$ teaspoon ground cinnamon

$\frac{1}{8}$ teaspoon ground nutmeg

$\frac{1}{8}$ teaspoon ground black pepper

$\frac{1}{2}$ cup chopped almonds, lightly toasted

1 cup fat-free chicken or vegetable broth

2 tablespoons Pomegranate Syrup (page 282)

SALMON

4 salmon fillets (5 ounces each)

1 teaspoon olive oil

$\frac{1}{4}$ teaspoon salt

$\frac{1}{8}$ teaspoon ground black pepper

$\frac{1}{4}$ cup chopped fresh cilantro, for garnish

Fresh pomegranate seeds (if available), for garnish

To make the sauce: Heat the oil in a nonstick sauté pan over medium heat. Add the onion and cook for 6 minutes, or until softened and light golden brown. Add the turmeric, cinnamon, nutmeg, and pepper and cook for 1 minute, or until fragrant. Remove from the heat.

Place the almonds in the bowl of a food processor and process until very finely ground. Add the cooked onion mixture, broth, and Pomegranate Syrup. Process until creamy and smooth. This may take 2 to 3 minutes. Return the sauce to the sauté pan. Bring to a boil, then reduce the heat, and simmer 3 minutes, or until the mixture is the consistency of thick cream. There will be about 1¼ cups sauce. Keep warm.

To make the salmon: Preheat a charcoal grill.

Brush the salmon lightly with the oil. Season with salt and ground black pepper. Arrange the fillets on a rack set about 6" over glowing coals. Grill about 3 minutes on each side, or until the fish is opaque. (Alternatively, salmon may be grilled on a hot, ridged grill pan over medium-high heat.)

Serve each fillet with 2 tablespoons of the sauce and garnish with the chopped cilantro and pomegranate seeds. Pass extra sauce at the table.

✳ **POMEGRANATE FACTOID:** Prime time to buy fresh pomegranates is from November to February. Look for deep-red coloring and smooth skin with few blemishes. Hard or dry, wrinkled skin signals old fruit.

NUTRIENT ANALYSIS PER SERVING

240 calories, 29 g protein, 2 g carbohydrates, 12 g total fat, 2 g saturated fat, 7 g monounsaturated fat, 2,460 omega-3s, 1 g fiber, 1 g sugar, 171 mg sodium

Lebanese Kebabs

MAKES 6 SERVINGS (2 SKEWERS EACH)

These moist little nuggets are loaded with flavor. The surprise ingredient of bulgur adds texture and fiber, though you can't tell it's there. This recipe is typically made with ground lamb, but this version is tasty, quick, and easy. You may even want to try serving the bite-size meatballs at your next party.

$\frac{1}{2}$ cup uncooked bulgur

1$\frac{1}{2}$ cups boiling water

1$\frac{1}{4}$ pound lean ground turkey (7 percent fat)

$\frac{1}{2}$ cup finely chopped yellow onion

1 tablespoon finely chopped garlic

1 tablespoon finely chopped mint

2 teaspoons ground cumin

1 teaspoon ground coriander

$\frac{1}{2}$ teaspoon ground mustard seed

$\frac{1}{2}$ teaspoon salt

$\frac{1}{2}$ teaspoon ground black pepper

12 skewers (6" each)

2 tablespoons chopped fresh cilantro, mint, or Italian parsley, for garnish

Place the bulgur and water in a small bowl and soak for 30 minutes.

While the bulgur is soaking, place the remaining kebab ingredients in a large mixing bowl. (If you've thawed the turkey from frozen, be sure to drain any juices before adding to the bowl.)

Drain the bulgur in a sieve to remove excess liquid. Transfer to the large mixing bowl; mix well. There will be about 3 cups of mixture. Form into 36 meatballs, about 1$\frac{1}{2}$" across, using about 1$\frac{1}{2}$ tablespoons of mixture per meatball.

Preheat oven to 400°F. Thread 3 meatballs per skewer, leaving about $\frac{1}{2}$" between each meatball. Place skewers on nonstick baking sheet. Skewers should be evenly spaced and not touching. Bake for 8 minutes, or until no longer pink.

To serve, place 2 skewers on each plate. Garnish with the fresh herbs. Serve with cucumber or tomato salad and hummus.

If there are any leftovers, try a kebab sandwich: Place 3 meatballs in a small whole wheat pita with shredded lettuce and tomato slices.

✳ **CUMIN FACTOID:** This pungent spice is commonly used in Mexican and Middle Eastern dishes. It has a nutty flavor and aroma, and its abundant phytochemicals have antioxidant as well as digestive properties.

NUTRIENT ANALYSIS PER SERVING
190 calories, 21 g protein, 12 g carbohydrates, 7 g total fat, 2 g saturated fat, 0 g monounsaturated fat, 0 mg omega-3s, 3 g fiber, 1 g sugar, 268 mg sodium

Southwest Salmon Burgers

MAKES 4 SERVINGS

You've run out of ways to cook salmon? Try this. Delish on a toasted whole grain bun or served with a crisp green salad.

1 tablespoon olive oil

½ cup finely chopped onion

2 small stone-ground corn tortillas

1 pound wild salmon fillets (without bones or skin)

¼ cup barbecue sauce

2 tablespoons chopped fresh cilantro

1 tablespoon fresh lime juice

1 teaspoon horseradish sauce

1 teaspoon Dijon mustard

4 whole grain burger rolls, toasted

Lettuce, tomato, and onion, for serving

Heat the oil in a medium pan over medium-high heat. Add the onions and cook, stirring frequently, until golden brown. Transfer to a mixing bowl.

Tear the tortillas into bite-size pieces and transfer to the bowl of a food processor. Process until finely ground. There will be about ½ cup. Transfer to the mixing bowl.

Place the salmon in the bowl of a food processor and pulse until the meat is just ground but still coarse. Add to the mixing bowl along with the barbecue sauce, cilantro, lime juice, horseradish, and mustard. Stir to combine. There will be about 2½ cups. Refrigerate for 1 hour, or until well chilled.

Lightly coat a grill rack with cooking oil spray. Preheat a barbecue grill to medium-hot.

Divide the salmon mixture into 4 balls and form into burger patties. Grill over medium-high heat for 3 to 4 minutes on each side, or until just cooked through. (Or you can cook the burgers in a nonstick sauté pan.)

Serve on the toasted rolls with lettuce, tomato, and onion. Serve with extra barbecue sauce.

✳ **SALMON FACTOID:** Wild Coho salmon is found in the Pacific as well as some fresh-water lakes, such as the Great Lakes. Four ounces of wild Coho salmon has 166 calories and 1,410 milligrams of omega-3s.

NUTRIENT ANALYSIS PER BURGER (WITHOUT BUN)
196 calories, 24 g protein, 11 g carbohydrates, 6 g total fat, 1 g saturated fat, 0 g monounsaturated fat, 1,110 mg omega-3s, 2 g fiber, 2 g sugar, 207 mg sodium

THE ORAC SCORE

POSITIVELY AGELESS
STOP THE CLOCK!TAILS WINE CHOICES

Red wine plays a vital role in the fight against aging. This is due to a group of phytochemicals it contains called polyphenols. The largest class of polyphenols is the flavonoids—which includes anthocyanins, ellagic acid, quercetin, and resveratrol, to name just a few. Scientists believe that many of these compounds are responsible for lowering blood cholesterol. But protection from heart disease isn't the only ben-efit of flavonoids. Their antioxidant properties are believed to fight against age-related mental decline, and they appear to minimize inflam-mation and discomfort from age-related diseases such as arthritis.

Red wine is well endowed with resveratrol, which has shown promise in slowing the growth of cancer in some studies. Resveratrol's concen-tration increases proportionately with the length of time the grape skins are present during the wine's fermentation process. That's why resvera-trol levels are significantly higher in red wine than white. Still, because wine also contains alcohol, enjoy its benefits in moderation with a glass or two a day.

WINE	ORAC PER 6 OZ
Red	4,585
White	702

Sesame Turkey Stir-Fry
with Cabbage and Green Beans

MAKES 4 SERVINGS

It's easy to whip up this colorful stir-fry. I actually enjoy the leftovers as a cold salad for lunch the next day with a splash of Tangy Mustard Dressing (page 281). Use any combination of your favorite veggies. Substitute lean beef or chicken for the pork, switch seasonings . . . the combinations are endless.

3 cups green beans, cut in 1" pieces

1 tablespoon olive oil

1 cup chopped yellow onion

1 red bell pepper, halved, seeded, and finely chopped

½ cup finely chopped carrot

1 tablespoon sesame oil

2 tablespoons chopped garlic

2 tablespoons peeled, chopped fresh ginger

¾ cup fat-free chicken broth

2 tablespoons low-sodium soy sauce

1 pound boneless turkey breast, cut in thin ½" × 1" strips (see note)

2 cups thinly sliced green cabbage

GARNISH

2 tablespoons chopped green onions

1 tablespoon chopped fresh cilantro

1 tablespoon toasted sesame seeds

Cook the beans for 2 minutes, or until bright green but still firm. Drain, rinse with cold water to stop cooking, drain again, and set aside. (If using frozen green beans, thaw them but omit this cooking step.)

Heat the olive oil in a large nonstick sauté pan over medium-high heat. Add the yellow onion, pepper, and carrot and cook, stirring frequently, for 5 minutes or until the vegetables are just tender. Transfer to a bowl and cover with a towel to retain the heat.

Add the sesame oil to the pan over medium-high heat. Add the garlic and ginger and cook, stirring constantly, for 30 seconds. Add ¼ cup of the broth and the soy sauce to the skillet. Add the turkey and cook, stirring constantly, for 4 minutes, or until the turkey is no longer pink. Add the remaining ½ cup broth and bring to a boil. Add the reserved onion mixture, cabbage, and green beans, cover, and simmer 3 minutes longer, or until the vegetables are just cooked. Divide among 6 plates and garnish with the green onions, cilantro, and sesame seeds. Serve immediately.

Note: It's easier to slice turkey thinly if you place it in the freezer for about 30 minutes first.

❄ **TURKEY FACTOID:** Skinless turkey breast has less fat than and twice the iron as the same amount of skinless chicken breast.

NUTRIENT ANALYSIS PER SERVING

167 calories, 11 g protein, 10 g carbohydrates, 6 g total fat, 1 g saturated fat, 3 g monounsaturated fat, 50 mg omega-3s, 4 g fiber, 4 g sugar, 209 mg sodium

Moroccan Fish Stew

MAKES 8 APPETIZER OR 6 MAIN-COURSE SERVINGS

This flavorful stew is a meal in itself. Loaded with fiber, it is rich in protein, too. The recipe adapts well to different beans or to using chicken instead of fish.

1 tablespoon olive oil

1 cup finely chopped yellow onion

1 teaspoon ground mustard seed

1 teaspoon ground turmeric

4 cups fat-free chicken or vegetable broth

1 cup chopped tomatoes

1 cup cooked black beans

1 cup cooked cannellini (white kidney) beans

1 cup edamame (uncooked)

1 pound bonelesss, skinless salmon (or other fish), cut in ³/₄" cubes

1 tablespoon chopped fresh dill (or 1 teaspoon dried)

2 tablespoons tahini (sesame paste)

Salt and ground black pepper to taste

2 tablespoons chopped fresh cilantro, for garnish

1 tablespoon grated lemon peel, for garnish

Add the oil to a large (5-quart) saucepan over medium heat. Add the onion and cook, stirring frequently, for 5 minutes, or until softened and just beginning to brown. Add the mustard seed and turmeric. Stir well. Add the broth and bring to a simmer.

Add the tomatoes and bring to boil. Reduce the heat to low and simmer for 3 minutes. Add the beans, edamame, salmon, and dill and simmer for 3 minutes longer, or until the fish is opaque. Remove from the heat. Whisk in the tahini. Season with salt and pepper if desired. Ladle the stew into bowls and garnish with the cilantro and lemon peel. Serve hot.

✳ **SESAME FACTOID:** Tahini, or ground sesame seed paste, is a great way to absorb the plentitude of vitamins and minerals in whole sesame seeds, which are more difficult to digest. Once opened, tahini should be refrigerated.

✳ **TURMERIC FACTOID:** Its vibrant, deep yellow-orange color gives turmeric double duty as a flavoring as well as a dye for textiles (and your clothes, if you're not careful!). This spice has powerful properties as an antioxidant and anti-inflammatory.

NUTRIENT ANALYSIS PER SERVING

223 calories, 19 g protein, 18 g carbohydrates, 9 g total fat, 1 g saturated fat, 3 g monounsaturated fat, 1,060 mg omega-3s, 8 g fiber, 2 g sugar, 293 mg sodium

Roast Pork Tenderloin with Citrus, Green Tea, and Spices

MAKES 8 SERVINGS

Serve this flavorful dish with wilted cabbage and polenta. If you're in the mood, you can grill the pork as opposed to oven roasting. Any leftovers will make a delicious sandwich or salad addition.

½ cup brewed green tea

½ cup red wine

¼ cup orange juice

¼ cup lime juice

1 tablespoon grated orange peel

1 tablespoon grated lime peel

1 tablespoon minced garlic

1 tablespoon Dijon mustard

¼ cup chopped fresh cilantro leaves

1 tablespoon chili powder

1 teaspoon ground cumin

½ teaspoon ground cinnamon

2 pounds lean pork tenderloin

Combine all the ingredients except the pork. Add the pork and marinate, covered and refrigerated, at least 2 hours.

Preheat oven to 400°F.

Drain the pork, reserving excess marinade to use for basting. Place the pork on a rack over a roasting pan. Roast for 25 minutes, or until a meat thermometer registers 160°F and the juices run clear (the pork should be barely pink inside). Turn the pork occasionally and baste with excess marinade. Slice ¼" thick to serve.

✳ **CITRUS FACTOID:** Citrus fruits are loaded with soluble fiber. The primary form, pectin, binds and dilutes carcinogenic substances in the intestinal tract, lowers cholesterol, and helps regulate blood glucose levels.

NUTRIENT ANALYSIS PER SERVING
162 calories, 24 g protein, 2 g carbohydrates, 5 g total fat, 2 g saturated fat, 2 g monounsaturated fat, 10 mg omega-3s, < 1 g fiber, < 1 g sugar, 69 mg sodium

Vegetables and Legumes

Gingered Edamame with Fire-Roasted Tomatoes

Black-Eyed Peas with Garlic

Sweet Potatoes with Onion Confit

Spaghetti (Squash) with Basil-Cress Pesto

Lima Beans with Parsley and Red Cabbage

Gingered Edamame
with Fire-Roasted Tomatoes

MAKES 6 SERVINGS

This is the perfect vegetable dish to serve with grilled chicken or fish or to take along to a potluck. Once the chopping's done, the cooking takes just minutes.

1 tablespoon olive oil

1 cup finely chopped yellow onion

2 tablespoons peeled and finely chopped fresh ginger

1 tablespoon minced garlic

1 can (14 ounces) fire-roasted tomatoes or 1 pound plum tomatoes, cored and cut into 4 wedges each + 1 tablespoon olive oil (see note)

2 tablespoons low-sodium soy sauce

¼ cup vegetable or chicken broth

2 cups shelled edamame

3 tablespoons chopped fresh cilantro, for garnish

Heat the oil in a large sauté pan over medium heat. Add the onion and cook, stirring, for 6 minutes, or until soft and translucent. Add the ginger and cook, stirring, 1 minute longer. Add the garlic and cook, stirring, 1 minute more. Do not brown the garlic.

Add the tomatoes, soy sauce, broth, and edamame to the pan. Bring the mixture to a boil, reduce the heat, and simmer for 3 to 4 minutes, or until the edamame are just cooked. Divide among 6 serving plates. Serve hot, garnished with the cilantro.

Note: If you are unable to find canned fire-roasted tomatoes, you can oven roast plum tomatoes. To roast tomatoes: Preheat oven to 400°F. Place the tomatoes on a 15" × 10" baking sheet. Drizzle with olive oil and toss to coat. Spread in an even layer on the prepared baking sheet. Roast about 30 minutes, turning once. Cool and chop roughly, transfer tomatoes and their juices to a bowl, and set aside.

✳ EDAMAME FACTOID: Edamame are soybeans that are harvested prematurely, when the beans are still green and sweet. Mature soybeans are tan in color and can be purchased dried or cooked (canned). Soybeans are the only vegetable that contains complete protein. They also contain a compound that helps lower LDL (least desirable cholesterol) levels.

NUTRIENT ANALYSIS PER SERVING
128 calories, 7 g protein, 16 g carbohydrates, 4 g total fat, 2 g saturated fat, 2 g monounsaturated fat, 20 mg omega-3s, 4 g fiber, 6 g sugar, 382 mg sodium

Black-Eyed Peas with Garlic

MAKES 4 SERVINGS (½ CUP EACH)

Black-eyed peas, also known as cowpeas, are an excellent source of protein and fiber. The added bonus is that they're loaded with antioxidants and, like other dried beans, they're very inexpensive. This recipe is equally delicious if you substitute cooked black beans for the black-eyed peas and green bell pepper for the red bell pepper.

1 tablespoon olive oil

½ cup finely chopped yellow onion

½ red bell pepper, finely chopped

1 tablespoon chopped garlic

1½ cups cooked black-eyed peas

½ cup chopped tomatoes

1 teaspoon ground cumin

1 teaspoon chopped fresh oregano (or ½ teaspoon dried)

½ teaspoon ground mustard seed

½ teaspoon salt

¾ cup fat-free, low-sodium chicken or vegetable broth

2 tablespoons chopped fresh cilantro, for garnish

Heat the oil in a sauté pan over medium heat. Add the onion and pepper and cook, stirring frequently, for 3 minutes. Add the garlic and cook for 1 minute longer. Do not brown the garlic. Add the black-eyed peas, tomatoes, cumin, oregano, mustard, salt, and broth. Reduce the heat and simmer for 5 minutes, or until the vegetables are just cooked through and the broth is reduced. Remove from the heat and garnish with the cilantro. Serve hot.

✳ **BLACK-EYED PEA FACTOID:** High in potassium and folic acid, ½ cup black-eyed peas also provides 4 grams of fiber and 3 grams of protein.

NUTRIENT ANALYSIS PER SERVING

133 calories, 6 g protein, 19 g carbohydrates, 4 g total fat, 1 g saturated fat, 3 g monounsaturated fat, 80 mg omega-3s, 7 g fiber, 4 g sugar, 366 mg sodium

Sweet Potatoes with Onion Confit

MAKES 8 SERVINGS

Sweet onion confit adds a homey flavor to creamy sweet potatoes. This is a great make-ahead dish for a potluck and a welcome addition to your holiday table.

2 sweet potatoes (about 2 pounds), peeled and cut in 1" cubes

1 tablespoon olive oil

2 medium yellow onions, chopped

¼ cup white wine or chicken broth

1 cup 1% low-fat milk or soy milk

1 tablespoon Pomegranate Syrup (page 282)

½ teaspoon salt

Preheat oven to 350°F.

In a 3-quart saucepan, cook the potatoes in boiling salted water until tender, about 15 minutes.

While the potatoes are cooking, heat the oil in a sauté pan over medium-high heat. Add the onions and cook until tender and lightly browned, about 8 minutes. Transfer to the bowl of a food processor. Add the wine or broth to the pan and cook for 2 minutes, scraping up any browned bits and allowing the liquid to reduce slightly. Add the liquid to the food processor and puree the onions until smooth. Add a few tablespoons of water, if necessary.

Drain the potatoes and return to the saucepan. Add the milk and heat until hot, but do not boil. Using a fork or a masher, mash the potatoes slightly. Pass the mixture through a food mill to remove lumps and transfer to a medium mixing bowl. Add the onion puree, Pomegranate Syrup, and salt. Mix well.

Transfer the mixture to a 1½-quart soufflé dish and bake for 20 minutes. Serve hot.

✳ **SOY MILK FACTOID:** Most soy milks have about the same amount of fat (and calories) as 2 percent dairy milk, *without* the cholesterol.

NUTRIENT ANALYSIS PER SERVING

110 calories, 3 g protein, 20 g carbohydrates, 2 g total fat, 0 g saturated fat, 3 g monounsaturated fat, 40 mg omega-3s, 3 g fiber, 8 g sugar, 205 mg sodium

Spaghetti (Squash) with Basil-Cress Pesto

MAKES 4 SERVINGS

This veggie is a creative replacement for white pasta. Add turkey meatballs and a salad and you have a meal.

1 medium spaghetti squash (about 1½ pounds)
1 packed cup fresh basil leaves, without stems
1 packed cup watercress leaves, without stems
1 tablespoon minced garlic
¼ cup chopped sun-dried tomatoes
2 tablespoons extra-virgin olive oil
2 tablespoons grated Romano cheese
¼ teaspoon salt (optional)
⅛ teaspoon ground black pepper

Preheat the oven to 375°F. Lightly coat a baking sheet with olive oil cooking spray.

Wash the outside of the squash and cut in half lengthwise. Remove the seeds. Pierce each half a few times with a fork. Place the squash cut side down on the baking sheet and bake 45 minutes, or until very tender when tested with a fork.

Meanwhile, prepare the pesto. Place the basil, watercress, garlic, and tomatoes in the bowl of a food processor or in a blender jar. Pulse until finely chopped. With the motor running, add the oil in a stream. Pulse to blend. Stop and scrape the sides down 2 or 3 times to puree evenly. Add the cheese and process for 10 to 15 seconds. Do not overprocess; the pesto should have some texture. Season with salt, if desired, and the pepper.

Remove the cooked squash from the oven and cool slightly. Using the tines of a fork, rake the spaghetti-like threads of the squash into a mixing bowl. Discard the skin. There will be about 3 cups of spaghetti squash. Pour the pesto over the squash and toss gently. Divide among serving plates and serve hot.

✻ SPAGHETTI SQUASH FACTOID: A member of the pumpkin family, spaghetti squash provides an excellent source of beta-carotene and folic acid. Extra cooked spaghetti squash can be served as a salad with vinaigrette or frozen in freezer bags. Thaw it partially before serving, and then steam it for about 5 minutes.

NUTRIENT ANALYSIS PER SERVING

77 calories, 2 g protein, 7 g carbohydrates, 5 g total fat, 1 g saturated fat, 3 g monounsaturated fat, 110 mg omega-3s, 2 g fiber, 3 g sugar, 287 mg sodium

Lima Beans with Parsley and Red Cabbage

MAKES 6 SERVINGS

Lima beans have a creamy texture and mild flavor. Try this simple preparation with roast chicken or grilled fish.

2 cups fresh shelled lima beans or 1 package (10 ounces) frozen lima beans (see note)

1 tablespoon olive oil

½ cup chopped yellow onion

2 teaspoons minced garlic

½ teaspoon curry powder

½ cup vegetable or fat-free chicken broth

1 cup thinly sliced red cabbage

½ teaspoon salt

¼ teaspoon ground black pepper

1 tablespoon chopped parsley

Cook the beans in a saucepan of boiling water for 6 minutes, or until barely tender. Transfer with a slotted spoon to a bowl of ice water to stop cooking and drain.

Heat the oil in a saucepan over medium high-heat. Add the onion and cook, stirring frequently, for 5 minutes, or until tender. Add the garlic and curry powder and cook, stirring, 1 minute longer, or until fragrant; do not brown the garlic.

Add the cooked beans, broth, and cabbage. Bring to a boil, then reduce the heat to a low simmer and cover the pan tightly. Allow the beans and cabbage to braise in the steam for 5 minutes, shaking the pan gently from time to time, until the cabbage is wilted. Season with salt and pepper; sprinkle with the parsley and serve hot.

Note: For 2 cooked cups of lima beans, start with about 1 cup of dried beans.

✳ **RED CABBAGE FACTOID:** Anthocyanins, the pigments that give red cabbage its vibrant color, are a type of plant chemical called flavonoids. These powerful antioxidants have been studied for conferring health benefits from improving vision, controlling diabetes, improving circulation, and preventing cancer to slowing the aging process.

NUTRIENT ANALYSIS PER SERVING

112 calories, 6 g protein, 17 g carbohydrates, 3 g total fat, < 1 g saturated fat, 2 g monounsaturated fat, 60 mg omega-3s, 6 g fiber, 1 g sugar, 240 mg sodium

Desserts

Spicy Strawberry Frozen Yogurt

Chocolate Almond Pudding

Sweet Pumpkin Polenta

Gingerbread with Dried Cherries
and Toasted Pecans

Rich Cocoa Sorbet

Ruby Lemon Sorbet

Orange and Blueberry Compote
in Green Tea–Ginger Syrup

Almond Berry Bars

Spicy Strawberry Frozen Yogurt

MAKES 4 SERVINGS OR 1 PINT

This recipe works well with other berries, too. If your fruit is supersweet, you may not need to add any sweetener. To retain optimal levels of ellagic acid and its antiaging benefits, do not strain the seeds from the berry puree.

1 pound strawberries, rinsed, hulled, and halved

1 tablespoon finely chopped or grated fresh ginger

1/4 cup fat-free or low-fat vanilla yogurt

2 tablespoons agave nectar, sorghum syrup, or dark honey (such as buckwheat)

1/4 teaspoon ground ginger

1/4 teaspoon pure vanilla extract

Place the strawberries and fresh ginger in the jar of a blender or the bowl of a food processor. Blend or process until very smooth. Add the yogurt, sweetener, ground ginger, and vanilla extract to the puree and stir to combine. Taste for sweetness. Cover and refrigerate until cold. Freeze in an ice-cream maker according to the manufacturer's instructions.

✳ **STRAWBERRY FACTOID:** With only 53 calories, a cup of sliced strawberries is the perfect low-cal dessert. It also provides over 3 grams of fiber and 160 percent of the RDA for vitamin C.

NUTRIENT ANALYSIS PER SERVING
80 calories, 2 g protein, 18 g carbohydrates, 0 g total fat, 0 g saturated fat, 0 g monounsaturated fat, 70 mg omega-3s, 2 g fiber, 14 g sugar, 20 mg sodium

Chocolate Almond Pudding

MAKES 4 SERVINGS (½ CUP EACH)

There are a variety of ready-to-drink nut milks on the market, which are made by soaking nuts or seeds in water, blending, and then straining the liquid. Served warm or cold, this silky crowd-pleaser takes just minutes to prepare. If you have a nut allergy, you can also prepare the pudding using low-fat milk or soy milk.

¼ cup unsweetened natural cocoa powder

¼ cup cornstarch

¼ teaspoon salt

2 cups unflavored almond milk, preferably unsweetened or sweetened with brown rice syrup

⅓ cup agave nectar

2 teaspoons pure vanilla extract

2 tablespoons toasted slivered almonds

In a 1-quart saucepan, combine the cocoa, cornstarch, and salt. Add just enough of the milk to make a smooth paste. Gradually stir in the agave and the remaining milk.

Cook over medium heat, stirring constantly, until the mixture begins to thicken. Remove from heat and stir in the vanilla extract. Pour into 4 serving dishes and cool. Sprinkle with the almonds just before serving.

✳ **ALMOND FACTOID:** Almonds are the best whole-food source of alpha-tocopherol, a form of antioxidant vitamin E, which may help prevent cancer.

NUTRIENT ANALYSIS PER SERVING

167 calories, 3 g protein, 32 g carbohydrates, 4 g total fat, 1 g saturated fat, 1 g monounsaturated fat, 0 mg omega-3s, 2 g fiber, 20 g sugar, 218 mg sodium

Sweet Pumpkin Polenta

MAKES 8 SERVINGS

The smell of sweet spices will fill the air while this creamy dessert is baking. It's divine straight from the oven but tastes heavenly the next day when it's cold—if there's any left the next day.

2 cups pumpkin puree, fresh or canned

1 large omega-3 egg, lightly beaten

$^2/_3$ cup agave nectar

1 teaspoon ground cinnamon

$^1/_2$ teaspoon ground ginger

$^1/_4$ teaspoon ground cloves

1 teaspoon pure vanilla extract

$^1/_3$ cup stone-ground cornmeal or polenta

2 cups water

1 cup low-fat, fat-free milk, or soy milk

$^1/_2$ teaspoon salt

toasted pecans (optional)

Preheat the oven to 350°F. Lightly coat a 2-quart soufflé dish or casserole with olive oil cooking spray. Set aside.

In a large mixing bowl, combine the pumpkin, egg, agave, cinnamon, ginger, cloves, and vanilla extract. Stir well to combine. Set aside.

In a 2-quart saucepan, combine the cornmeal, water, milk, and salt; mix well. Bring to a boil over medium-high heat, stirring constantly. Cook, stirring, 10 minutes or longer until thick and smooth. Remove from the heat. Carefully pour in the reserved pumpkin mixture and stir to combine. Pour into the prepared baking dish. Bake for 50 minutes, stirring well once, halfway through.

The mixture will be thick and bubbly. Serve warm, sprinkled with toasted pecans, if desired.

✳ **PUMPKIN FACTOID:** Pumpkin's high concentration of antioxidants and beta-carotene make it a favorite antiaging ingredient for skin-care products.

NUTRIENT ANALYSIS PER SERVING

127 calories, 3 g protein, 26 g carbohydrates, 2 g total fat, 0 g saturated fat, 5 g monounsaturated fat, 30 mg omega-3s, 2 g fiber, 17 g sugar, 254 mg sodium

Gingerbread with Dried Cherries and Toasted Pecans

MAKES 16 SERVINGS

It's easy to increase your omega-3 intake when you hide ground flaxseed in unsuspecting places. This irresistibly moist cake is flecked with chewy bits of fruit and crunchy pecans. It's equally delicious with dried blueberries or dried cranberries, or toasted almond slivers.

2 cups stone-ground whole wheat flour

2 tablespoons ground flaxseed

2 teaspoons baking soda

1/4 teaspoon salt

2 teaspoons ground ginger

1 teaspoon ground cinnamon

1/4 teaspoon ground cloves

1/8 teaspoon ground nutmeg

1/3 cup olive or canola oil

2 large omega-3 eggs

2/3 cup sorghum syrup or unsulfured molasses

2/3 cup soy or low-fat milk

1 teaspoon pure vanilla extract

1/2 cup chopped dried cherries

1/4 cup chopped toasted pecans

Preheat the oven to 350°F. Lightly coat an 8" × 8" square baking pan with olive oil cooking spray.

In a bowl, measure the flour, flaxseed, baking soda, salt, ginger, cinnamon, cloves, and nutmeg. Set aside.

In another bowl, whisk together the oil, eggs, sweetener, milk, and vanilla extract. Make a well in the reserved dry ingredients and pour in the liquid mixture. Stir until just combined. Fold in the fruit and nuts.

Pour the batter into the prepared pan. Bake for 10 minutes. Reduce the oven temperature to 325°F and bake for 30 to 35 minutes longer, or until a toothpick used to test doneness comes out clean.

✳ **GINGER FACTOID:** Ginger contains a bundle of plant chemicals that can aid digestion and ease motion sickness. It promotes production of bile in the liver and gallbladder, which helps digest fats. This, in turn, helps lower cholesterol levels.

NUTRIENT ANALYSIS PER SERVING
176 calories, 4 g protein, 25 g carbohydrates, 7 g total fat, 1 g saturated fat, 5 g monounsaturated fat, 60 mg omega-3s, 4 g fiber, 10 g sugar, 154 mg sodium

THE ORAC SCORE

DRIED FRUITS: ARE THEY EVEN BETTER THAN FRESH?

Since dried fruits have much less water than their original form, their size, flavor, and calories are much more concentrated. That means a little has a lot of calories! Dried fruits are great on occasion, however, to add texture to a salad or a chewy bite to muffins or breads. Whole fruits are the ultimate antiagers.

DRIED FRUIT PER 1/4 CUP	ORAC
Prunes	3,646
Dates (Deglet Noor)	1,734
Figs	1,269
Raisins	1,245
Date (Medjool)	1,062

Rich Cocoa Sorbet

MAKES ABOUT 1 QUART (8 SERVINGS; ½ CUP EACH)

In any recipe, the end result is a function of the quality of the ingredients used. This sorbet is a perfect example, as the finished product really depends on the caliber of the cocoa powder you use (see the Shopping Resources on page 351 for recommendations). Buy the best you can afford.

1 cup natural cocoa powder

1¾ cups water

¾ cup agave nectar

pinch salt

1½ teaspoons pure vanilla extract

Measure the cocoa into a small saucepan. Slowly whisk in ¾ cup of the water until the cocoa is dissolved and there are no lumps. Whisk in the agave, salt and remaining 1 cup water. Over medium heat, bring the mixture to a boil, stirring frequently. Remove from the heat and stir in the vanilla extract. Chill in the refrigerator until very cold. Freeze in an ice-cream maker according to the manufacturer's instructions.

Note: Need a mini treat for your nighttime sweet tooth? Finished sorbet may be frozen in individual 1-ounce portions in flexible ice-cube trays or silicone flexible mini baking pans.

✳ **COCOA FACTOID:** Cocoa beans contain antioxidants called flavonoids, similar to those found in wine. These compounds help reduce the blood's ability to clot and this lowers the risk of heart attacks and stroke.

NUTRIENT ANALYSIS PER SERVING

95 calories, 2 g protein, 24 g carbohydrates, 1 g total fat, 0 g saturated fat, 0 g monounsaturated fat, 30 mg omega-3s, 4 g fiber, 18 g sugar, 21 mg sodium

Ruby Lemon Sorbet

MAKES ABOUT 1 QUART (8 SERVINGS; ½ CUP EACH)

This vibrant and tangy sorbet gets its pucker from lots of lemon and pomegranate juices. Get a real antioxidant blast from this frosty treat.

1 cup Pomegranate Syrup (page 282)

1 cup fresh lemon juice (from about 6 lemons)

2 tablespoons grated lemon peel (from 4 lemons)

1 cup water

¼ cup agave nectar

Combine all the ingredients; mix well. Chill the mixture for 30 minutes, then freeze according to the manufacturer's instructions for your ice-cream maker.

If you do not have an ice-cream maker, place the mixture in a medium mixing bowl and freeze until partially frozen, about 1 hour. Remove from the freezer and mix well with a hand mixer or pulse with a food processor to break up ice crystals. Repeat the freezing and mixing steps one or two times.

✳ **POMEGRANATE FACTOID:** Seems the peel of pomegranates has even more antioxidant brawn than the powerful juice. Though it's not edible, scientists hope to create extracts from the peel so we can benefit from the entire fruit, not just the pulp.

NUTRIENT ANALYSIS PER SERVING

95 calories, 3 g protein, 25 g carbohydrates, 0 g total fat, 0 g saturated fat, 0 g monounsaturated fat, 0 mg omega-3s, < 1 g fiber, 23 g sugar, 22 mg sodium

Orange and Blueberry Compote in Green Tea–Ginger Syrup

MAKES 6 SERVINGS

Yes, it is possible to have luscious desserts without sugar or white flour. This sophisticated indulgence is as pretty as it is delicious.

1 cup water

¼ cup grated, peeled fresh ginger

2 green tea bags

2 tablespoons light agave nectar

2 large seedless navel oranges

2 cups fresh blueberries

2 tablespoons fresh lemon juice

1 teaspoon pure vanilla extract

GARNISH

1 tablespoon toasted almond slices

1 tablespoon thinly sliced mint, chiffonade

1 tablespoon Pomegranate Syrup (page 282), optional

In a small saucepan, bring the water and ginger to a boil over high heat. Reduce the heat, add the tea bags, and simmer for 2 minutes. Remove from the heat. Remove the tea bags. Cool the ginger-water mixture completely. Strain into a liquid measuring cup. There should be about ½ cup of liquid. Add the agave and additional water if needed to make ¾ cup.

Remove the peel from the oranges with a zester or citrus grater. Set aside the peel from 1 of the oranges and reserve the rest for another use, if you want. Peel the oranges. Slice the oranges horizontally into ½"-thick, round slices. Place in a medium mixing bowl. Add the blueberries.

Stir the lemon juice and vanilla extract into the ginger infusion. Pour the syrup over the fruit and toss carefully. Divide among 6 dessert bowls. Garnish with almonds, mint, and reserved orange peel. Drizzle with the Pomegranate Syrup.

✳ **ORANGE FACTOID:** In addition to folate, potassium, and fiber, one medium orange provides 130 percent of a day's requirement for vitamin C.

NUTRIENT ANALYSIS PER SERVING
123 calories, 1 g protein, 30 g carbohydrates, 1 g total fat, 0 g saturated fat, 1 g monounsaturated fat, 40 mg omega-3s, 22 g sugar, 6 g fiber, 9 mg sodium

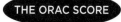

THE ORAC SCORE

SWEET SUBSTITUTES

With the explosive rise of obesity and diabetes, artificial sweeteners are wildly popular, distinctly for their lack of calories. This is certainly a seductive alternative for many in their battle at losing weight or keeping blood sugars in check. But if you're looking for a more natural, potentially healthier option, there are other choices you may not have considered. They do have calories, but this handful of sweeteners offers other healthy attributes, such as antioxidant oomph which is not found in nutrient-void sugars or artificial ingredients. Before you grab a supersize spoon, remember, moderation is always key.

SWEETENER PER TBSP	ORAC
Blackstrap molasses	5,366
Sorghum syrup	1,206
Brown rice syrup	857
Tupelo honey	512
Agave nectar	320

Almond Berry Bars

MAKES 32 BARS

Great for breakfast on the go, these wheat-free bars are a terrific anytime snack. There are unlimited variations to this recipe, using different nuts, nut butters, and dried fruits.

3 cups old-fashioned rolled oats

$\frac{1}{2}$ cup soy flour

$\frac{1}{4}$ cup sorghum flour or whole wheat flour

$\frac{1}{4}$ cup nonfat dry milk powder

$\frac{1}{2}$ cup oat bran

$\frac{1}{2}$ cup ground flaxseed

$\frac{1}{2}$ cup toasted chopped almonds

$\frac{1}{2}$ cup dried blueberries

$\frac{1}{2}$ cup chopped dried cherries

$\frac{1}{2}$ teaspoon salt

1 cup agave nectar

$\frac{1}{3}$ cup natural almond butter, stirred well before measuring

$\frac{1}{4}$ cup almond milk

2 teaspoons pure vanilla extract

Preheat the oven to 325°F. Lightly coat a 13" × 9" baking pan with olive oil cooking spray.

In a large mixing bowl, combine the oats, flours, milk powder, bran, flaxseed, almonds, blueberries, cherries, and salt. Stir to combine well. Set aside.

In a small saucepan, warm the agave nectar, nut butter, and almond milk over low heat until blended. Do not boil. Remove from the heat and stir in the vanilla extract.

Add the warm nut butter mixture to the dry ingredients and quickly stir the mixture until it is well combined. Pat into the prepared pan. Press firmly with your hands to remove any air pockets. Bake for 30 minutes, or until light golden brown.

Cool for 10 minutes, then cut into 32 bars.

When just cool enough to handle, remove the bars from the pan to a cooling rack. Store in airtight containers in the refrigerator for optimal freshness.

✳ **OATMEAL FACTOID:** This incredible edible grain is a staple in kitchens as well as in beauty products. The anti-inflammatory properties of oats provide relief from dry and itchy skin, so it's often used in soaps, bath products, and skin scrubs.

NUTRIENT ANALYSIS PER BAR
130 Calories, 4 g protein, 20 g carbohydrates, 4 g total fat, 0 g saturated fat, 0 g monounsaturated fat, 52 mg omega-3s, 3 g fiber, 9 g sugar, 63 mg sodium

Aging Research/Support/Resources

- AARP: www.aarp.org
- American Aging Association: www.americanaging.org
- International Council on Active Aging: www.icaa.cc
- National Institute on Aging: www.nia.nih.gov
- Okinawa Centenarian Study: www.okicent.org

ALZHEIMER'S DISEASE

- Alzheimer's Association: www.alz.org
- Alzheimer's Foundation of America: www.alzfdn.org

BONE HEALTH

- National Osteoporosis Foundation: www.nof.org; 800-223-9994

CANCER

- American Cancer Society: www.cancer.org

CALORIE RESTRICTION

- Calorie Restriction Society: www.calorierestriction.org

DIABETES

- American Association of Diabetes Educators: www.aadenet.org
- American Diabetes Association: www.diabetes.org
- CDC diabetes public health resource: www.cdc.gov/diabetes

HEART HEALTH

- American Heart Association: www.americanheart.org

MENOPAUSE

- Template for a menstrual journal: www.pms.org.uk Menstrual%20Chart.doc or www.mymonthlycycles.com
- Home menopause test kit: www.boomersexualhealth.com
- www.myscentuelle.com
- North American Menopause Society: www.menopause.org

MUSCLES AND EXERCISE

- American College of Sports Medicine: www.acsm.org

NUTRITION

- American Dietetic Association: www.eatright.org
- Center for Science in the Public Interest: www.cspinet.org
- Office of Dietary Supplements: http://dietary-supplements.info.nih.gov
- USDA Food and Nutrition Information Center: www.nal.usda.gov/fnic (recommended dietary intakes)
- USDA Food Composition Database: www.nal.usda.gov/fnic/foodcomp/Data/index.html

ORAC TESTING

- Brunswick Labs: www.brunswicklabs.com

STROKE

- American Stroke Association: www.strokeassociation.org

TEETH

- American Dental Association: www.ada.org

VISION

- National Eye Institute: www.nei.nih.gov

BODY-FAT SCALE

Tanita
847-640-9241
www.tanita.com
Body fat and body composition monitors

CALCIUM SUPPLEMENTS

www.cherylforberg.com
Calcium supplementation information and supplements

OMEGA-3 SUPPLEMENTS

www.cherylforberg.com
Omega-3 supplementation information and supplements

POSITIVELY AGELESS FOODS

Madhava
800-530-2900
www.wildorganics.net
Organic agave nectar, honey

Melissa's/World Variety Produce
PO Box 21127
Los Angeles, CA 90021
800-588-0151
www.melissas.com
Organic agave nectar, organic and exotic fruits and vegetables, whole grains, organic
    food products, herbs, nuts, gift baskets

Efoodpantry
PO Box 3483
Springfield, IL 62708
866-372-6879 (866-epantry)
www.efoodpantry.com
custsvc@efoodpantry.com
Organic natural cocoa powder, spices, natural products, gluten-free products,
   sugar-free products, low-sodium products

Scharffen Berger Chocolate Maker
914 Heinz Avenue
Berkeley, CA 94710
800-930-4528
www.scharffenberger.com
Unsweetened natural cocoa powder

Heintzman Farms
RR 2, Box 265
Onaka, SD 57466
605-447-5813
www.heintzmanfarms.com
Flaxseed

Bob's Red Mill Natural Foods
5209 SE International Way
Milwaukie, OR 97222
800-349-2173
www.bobsredmill.net
Whole grain flours, gluten-free flours, seeds, beans, bulk grains

Ezekiel 4:9
www.foodforlife.com
Whole grain breads and cereals

Hodgson Mill
1100 Stevens Avenue
Effingham, IL 62401
800-347-0105
www.hodgsonmill.com
Whole grains

Sun Organic Farm
888-269-9888
www.sunorganic.com
Grains and flours; organic food products including beans and legumes, flax, nuts and
   seeds, and oils

The Nut Factory
PO Box 815
Greenacres, WA 99016
888-239-5288
www.thenutfactory.com
Year-round supply of nuts in shell—walnuts, almonds, filberts, and Brazil nuts

Nuts Online
www.nutsonline.com
800-558-6887; 908-523-0333
Year-round supply of nuts in shell—walnuts, almonds, filberts, Brazil nuts, pecans, pistachios, and peanuts

Living Tree Community Foods
800-260-5534; 510-526-7106
www.livingtreecommunity.com
Nuts, nut butters, oils, agave nectar

Alaskan Harvest
8040 SE Stark Street
Portland, OR 97215
800-824-6389; 888-824-4278
www.alaskanharvest.com
Sustainably harvested wild ivory king salmon; king, silver, and sockeye salmon; and Alaskan Black Cod available year-round

Vital Choice Seafood
605 30th Street
Anacortes, WA 98221
www.vitalchoice.com
800-608-4825
Sustainably harvested wild salmon, sablefish, scallops, tuna, and more

Kalustyan's
123 Lexington Avenue
New York, NY 10016
800-352-3451; 212-685-3451
www.kalustyans.com
Spices, teas, beans, grains, chipotle chiles, pomegranate syrup, tahini, natural cocoa powder

Penzey's Spices
800-741-7787
www.penzeys.com
Unsweetened natural cocoa powder, spices

Twin Valley Mills
RR 1, Box 45
Ruskin, NE 68974
402-279-3965
www.twinvalleymills.com
Sorghum flour

Making Tracks Sorghum syrup
P.O. Box 4898
Chatsworth, CA 91313-4898
800-488-8898
www.makingtracks.com
makingtracks@hotmail.com
Sorghum syrup

SpecialTeas
500 Long Beach Boulevard
Stratford, CT 06615
888-365-6983 (888-enjoy-tea)
www.specialteas.com
Matcha green tea

Stash Tea Company
PO Box 910
Portland, OR 97207
800-826-4218
www.stashtea.com
Specialty teas including black teas, herbals, green, white, matcha, decaf, and
    organic teas

Though this book was written using the most recent research available, new studies
emerge every day on the health benefits conferred by a wide variety of foods and
beverages. Please visit our companion website, www.cherylforberg.com, for research
updates as well as additional resources.

SOURCES

INTRODUCTION

1. www.census.gov/prod/99pubs/p23-199.pdf

2. www.cdc.gov/nchs/data/hus/hus05.pdf#027

3. http://webapp.cdc.gov/sasweb/ncipc/leadcaus10.html.

4. T. Perls, "The Different Paths to Age One Hundred," *Annals of the NY Academy of Sciences* 2005;1055:13–25.

5. Bradley J. Willcox and D. Craig Willcox, *The Okinawa Program*. New York: Clarkson Potter (2001).

6. A. Manning, "Aging Gracefully Is the Biggest Concern," *USA Today*, http://www.usatoday.com/news/health/2005-10-23-aging-side_x.htm.

7. Sohal, et al., "Mechanisms of Aging: An Appraisal of the Oxidative Stress Hypothesis," *Free Radical Biology & Medicine* September 1, 2002;33(5):575–86.

8. J. Vina, et al., "Mitochondrial Theory of Aging: Importance to Explain Why Females Live Longer Than Males," *Antioxidants & Redox Signaling* October 2003;5(5):549–56.

9. J. Vina, "Why Females Live Longer Than Males: Control of Longevity by Sex Hormones," *Science of Aging Knowledge Environment* June 8, 2005;(23):17

10. www.americanheart.org/presenter.jhtml?identifier=2876

11. http://circ.ahajournals.org/cgi/content/full/113/6/e85/TBL32

12. www.americanheart.org/presenter.jhtml?identifier=4756

13. www.americanheart.org/presenter.jhtml?identifier=2876

14. www.americanheart.org/presenter.jhtml?identifier=2876

15. L. K. Heilbronn and E. Ravussin, "Calorie Restriction and Aging: Review of the Literature and Implications for Studies in Humans," *American Journal of Clinical Nutrition* 78;(2003):361–69.

16. E. N. Whitney and E. R. Rolfes, *Understanding Nutrition* (Wadsworth, 2002).

17. M. E. Shils, et al., *Modern Nutrition in Health and Disease*. Lippincott Williams and Wilkins (2006).

18. B. J. Merry, "Oxidative Stress and Mitochondrial Function with Aging—the Effects of Calorie Restriction," *Aging Cell* 3: (2004):7–12.

19. H. Vlassara and M. R. Palace, "Glycoxidation: The Menace of Diabetes and Aging," *Mount Sinai Journal of Medicine* September 4, 2003;70(4):232–41.

20. T. Goldberg, et al., "Advanced Glycoxidation End Products in Commonly Consumed Foods," *Journal of the American Dietetic Association* August 2004;104(8):1287–91.

21. Uribarri, J. et al., "Diet-Derived Advanced Glycation End Products Are Major Contributors to the Body's AGE Pool and Induce Inflammation in Healthy Subjects," *Annals of the New York Academy of Science* 1043 (2005): 461–466.

22. Heart Disease and Stroke Statistics—2006 Update, *Circulation* 113 (2006): e85–e151.

23. www.cancer.org/downloads/STT/CAFF2006PWSecured.pdf

24. http://diabetes.niddk.nih.gov/dm/pubs/statistics/index.htm#13

25. www.nof.org/osteoporosis/diseasefacts.htm

26. www.nei.nih.gov/eyedata/pdf/VPUS.pdf

27. http://apps.nccd.cdc.gov/nohss/ListV.asp

28. D. Sarkar and P. B. Fisher, "Molecular Mechanisms of Aging-Associated Inflammation," *Cancer Letters* 236, no. 1 (2006)13–23.

29. http://apps.nccd.cdc.gov/brfss/Trends/trendchart.asp?qkey=10150&state=US

30. www.healthypeople.gov/document/html/volume2/19nutrition.htm#_ednref45

31. G. S. Roth,D. K. Ingram, and M. A. Lane, "Caloric Restriction in Primates and Relevance to Humans," *Annals of the New York Academy of Sciences* April 2001;928:305–15.

32. H. K. Heilbronn, et al., "Effect of 6-Month Calorie Restriction on Biomarkers of Longevity, Metabolic Adaptation, and Oxidative Stress in Overweight Individuals," *Journal of the American Medical Association* April 5, 2006; 295(13):1539–48.

WEEK ONE:

1. http://texasheart.org/HIC/Anatomy/coroanat.cfm

2. Heart, How it Works, www.americanheart.org/presenter.jhtml?identifier=4642.

3. R. C. Tallis and H. M. Fillet, *Geriatric Medicine and Gerontology.*

4. Heart, How it Works, www.americanheart.org/presenter.jhtml?identifier=4642.

5. Angina, www.americanheart.org/presenter.jhtml?identifier=4472

6. Heart Attack, www.americanheart.org/presenter.jhtml?identifier=4578

7. Congestive Heart Failure, www.americanheart.org/presenter.jhtml?identifier=4585

8. Cholesterol, www.americanheart.org/presenter.jhtml?identifier=4488

9. Risk Factors and Coronary Heart Disease, www.americanheart.org/presenter.jhtml?identifier=4726

10. www.nature.com/nm/journal/v8/n11/full/nm1102-1211.html

11. A. Lapoint, et al., "Effects of Dietary Factors on Oxidation of Low-Density Lipoprotein Particles," *Journal of Nutritional Biochemistry* October 2006;17(10):645–58.

12. Diabetes Mellitus, www.americanheart.org/presenter. jhtml?identifier=4546

13. Metabolic Syndrome, www.americanheart.org/presenter. jhtml?identifier=4756

14. High Blood Pressure, www.mayoclinic.com/health/high-blood-pressure/DS00100/DSECTION=2

15. What Is High Blood Pressure? www.nhlbi.nih.gov/health/dci/Diseases/ Hbp/HBP_WhatIs.html, www.americanheart.org/presenter. jhtml?identifier=4756

16. www.nhlbi.nih.gov/health/public/heart/hbp/dash/new_dash.pdf

17. www.nhlbi.nih.gov/guidelines/hypertension/express.pdf

18. M. E. Shils, et al., *Modern Nutrition in Health and Disease*: 1099–1101.

19. Y-C Yang, et al., "The Protective Effect of Habitual Tea Consumption on Hypertension, *Archives of Internal Medicine* July 26, 2004;164(14):1534–40.

20. What Are Healthy Levels of Cholesterol? www.americanheart.org/ presenter.jhtml?identifier=183

21. Lowering Your Cholesterol with TLC, www.nhlbi.nih.gov/health/ public/heart/chol/chol_tlc.pdf

22. www.hsph.harvard.edu/nutritionsource/fats.html

23. Fish and Omega-3 Fatty Acids, www.americanheart.org/presenter. jhtml?identifier=4632

24. L. Fontana, et al., "Long-Term Calorie Restriction Is Highly Effective in Reducing the Risk for Atherosclerosis in Humans," *Proceedings of the National Academy of Sciences USA* April 27, 2004;101(17):6659–63.

25. Markers of Inflammation and Cardiovascular Disease, www.american-heart.org/downloadable/heart/1043429236960hc0303000499.pdf

26. Inflammation, Heart Disease and Stroke, www.americanheart.org/ presenter.jhtml?identifier=4648

27. AHA/CDC panel issues report, www.americanheart.org/presenter. jhtml?identifier=3007984

28. K. Niu, et al., "Dietary Long-Chain n-3 Fatty Acids of Marine Origin and Serum C-Reactive Protein Concentrations are Associated in a Population with a Diet Rich in Marine Products," *American Journal of Nutrition* July 2006;84:223–29.

29. C. Chrysohoou, et al., "Adherence to the Mediterranean Diet Attenuates Inflammation and Coagulation Process in Healthy Adults: The ATTICA Study," *Journal of the American College of Cardiology* July 7, 3004;44(1):152–58.

30. D. B. Panagiotakos, et al., "The Associations between Physical Activity, Inflammation, and Coagulation Markers, in People with Metabolic Syndrome: The ATTICA study," *European Journal of Cardiovascular Prevention and Rehabilitation* April 2005;12:151–58.

31. What Is Cancer? www.cancer.org/docroot/CRI/content/CRI_2_4_1x_What_Is_Cancer.asp?sitearea=

32. D. Warshawsky and J. R. Landolph, *Molecular Carcinogenesis and the Molecular Biology of Human Cancer.*

33. Who Gets Cancer? www.cancer.org/docroot/CRI/content/CRI_2_4_1x_Who_gets_cancer.asp?sitearea=.

34. Known and Probable Carcinogens, www.cancer.org/docroot/PED/content/PED_1_3x_Known_and_Probable_Carcinogens.asp?sitearea=PED.

35. R. C. Tallis and H. M. Fillit, *Geriatric Medicine and Gerontology.*

36. M. E. Shils, et al., *Modern Nutrition in Health and Disease.*

37. G. Block, B. Patterson, and A. Subar, "Fruit, Vegetables, and Cancer Prevention: A Review of the Epidemiological Evidence," *Nutr Cancer* 1992;18(1):1–29.

38. A. Basu, et al., "Tomatoes versus Lycopene in Oxidative Stress and Carcinogenesis: Conclusions from Clinical Trials," *European Journal of Clinical Nutrition* March 2007;61(3):295–303.

39. S. Gallus, et al., "Mediterranean Diet and Cancer Risk," *European Journal of Cancer Prevention* 2004;13:447–52.

40. N. J. Temple, et al., *Nutritional Health: Strategies for Disease Prevention.*

41. S. D. Hursting, et al., "Calorie Restriction, Aging, and Cancer Prevention," *Annual Review of Medicine* 2003;54:131-52).

42. Samad, AK et all"A Meta-Analysis of the Association of Physical Activity with Reduced Risk of Colorectal Cancer." 2005 May;7(3):204-13

43. Stomach Cancer, www.mayoclinic.com/health/stomach-cancer/DS00301/DSECTION=1.

44. Heterocyclic Amines in Cooked Meats, www.cancer.gov/cancertopics/factsheet/Risk/heterocyclic-amines.

45. What Are the Risk Factors for Breast Cancer? www.cancer.org/docroot/CRI/content/CRI_2_4_2X_What_are_the_risk_factors_for_breast_cancer_5.asp?rnav=cri.

46. Risk Factors and Prevention. www.komen.org/intradoc-cgi/idc_cgi_isapi.dll?IdcService=SS_GET_PAGE&ssDocName=AbcGettingOlder.

47. Breast Cancer: Risk Factors, www.mayoclinic.com/health/breast-cancer/DS00328/DSECTION=4.

48. Genetic Testing for BRCA1 and BRCA2, www.cancer.gov/cancertopics/factsheet/Risk/BRCA

49. Breast cancer screening, www.cancer.gov/cancertopics/pdq/screening/breast/Patient/page3.

50. What Causes Endometrial Cancer? www.cancer.org/docroot/CRI/content/CRI_2_2_2x_What_causes_endometrial_cancer.asp?rnav=cri.

51. Endometrial Cancer Screening, www.cancer.gov/cancertopics/pdq/screening/endometrial/Patient/page3.

52. P. L. Horn-Ross, et al., "Phytoestrogen Intake and Endometrial Cancer

Risk," *Journal of the National Cancer Institute* (J Natl Cancer Inst. 2003 Aug 6;95(15):1158-64).

53. Shin, MH et al "Intake of Dairy Products, Calcium, and Vitamin D and Risk of Breast Cancer" J Natl Cancer Inst. 2002 Sep 4;94(17):1301-11

54. What Causes Colorectal Cancer? www.cancer.org/docroot/CRI/content/CRI_2_2_2X_What_causes_colorectal_cancer.asp?rnav=cri.

55. What Is Colorectal Cancer? www.cancer.org/docroot/CRI/content/CRI_2_2_1X_What_is_colon_and_rectum_cancer_10.asp?rnav=cri.

56. Colorectal Cancer Screening, www.cancer.gov/cancertopics/pdq/screening/colorectal/Patient/page3.

57. *Geriatric Medicine and Gerontology* (2003): 943, 1027, 1038.

58. http://digestive.niddk.nih.gov/ddiseases/pubs/yrdd/

59. *Merck Manual—home edition.*

60. Merck, www.merck.com/mrkshared/CVMHighLight?file=/pubs/mmanual_ha/sec3/ch54/ch54c.html%3Fregion%3Dmerckcom&word=reflux&domain=www.merck.com#hl_anchor.

61. National Institutes of Health, http://digestive.niddk.nih.gov/ddiseases/pubs/gerd/#6.

62. Mayo. www.mayoclinic.com/health/heartburn-gerd/DS00095/DSECTION=3.

63. Mayo Clinic, www.mayoclinic.com/health/gallstones/DS00165/DSECTION=9.

64. www.aafp.org/afp/990301ap/1161.html

65. Mayo. www.mayoclinic.com/health/heartburn-gerd/DS00095/DSECTION=5.

66. National Institutes of Health, http://digestive.niddk.nih.gov/ddiseases/pubs/gerd/#4.

67. *Modern Nutrition in Health and Disease*: 1185, 1523, 1194–96.

68. Merck. www.merck.com/mrkshared/CVMHighLight?file=/pubs/mmanual_ha/sec1/ch02/ch02k.html%3Fregion%3Dmerckcom&word=lactose&domain=www.merck.com#hl_anchor.

69. Mayo, www.mayoclinic.com/health/lactose-intolerance/DS00530/DSECTION=3.

70. http://digestive.niddk.nih.gov/ddiseases/pubs/lactoseintolerance/

71. http://digestive.niddk.nih.gov/ddiseases/pubs/lactoseintolerance/#diagnosed

72. Mayo, www.mayoclinic.com/health/celiac-disease/DS00319/DSECTION=8.

73. National Institutes of Health, http://digestive.niddk.nih.gov/ddiseases/pubs/celiac/

74. http://digestive.niddk.nih.gov/ddiseases/pubs/celiac/#5

75. Celiac Sprue Association, www.csaceliacs.org/gluten_choices.php

76. "Physical Activity and Decreased Risk of Clinical Gallstone Disease among Post-Menopausal Women"

77. NIH, http://digestive.niddk.nih.gov/ddiseases/pubs/gallstones/index.htm#diagnosed

78. www.mayoclinic.com/health/gallstones/DS00165/DSECTION=6

79. *Merck Manual of Health and Aging*

80. Mayo Clinic, www.mayoclinic.com/health/constipation/DS00063/DSECTION=1.

81. Eiirenpreis E et al, Irritable bowel syndrome. 10% to 20% of older adults have symptoms consistent with diagnosis. Geriatrics. 2005 Jan;60(1):25-8.

82. National Institutes of Health, http://digestive.niddk.nih.gov/ddiseases/pubs/ibs_ez/.

83. www.mayoclinic.com/health/irritable-bowel-syndrome/DS00106/DSECTION=10

84. National Institutes of Health. http://digestive.niddk.nih.gov/ddiseases/pubs/diverticulosis/

85. www.mayoclinic.com/health/diverticulitis/DS00070/DSECTION=8

86. Marlett, J. A., et al., "Health Implications of Dietary Fiber," *Journal of the American Dietitians Association* July 2002;102(7):993-1000

87. http://digestive.niddk.nih.gov/ddiseases/pubs/hpylori/index.htm

88. www.niaid.nih.gov/publications/immune/the_immune_system.pdf

89. www.merck.com/mmhe/sec16/ch186/ch186a.html?qt=autoimmune&alt=sh

90. www.merck.com/mmhe/sec16/ch183/ch183d.html

91. *Geriatric Medicine and Gerontology*: 115–116.

92. Christian R, Gomez, 1, 2, Eric D Boehmer,1 and Elizabeth J Kovacs, *The Aging Innate Immune System.*

93. *Medical Immunology Made Memorable*:11.

94. Devan Sakara and Paul B. Fisher, "Molecular Mechanisms of Aging-Associated Inflammation."

95. Marx J. "Inflammation and Cancer: The Link Grows Stronger," *Science* 2004 Nov 5;306(5698):966-8

96. www.nlm.nih.gov/medlineplus/ency/article/003356.htm

97. www.arthritis.org/conditions/diseasecenter/ra/ra_diagnosis2.asp

98. www.nlm.nih.gov/medlineplus/ency/article/003638.htm

99. www.nlm.nih.gov/medlineplus/ency/article/003643.htm

100. www.nlm.nih.gov/medlineplus/ency/article/003516.htm

101. www.nlm.nih.gov/medlineplus/ency/article/003329.htm

102. Simopoulos, A. P., "Omega-3 Fatty Acids in Inflammation and Autoimmune Diseases," *Journal of the American College of Nutrition* December 2002;21(6):495–505

103. Stamp, L. K., et al., "Diet and Rheumatoid Arthritis: A Review of the Literature," *Semin Arthritis and Rheumatology* October 2005;35(2):77–94

104. Haglund O. "Effects of a New Fluid Fish Oil Concentrate, Eskimo-3, on Triglycerides, Cholesterol, Fibrinogen and Blood Pressure," *Journal of Internal Medicine* May 1990;227(5):347–53

105. Simopoulos, A. P. "Omega-3 Fatty Acids in Inflammation and Autoimmune Diseases." *Journal of the American College of Nutrtition* 21 (December 2002): 495–505.

106. Mischoulon, D., et al. "Docosahexanoic Acid and Omega-3 Fatty Acids in Depression," *The Psychiatric Clinics of North America* 23 (2000): 785–94.

107. Jae SY et al "Effects of Lifestyle Modifications on C-Reactive Protein: Contribution of Weight Loss and Improved Aerobic Capacity." *Metabolism* 2006 Jun;55(6):825-31

108. Arpita Basu, Sridevi Devaraj, Ishwarlal Jialal, and Margo Denke, series ed., *Dietary Factors That Promote or Retard Inflammation.*

109. I. Rahman, S. K. Biswas, and P. A. Kirkham, "Regulation of Inflammation and Redox Signaling by detary Polyphenols," *Biochemical Pharmacology* 72, no. 2 (November 30, 2006):1439–52.

110. "Low Serum Selenium and Total Carotenoids Predict Mortality among Older Women Living in the Community: The Women's Health and Aging Studies."

111. Catherine J. Field, Ian R. Johnson, and Patricia D. Schley, "Nutrients and Their Role in Host Resistance to Infection." *Journal of Leukoc Biology* January 2002;71(1):16–32.

112. Institute of Medicine, *Dietary Reference Intakes (DRIs): Recommended Intakes for Individuals Food and Nutrition Board,* Washington, DC: National Academies Press.

113. U. Singh, et al., "Vitamin E, Oxidative Stress, and Inflammation," *Annual Review of Nutrition* 25(2005):151–74.

114. A. L. Ray, et al., "Low Serum Selenium and Total Carotenoids Predict Mortality among Older Women Living in the Community: The Women's Health and Aging Studies," *The Journal of Nutrition* 136 (2006): 172–6.

115. *Understanding Nutrition*: 446.

116. Gibney, *Clinical Nutrition*: 259, 256

117. Gill, H S1; Guarner, F2. "Probiotics and Human Health: A Clinical Perspective." *Postgrad Med J.* 2004 Sep;80(947):516-26

118. Tomoi Sato and Go Miyata, The Nutraceutical Benefit, Part I: Green Tea. April 2000;16(4):315-7

119. www.nlm.nih.gov/medlineplus/ency/article/007165.htm

120. M. L. Sopori and W. Kozak, "Immunomodulatory Effects of Cigarette Smoke," *Journal of Neuroimmunology* 1998 Mar 15;83(1-2):148-56.

121. Robert Brown Taylor and Alan K. David, *Family Medicine—Principles and Practice*

122. www.mayoclinic.com/health/fatigue/HQ00673

123. www.cdc.gov/cfs/cfsbasicfacts.htm

124. www.nlm.nih.gov/medlineplus/ency/article/003088.htm

125. www.mayoclinic.com/health/hypothyroidism/DS00353/DSECTION=1

126. www.mayoclinic.com/health/hyperthyroidism/DS00344

127. www.nlm.nih.gov/medlineplus/ency/article/000584.htm

128. www.sleepfoundation.org/hottopics/index.php?secid=9&id=31

129. http://familydoctor.org/212.xml

WEEK TWO:

1. http://diabetes.niddk.nih.gov/dm/pubs/statistics/index_dtag. htm#age

2. http://diabetes.niddk.nih.gov/dm/pubs/statistics/index.htm#7

3. http://diabetes.niddk.nih.gov/dm/pubs/overview/index.htm#what

4. http://diabetes.niddk.nih.gov/dm/pubs/stroke/index.htm

5. http://diabetes.niddk.nih.gov/dm/pubs/complications_heart/index. htm

6. http://diabetes.niddk.nih.gov/dm/pubs/complications_eyes/index. htm#hurt

7. http://diabetes.niddk.nih.gov/dm/pubs/complications_kidneys/index. htm#6

8. http://diabetes.niddk.nih.gov/dm/pubs/complications_feet/index. htm#3

9. http://diabetes.niddk.nih.gov/dm/pubs/insulinresistance/index.htm#2

10. http://www.merck.com/mmhe/sec13/ch165/ch165a.html#sec13-ch165-ch165a-289

11. http://www.diabetes.org/pre-diabetes/pre-diabetes-symptoms.jsp

12. http://www.diabetes.org/type-2-diabetes/blood-glucose-checks.jsp

13. http://diabetes.niddk.nih.gov/dm/pubs/type1and2/Daily.htm#4

14. http://www.diabetes.org/type-1-diabetes/a1c-test.jsp

15. "Reduction in the Incidence of Type 2 Diabetes with Lifestyle Intervention or Metformin"

16. "Evidence-Based Nutrition Principles and Recommendations for the Treatment and Prevention of Diabetes and Related Complications"

17. Lydia A. Bazzano, Mary Serdula, and Simin Liu, *Prevention of Type 2 Diabetes by Diet and Lifestyle Modification.*

18. "Chromium Picolinate Supplementation Attenuates Body Weight Gain and Increases Insulin Sensitivity in Subjects with Type 2 Diabetes."

19. Food and Nutrition Board, Institute of Medicine, *Dietary Reference Intakes (DRIs): Recommended Intakes for Individuals*, Washington, DC: National Academies Press.

20. Study quoted in "Role of Sleep Duration and Quality in the Risk and Severity of Type 2 Diabetes Mellitus."

21. I. Shai, et al., "Ethnicity, Obesity, and Risk of Type 2 diabetes in Women: A 20-Year Follow-Up Study," *Diabetes Care* 29, no. 7 (July 2006): 1585–90.

22. Y. Ma, et al., "Association between Carbohydrate Intake and Serum Lipids." *J Am Coll Nutr.* 25, no 2 (April 2006): 155–63.

23. Jennie Brand-Miller, Thomas Wolever, Kaye Foster-Powell, and Stephen Colagiuri, *The New Glucose Revolution*, New York: Marlowe & Company, 2003.

24. http://www.mayoclinic.com/health/menopause/DS00119/DSECTION=1

25. http://www.niapublications.org/agepages/menopause.asp

26. *Current Obstetric and Gynecologic Diagnosis and Treatment*, 2003.

27. "Menopause Guidebook," North American Menopause Society, http://www.menopause.org/edumaterials/guidebook/mgtoc.htm.

28. http://www.nhlbi.nih.gov/health/women/pht_facts.pdf

29. Dana G. Carroll, *Nonhormonal Therapies for Hot Flashes in Menopause.*

30. A. Vincent, "Soy Isoflavones: Are They Useful in Menopause?" *Mayo Clinic Proceedings* 75, no. 11 (November 2000): 1174–84.

31. M. Messina and C. J. Hughes, "Efficacy of Soyfoods and Soybean Ioflavone Supplements for Alleviating Menopausal Symptoms Is Positively Related to Initial Hot Flush Frequency," *Journal of Medicinal Food* 6, no. 1 (Spring 2003):1–11.

32. Laura Harkness, Soy and Bone: Where Do We Stand?

33. Pamela Peeke, *Body for Life for Women.*

34. D. Mischoulon, et al., "Docosahexanoic Acid and Omega-3 Fatty acids in Depression," *Psychiatric Clinics of North America* 23, no. 4 (December 2000): 785–94.

35. V. Lerner, et al., "Vitamin B_{12} and Folate Serum Levels in Newly Admitted Psychiatric Patients," *Clinical Nutrition* 25, no. 1 (February 2006): 6–7.

36. Y. Osher, et al., "Clinical Trials of PUFAs in Depression: State of the Art," *World Journal of Biological Psychiatry* 7, no. 4 (2006): 223–30.

37. Lee, S., et al., "Current Clinical Applications of Omega-6 and Omega-3 Fatty Acids. *Nutrition in Clinical Practice* 21, no. 4 (August 2006): 323–41.

38. B. L. Seaward, *Managing Stress.*

39. http://www.mayoclinic.com/health/stress/SR00001

40. "Stress Hormones in Health and Illness: The Roles of Work and Gender."

41. "Stress, Breakfast Cereal Consumption and Cortisol," *Nutritional Neuroscience* 5, no. 2 (April 2002): 141–4.

42. http://www.alz.org/brain/overview.asp

43. http://www.nia.nih.gov/Alzheimers/Publications/UnravelingTheMystery/Part1/NeuronsAndTheirJobs.htm

44. http://www.strokeassociation.org/downloadable/stroke/1095278734638What_Is_a_Stroke_Final%20Science%20review%206-03-03%20vF3.pdf

45. http://www.alz.org/Resources/FactSheets/basics_of_alz_low.pdf

46. http://www.nlm.nih.gov/medlineplus/tutorials/preventingstrokes/hp139102.pdf

47. http://www.ninds.nih.gov/disorders/stroke/preventing_stroke.htm#Treatable%20Risk%20Factors

48. T. J. Moore, et al., "DASH (Dietary Approaches to Stop Hypertension) Diet Is Effective Treatment for Stage 1 Isolated Systolic Hypertension." *Hypertension* 38, no. 2 (August 2001): 155–8.

49. K. C. McDonald, "Clinical inquiries: What Lifestyle Changes Should We Recommend for the Patient with Newly Diagnosed Hypertension?" *Journal of Family Practice* 55, no. 11 (November 2006): 991–3.

50. J. David Spence, *Nutrition and Stroke Prevention*

51. http://www.americanheart.org/presenter.jhtml?identifier=535

52. http://www.americanheart.org/presenter.jhtml?identifier=4742

53. http://www.americanheart.org/presenter.jhtml?identifier=4742

54. http://www.alz.org/Resources/FactSheets/basics_of_alz_low.pdf

55. Kaj Blennow, Mony J.de Leon, and Henrik Zetterberg, *Alzheimer's disease,*

56. http://www.nia.nih.gov/Alzheimers/Publications/UnravelingTheMystery/Part1/Hallmarks.htm

57. Jeffrey L. Cummings, *Alzheimer's Disease.*

58. "Reduced Risk of Alzheimer Disease in Users of Antioxidant Vitamin Supplements: The Cache County Study."

59. http://www.alz.org/icad/newsreleases/071606_noon_diabtesandad.asphttp://www.alz.org/icad/newsreleases/071606_noon_diabtesandad.asp

60. "Aggregation of Vascular Risk Factors and Risk of Incident Alzheimer Disease."[Articles]

61. Nikolaos Scarmeas, *Mediterranean Diet and Risk for Alzheimer's Disease.*

62. Sudha Seshadri, "Plasma Homocysteine as a Risk Factor for Dementia and Alzheimer's Disease."

63. http://www.alz.org/maintainyourbrain/mactive.asp

64. "Late-Life Engagement in Social and Leisure Activities Is Associated with a Decreased Risk of Dementia: A Longitudinal Study from the Kungsholmen Project."

65. http://www.alz.org/maintainyourbrain/socially.asp

WEEK THREE:

1. *Understanding Nutrition*, 2002: 403, 421.
2. *Geriatric Medicine and Gerontology.* 2003: pages 863, 865–866.
3. "Management of Osteoporosis in Postmenopausal Women: 2006 Position Statement of the North American Menopause Society"
4. http://www.niams.nih.gov/bone/hi/overview.htm
5. http://www.nof.org/osteoporosis/diseasefacts.htm
6. http://www.niams.nih.gov/bone/hi/prevent_fracture.htm
7. *Current Obstetric and Gynecologic Diagnosis and Treatment,* 200.3
8. *Family Medicine: Principles and Practice,* 2003.
9. http://dietary-supplements.info.nih.gov/factsheets/calcium.asp#h5
10. *Modern Nutrition in Health and Disease*
11. http://www.nof.org/osteoporosis/bmdtest.htm
12. http://www.niams.nih.gov/bone/hi/osteoporosis_diagnosis.htm
13. http://www.mayoclinic.com/health/bone-density-tests/WO00024
14. Food and Nutrition Board, Institute of Medicine, "Dietary Reference Intakes (DRIs): Recommended Intakes for Individuals," Washington, DC: National Academies Press.
15. http://www.nof.org/prevention/calcium.htm
16. "Effects of High-Intensity Strength Training on Multiple Risk Factors for Osteoporotic Fractures: A Randomized Controlled Trial."
17. "Exercise for Prevention of Osteoporotic Fracture"
18. http://www.niams.nih.gov/bone/hi/prevent_fracture.htm
19. http://www.nof.org/prevention/exercise.htm
20. http://www.niams.nih.gov/bone/hi/prevent_falls.htm
21. http://www.niams.nih.gov/bone/hi/calcium_supp.htm
22. www.guideline.gov/summary/summary.aspx?doc_id=8151&nbr=4544&ss=6&xl=999
23. Dreyer, HC, et al, "Role of Protein and Amino Acids in the Pathophysiology and Treatment of Sarcopenia," *Journal of the American College of Nutrition*, April 2005, Apr;24(2):140S-145S.
24. Volpi, E, et al, "Muscle Tissue Changes with Aging," *Curr Opin Clin Nutr Metab Care*, July 2004 , 7(4):405-10.
25. Doherty, TJ, "Invited Review: Aging and Sarcopenia," *Journal of Applied Physiology*," Oct. 2003, 95(4):1717-27.
26. Evans, WJ, "Effects of Exercise on Senescent Muscle," *Clin Orthop Relat Res*, Oct. 2002, ;(403 Suppl):S211-20.
27. Evans, WJ, "Protein Nutrition, Exercise and Aging," *Journal of the American College of Nutrition*, Dec. 2004, 23(6 Suppl):601S-609S.
28. Hunter, GR, et al, "Effects of Resistance Training on Older Adults," *Sports Medicine*, 2004, 34(5):329-48.
29. Hans C. Dreyer and Elena Volpi, "Role of Protein and Amino Acids in the Pathophysiology and Treatment of Sarcopenia."

WEEK FOUR:

1. *The Perricone Prescription*
2. Tallis and Fillit, *Geriatric Medicine and Gerontology*, 2003: 1269–71.
3. http://www.skincarephysicians.com/agingskinnet/basicfacts.html
4. *Prevention and Treatment of Skin Aging*
5. http://www.niapublications.org/agepages/skin.asp
6. "The Receptor for Advanced Glycation End Products Is Highly Expressed in the Skin and Upregulated by Advanced Glycation End Products and Tumor Necrosis Factor-Alpha"
7. "Estrogen and Skin: The Effects of Estrogen, Menopause, and Hormone Replacement Therapy on the Skin."
8. Photoaging: Mechanisms and Repair
9. Oxidative Stress in the Pathogenesis of Skin Disease
10. H. Sies and W. Stahl, "Nutritional Protection against Skin Damage from Sunlight," *Annual Review of Nutrition* 24 (2004) :173–200
11. Chemoprevention of Nonmelanoma Skin Cancer
12. http://dietary-supplements.info.nih.gov/factsheets/vitamina.asp
13. *Geriatric Medicine and Gerontology*: 1273, 1171.
14. *Griffith's 5-Minute Medical Consult*
15. *Fitzpatrick's Color Atlas and Synopsis of Clinical Dermatology*
16. http://www.mayoclinic.com/health/gray-hair/AN00310
17. http://www.webmd.com/content/article/78/95827.htm
18. Nutritional Factors and Hair Loss
19. *Geriatric Medicine and Gerontology*
20. http://www.ada.org/prof/resources/topics/science_perio_coronary.asp
21. http://www.perio.org/consumer/mbc.heart.htm
22. http://www.perio.org/consumer/smileforlife.htm
23. Shils, et al., *Modern Nutrition in Health and Disease,* 2006.
24. http://www.umm.edu/patiented/articles/what_will_confirm_diagnosis_of_periodontal_disease_000024_7.htm
25. http://www.ada.org/public/topics/periodontal_diseases_faq.asp
26. http://www.nlm.nih.gov/medlineplus/ency/article/001055.htm
27. http://www.ada.org/public/topics/plaque.asp
28. http://www.ada.org/public/topics/cleaning.asp
29. http://diabetes.niddk.nih.gov/dm/pubs/complications_teeth/index.htm
30. http://www.cdc.gov/OralHealth/factsheets/adult.htm
31. http://www.nei.nih.gov/health/maculardegen/armd_facts.asp#2b
32. http://www.mayoclinic.com/health/macular-degeneration/DS00284/DSECTION=8

33. http://www.nei.nih.gov/health/diabetic/retinopathy.asp#1a

34. http://www.mayoclinic.com/health/diabetic-retinopathy/DS00447/DSECTION=4

35. http://www.nei.nih.gov/health/cataract/cataract_facts.asp#2a

36. Sybille Franke, "Increased Levels of Advanced Glycation End Products in Human Cataractous Lenses"

37. W. Stahl, "Macular Carotenoids: Lutein and Zeaxanthin," *Developments in Ophthalmology* 38 (2005): 70–88.

38. http://www.nei.nih.gov/news/statements/lutein.asp

WEEK FIVE: *POSITIVELY AGELESS* RECIPES

1. P. Ninfali, et al., "Antioxidant Capacity of Vegetables, Spices and Dressings relevant to Nutrition," *British Journal of Nutrition* 93, no. 2 (2005): 257–66.

2. Values from X. Wu, G. R. Beecher, J. M. Holden, D. B. Haytowitz, S. E. Gebhardt, and R. L. Prior, "Lipophilic and Hydrophilic Antioxidant Capacities of Common Foods in the United States," *Journal of Agriculture and Food Chemistry* 52, no. 12 (2004): 4026–37.

Underscored page references indicate sidebar notes. Boldfaced page references indicate photographs.

A

Advanced glycation end products
    (AGEs)
 about, 10
 Alzheimer's risk and, 166
 content of foods (table), 11
 created by glycation, 10
 diseases associated with, 10
 high blood sugar and, 130
 median daily intake of, 11
 outside sources of, 12
 in overcooked meats, 60
 prediabetes and buildup of, 10
 proteins cross-linked by, 10
 skin damage from, 222
 as wrinkling process contributors,
    10
Agave nectar, 28
Age-related macular degeneration
    (AMD), 18, 238–39, 240
Aging. See also Antiaging
 AGEs linked to diseases associated
    with, 10
 free radical damage as cause of, 5, 6
 growing numbers of centenarians, 1
 immune system and, 84
 longevity as measure of health, 2
 research growing in, 2–3
 risks increasing with
    autoimmune diseases, 85
    cancer, 16–17, 54, 55, 60–61, 68, 86
    dental problems, 234–35
    diabetes, 17, 127
    heart disease, 16, 38–39
    inflammation, 85–86
    muscle loss, 18, 195
    osteoporosis, 17–18, 187
    skin changes, 18, 231–32

 stroke, 17
 vision problems, 18, 238–39
 slowed by omega-3s, 64
 surgical and nonsurgical procedures
    postponing, 5
 top concerns about, 2
ALA omega-3s. See also Omega-3s
 conversion of, 64, 88, 260, 283
 sources of, 90, 111, 260, 283, 288
Alcohol. See also Wine
 avoiding during stress, 154
 cancer risk increased by, 58–59, 62
 diabetes risk reduced by, 140–41
 drinking in moderation, 31, 47,
    58–59, 101, 140–41
 fatigue increased by, 101
 high blood pressure linked to, 47
 osteoporosis risk and, 188, 193
Allium compounds, 58
Almond Berry Bars, 346–47
Almonds, 13, 338
Alopecia areata, 232
Alpha-linolenic acid. See ALA omega-
    3s
Alpha-tocopherol. See Vitamin E
Alzheimer's disease
 aging and risk of, 164, 165
 biomarkers, 166–67
 family history and risk of, 165
 free radical damage with, 13
 plaques and tangles with, 165
 prevalence of, 164
 preventing, 167–69
 risk factors that can be changed,
    165–66
 Symptoms of, 164
AMD. See Age-related macular
    degeneration

Amenorrhea, 187–88
Angina, 40, 41
Anthocyanin antioxidants, <u>44</u>, 299
Antiaging. *See also* Aging
  beet benefits for, 299
  defined, 2
  never to late to start, 4
  pumpkin benefits for, 339
Anticonvulsant drugs, <u>186</u>
Anti-inflammatory substances, 90, 347
Antioxidants. *See also* Oxygen radical
    absorbency capacity (ORAC);
    specific kinds
  as Alzheimer's protection, 165–66
  benefits of foods containing, <u>14–15</u>
  example of need for, <u>8</u>
  free radicals fought by, 8–9, <u>8</u>, <u>14</u>
  as inflammation protection, 13, 89–90
  Shopping with them in mind, 110
  for skin health, 225, 228–29
  Sources of
    alternative sweeteners, <u>28–29</u>
    bay leaves, 303
    beans and legumes, <u>80</u>
    beets, 299
    berries, <u>44</u>
    black tea, <u>15</u>
    blueberries, <u>44</u>, 288
    broccoli, 317
    chili powder, 285
    citrus fruits, <u>44</u>
    cocoa, <u>104</u>
    extra-virgin olive oil, <u>150</u>, 295
    fruits (table), <u>44–45</u>
    grapes, purple, <u>44</u>
    honey, <u>15</u>, <u>29</u>
    mint family, 271
    mustard, 281
    nuts, <u>111</u>
    oils, <u>150</u>
    oregano, <u>274</u>, 302
    overview, 9
    plums, <u>44</u>
    pomegranate, <u>15</u>, 343
    pumpkin, 339
    red beans, 301
    red wine, <u>15</u>, 112, 309
    sorghum flour, 307
    spinach, <u>14</u>
    strawberries, <u>14</u>
    supplements vs. food, 9
    top foods (table), <u>19</u>
    turmeric, <u>274</u>, 328
    vegetables, <u>14</u>
  for stroke prevention, 163

Apoptosis, 57
Arthur's Tomato Salad, 311
Asian-style Fish, 319
Asparagus Spears with Smoked
    Salmon and Tangy Mustard
    Dressing, 293
Atherosclerosis. *See also* Heart disease
  beginnings of, 40
  cholesterol's role in, 41–42
  described, 40
  diabetes' role in, 42–43, 128–29
  high blood pressure's role in, 42
  metabolic syndrome's role in, 42–43
  Smoking's role in, 43
Autoimmune diseases, 84, 85, 87–90.
    See also specific diseases
Avocados, 316

B

Baby Spinach Salad, 314
Bacon, turkey, 60
Baked Eggs in Savory Turkey Cups, 266
Barbecue Sauce, 285
Barley, 305
Barley Risotto with Wilted Greens, 305
Bay leaves, 303
B cell count, 87
Beans
  antiaging benefits of, <u>80</u>
  as antioxidant source, 301
  as fiber source, 170
  garbanzo, 294
  ORAC content of, <u>80</u>
Beets, 299
Bell peppers, 13, 263
Berries, 170. *See also* Blueberries;
    Strawberries
Beta-carotene. *See also* Vitamin A
  sources of, <u>58</u>, 272, <u>312</u>, 334, 339
  from supplements vs. food, 9
Beta-sitosterol, 291
Beverages. *See also* Alcohol; Fluids or
    water; Wine
  caffeine content of (table), <u>103</u>
  Grapefruit Lassi, 278
  Hot Chocolate, 277
  Mango Mint Smoothie, 269
  Nutty Chocolate Shake, 270
  Pinolillo (Spanish Chocolate Shake),
    273
  Sparkling Melon Agua Fresca, 272
  Spicy Chai, 276
  Zinger Green Tea, 271
Bioelectrical impedance analysis (BIA),
    199–200

Biomarkers
    about, 31
    for conditions
        Alzheimer's disease, 166–67
        cancer, 55–56
        constipation, 79
        diabetes and prediabetes, 131–33
        diverticulosis and diverticulitis, 82
        fatigue, 98
        gallstones, 78
        GERD, 74
        gluten intolerance, 77
        hair loss, 232
        heartburn, 74
        heart disease, 43, 46, 47–48, 52,
            53
        IBS, 81
        immune system impairment,
            86–87
        lactose intolerance, 75–76
        menopause, 146
        muscle loss, 198–200
        osteoporosis, 189–90
        periodontal disease, 235
        skin aging, 222–23
        vision problems, 239
    defined, 23, 31
    for longevity, 23, 42
Birth control pills, 42
Black-Eyed peas, 332
Black-Eyed Peas with Garlic, 332
Blackstrap molasses, 29
Black tea. See Tea
Blindness, diabetes and risk of, 129
Blood pressure
    biomarkers for heart disease, 43, 46
    low, defined, 46
    normal levels, 43
    prehypertension levels, 43
    Stroke prevention and, 159
    Systolic, heart disease risk and, 38–39
    Systolic, menopause linked to
        elevation of, 42
Blood pressure, high
    arterial damage from, 40
    biomarkers for heart disease, 43, 46
    DASH diet for, 46
    defined, 43
    with diabetes, defined, 46
    heart failure risk from, 42
    lowering, 46–47, 159
    medical advice for, 51
    risk factors for, 42
    role in atherosclerosis, 42
    as silent killer, 42
    Sodium intake and, 27

Blood sugar. See also Diabetes; Insulin
    at-home monitoring, 132
    chili powder for control of, 285
    dental health and, 237
    diabetic retinopathy and, 240
    fatigue and, 100
    fiber for regulating, 170
    glycation of, 10
    glycemic index, 137, 138–39
    glycemic load, 138–39
    high, problems from, 42, 128–30
    insulin's role for, 128
    meal timing and, 27
    tests for, 114, 131–32
    white carbohydrates' effect on, 25
Blueberries, 44, 288
Bod Pod machine, 200
Body mass index (BMI) chart, 134–35
Body temperature, lowering, 23
Bones. See also Osteoporosis
    about, 185
    avoiding injury, 193–94
    medications robbing calcium from,
        186, 188–89
Breakfast. See also Menu plans
    Baked Eggs in Savory Turkey Cups,
        266
    Bran Yogurt Muffins, 264–65
    Breakfast Polenta with Berries and
        Vanilla, 267
    Cheesy Vegetable Frittata, 262–63
    Creamy Almond Kasha, 261
    Old-Fashioned Breakfast Sausage, 259
    Positively Ageless Flax Cereal, 260
    protein needed for, 259
    stress hormones reduced by, 154
Breakfast Polenta with Berries and
    Vanilla, 267
Breast cancer
    examining your breasts, 62–63, 114
    hormones linked to, 55
    prevalence of, 16
    reducing risk for, 65–67
    risk factors for, 16, 60–62, 145–46
    screening methods for, 62–63
Broccoli, 60, 317
Broccoli Salad with Caramelized Onions
    and Toasted Almonds, 317
Brown rice syrup, 28–29
Buckwheat, 261
Bulgur, 308
B vitamins. See also specific vitamins
    depression from deficiency of, 149
    fatigue reduced by, 100
    homocysteine lowered by, 53, 163
    sources of, 284, 317

C

Caffeine
  about, 103
  avoiding during stress, 154, 170
  content of beverages, 103
  exercise and, 205
  fatigue cycle from, 102
  limiting to prevent osteoporosis, 193
  steeping time for tea and, 276
Calcium
  cancer risk reduced by, 66–67, 71
  sources of, 66–67, 71, 190, 284
  stored in bones, 185
  supplements, 191
Calipers, body fat, 199
Calories
  adding 100 to menu plans, 116, 174,
    208, 246
  in American diet, 21
  base for menu plans, 116, 174, 208,
    246
  benefits of restricting, 9, 22–24, 51
  caloric density in fruits and
    vegetables, 25
  cholesterol reduced by restricting, 51
  counting, 110
  estimating your needs, 30
  free radicals reduced by restricting, 9
  in nutritional analyses, 257
  percent from fat, 21, 50, 57
Cancer. See also specific kinds
  aging and risk of, 16–17, 54, 55,
    60–61, 68, 86
  biomarkers, 55–56
  breast, 16, 55, 60–63, 65–67
  colorectal, 16, 26, 57, 68–71, 114
  common types of, 54
  dietary factors in, 55
  DNA damage and, 54, 55
  endometrial, 55, 63, 65–67
  fatal, 54
  free radicals and risk of, 6
  hormones linked to, 55, 61, 63
  hormone therapy and risk of, 145–46
  lung, 16, 17
  reducing risk for, 56–60, 65–67, 70–71
  resveratrol for slowing growth of, 325
  risk in women, 16–17
  screening methods for, 62–63, 65, 70
  smoking and risk of, 55
  stomach, 59–60
Candied Pecans, 291
Cantaloupe, 272
Carbohydrates, 25, 170, 257
Cardiovascular disease. See Heart
  disease

Carotenoids, 58, 91, 299. See also
  specific kinds
Cataracts, 10, 18, 129, 239
Catechins, 58
Celiac disease from gluten intolerance,
  76–78
Centenarians, 1, 3, 4, 20, 23
CFS (chronic fatigue syndrome), 98
Cheesy Vegetable Frittata, 262–63
Chicken, 49, 259, 327
Chickpeas, 294
Chili powder, 285
Chinese parsley, 319
Chlorophyll, 299
Chocolate Almond Pudding, 338
Chocolate and cocoa, 104, 277, 342
Cholesterol. See also HDL cholesterol;
  LDL cholesterol
  about, 41
  aids in lowering
    calorie restriction, 51
    flavonoids, 325
    ginger, 341
    overview, 48–49, 51–52
    pecans, 291
    phytosterols, 316
    soybeans, for LDL, 331
  as biomarker for heart disease,
    47–48
  categories of levels, 47, 48
  diabetes and elevation of, 130
  dietary, 49, 163, 333
  heart disease risk and, 38–39
  medical advice for, 51
  oxidized by free radicals, 6
  ratio of HDL to total, 48
  reducing intake of, 49
  role in atherosclerosis, 41–42
  in soy milk vs. dairy milk, 333
  stroke prevention and, 159, 162
Chromium, 140, 140
Chronic fatigue syndrome (CFS), 98
Cilantro, 319
Cinnamon, 274
Citrus fruits, 44, 329. See also specific
  kinds
Cobalamin (B₁₂), 53, 163
Cocoa and chocolate, 104, 277, 342
Collagen, 221, 222
Colorectal cancer
  fiber as protection against, 26
  prevalence of, 16
  reducing risk for, 70–71
  risk factors for, 16, 57, 68–70
  screening methods for, 70, 114
Concentration, lack of, 144

Condiments
   Barbecue Sauce, 285
   Curried Tomato Dipping Sauce, 280
   Easy Blueberry Jam, 288
   Mango Butter, 286
   Miso Marinade, 287
   Pomegranate Syrup, 282
   Tahini Yogurt Sauce, 284
   Tangy Mustard Dressing, 281
   Tomato Ginger Vinaigrette, 283
   Watercress Sauce, 289
Constipation, 79–80
Cooked foods, cancer risk and, 60
Cornmeal, 267, 273
Corticosteroids, 186
Cortisol, 152–53, 154
C-reactive protein (CRP), 52, 86, 88
Creamy Almond Kasha, 261
Cumin, 323
Cumin-Spiced Bulgur and Lentils, 308
Cured foods, avoiding, 60
Curried Tomato Dipping Sauce, 280
Cytokines, 85

D

Dairy foods
   as calcium sources, 66–67, 71
   cholesterol in, 49
   low-fat, choosing, 46–47
   milk, 277, 333
   primary guidelines for, 26
   servings per day, 112, 204
   for skin protection, 220
DASH (Dietary Approaches to Stop
   Hypertension), 46
Dementia, causes of, 157
Dental health
   age-related problems, 234–35
   biomarkers for periodontal disease,
   235
   heart disease risk and, 20
   importance of, 19–20
Depression during menopause, 144,
   149, 172
Desserts
   Almond Berry Bars, 346–47
   Chocolate Almond Pudding, 338
   Gingerbread with Dried Cherries and
     Toasted Pecans, 340–41
   Orange and Blueberry Compote in
     Green Tea-Ginger Syrup, 344–45
   Rich Cocoa Sorbet, 342
   Ruby Lemon Sorbet, 343
   Spicy Strawberry Frozen Yogurt, 337
   Sweet Pumpkin Polenta, 339

DEXA (dual energy x-ray
   absorptiometry), 189, 205
DHA omega-3s
   about, 64
   conversion of ALA form to, 260, 283
   food sources of (table), 90
Diabetes. See also Blood sugar; Insulin
   alternatives to artificial sweeteners,
   345
   arterial damage from, 40
   biomarkers, 131–33
   chili powder for blood sugar control,
   285
   forms of, 128
   high blood pressure with, 46
   ORAC content of sweeteners, 345
   overview, 127–30
   prediabetes, 10, 130–33
   preventing and treating, 133–41, 163
   problems from high blood sugar,
   128–30
   risk factors for, 17, 42, 127, 128
   role in atherosclerosis, 42–43
   tests for, 114, 131–33
Diabetic retinopathy, 239, 240
Diet
   American, ills of, 20–22
   DASH, 46
   factors increasing cancer risk, 55
   guidance for health conditions
     Alzheimer's disease, 167–68
     cancer, 57, 59–60, 65–67, 70–71
     cholesterol and triglycerides,
       48–49, 51–52
     constipation, 79–80
     dental health, 235, 236
     diabetes, 133, 137, 140
     diverticulosis and diverticulitis,
       82–83
     fatigue, 99–102
     gallstones, 79
     gluten intolerance, 77–78
     hair loss, 233
     heartburn and GERD, 74–75
     heart disease, 147–48
     high blood pressure, 46–47
     IBS, 81–82
     lactose intolerance, 76
     menopause, 147
     skin, 220, 221, 225, 228–30
     stress, 154–55
     vision problems, 240–41
   history, osteoporosis and, 188
   for immune system strength, 90–96
   Mediterranean, 167–68

of Okinawan centenarians, 20, 23
primary guidelines for, 24–29, 31
Dietary Approaches to Stop
Hypertension (DASH), 46
Digestive system
constipation, 79–80
diverticulosis and diverticulitis,
82–83
gallstones, 78–79
gluten intolerance, 76–78
heartburn and GERD, 73–75
irritable bowel syndrome (IBS),
81–82
lactose intolerance, 75–76
overview, 72–73
protecting with beans and legumes,
80
ulcers, 74
Diverticulosis and diverticulitis, 82–83
DNA damage
cancer risk and, 54, 55
by free radicals, 6, 7, 23
reduced by calorie restriction, 23
Docosahexaenoic acid. See DHA
omega-3s
Dried fruits, 341
Drinking. See Alcohol; Fluids or water
Dual energy x-ray absorptiometry
(DEXA), 189, 205

E

Easy Blueberry Jam, 288
Edamame, 331
EGCG (Epigallocatechin-3-gallate), 58
Eggs, 49, 93, 266
Eicosapentaenoic acid. See EPA
omega-3s
Ellagic acid, 58
Endometrial cancer
hormones linked to, 55
reducing risk for, 65–67
risk factors for, 63, 65
screening methods for, 65
Entrées
Asian-Style Fish, 319
Grilled Salmon with Almond
Pomegranate Sauce, 320–21
Lebanese Kebabs, 322–23
Moroccan Fish Stew, 328
Roast Pork Tenderloin with Citrus,
Green Tea, and Spices, 329
Sesame Turkey Stir-Fry with
Cabbage and Green Beans,
326–27
Southwest Salmon Burgers, 324–25

EPA omega-3s
about, 64
conversion of ALA form to, 260, 283
food sources of (table), 90
inflammation reduced by, 88
Epigallocatechin-3-gallate (EGCG), 58
Estrogen, 8, 61, 63
Ethnicity. See Racial and ethnic
background
Exercise
amenorrhea from, 187–88
blood pressure lowered by, 47
brain, 169, 173
cancer risk reduced by, 57
changing schedule for, 171
cholesterol levels improved by, 52
constipation reduced by, 79
diverticulosis and diverticulitis
reduced by, 83
fatigue reduced by, 102
gallstone risk reduced by, 78–79
immune system strengthened by, 96
increasing, 244–45
journal for, 114
lack, osteoporosis risk and, 188
maintaining and building muscle,
201–3, 206–7
for osteoporosis prevention, 148,
192–93
sports for, 173
starting, 113, 172, 206–7
for stress reduction, 155
warming up before, 206
Eyebrows, 233, 244

F

Family history
Alzheimer's and, 165
cancer and, 61, 69
diabetes and, 127
osteoporosis and, 188
Fat, body. See also Obesity or
overweight; Triglycerides
cortisol and accumulation of, 153
damaged by free radicals, 6, 23
measuring, 199–200
table of ranges, 200
Fat, dietary. See also Omega-3s;
Saturated fat; Triglycerides
AGE content of foods containing, 12
in American diet, 21
animal, avoiding, 57
cancer risk increased by, 63, 69, 71
gallstone formation and, 78, 79
ginger for aid in digesting, 341

Fat, dietary *(cont.)*
    inflammation increased by, 88–89
    low-fat dairy foods, 46–47
    maximum daily amount (table), <u>50</u>
    nonstick pans for avoiding, 107
    in nutritional analyses, 257
    percent of calories from, 21, <u>50</u>, 57
    in pork tenderloin vs. chicken, 259
    primary guidelines for, 26
    reducing intake of, 48–49
    for skin protection, <u>220</u>
    stroke prevention and, 159
    in turkey vs. chicken, 327
    unsaturated, choosing, 49
Fatigue
    biomarkers, 98
    chronic fatigue syndrome (CFS),
       98
    medical advice for, 98
    medical conditions involving, 97
    prevalence of, 97
    preventing, 99–105
Fatty acids. *See* Omega-3s
Fiber
    adding gradually to diet, 27, 110–11
    blood sugar regulated by, 170
    cancer risk reduced by, 66, 70–71
    content of foods (table), <u>32</u>
    diverticulosis and diverticulitis
       reduced by, 82–83
    good and excellent sources of, <u>32</u>
    health benefits of, 51, 66
    IBS reduced by, 81–82
    in nutritional analyses, 257
    primary guidelines for, 26–27
    soluble, 51–52
    sources of, 52, 260, 329, 332, 337, 345
Fish
    avoiding pickled, salted, or cured, 60
    primary guidelines for, 26
    salmon, 293, 325
    for skin protection, <u>220</u>
Flavonoids, <u>59</u>, <u>325</u>, 335, 342
Flaxseed
    as ALA omega-3s source, <u>90</u>, 283
    conversion of ALA omega-3s from,
       260, 283
    as lignans source, <u>59</u>
Fluids or water. *See also* Beverages
    beverage recipes, 268–78
    constipation reduced by, 79, 80
    daily water intake, 27, 111–12
    diverticulosis and diverticulitis
       reduced by, 83
    exercise and, 205

    health benefits of drinking, 27
    IBS reduced by, 82
    immune system strengthened by, 96
    primary guidelines for, 27
    for skin health, 225
    for stress reduction, 154
Folic acid or folate
    cancer risk reduced by, 71
    homocysteine lowered by, 53, 163, 168
    sources of, 71, 332, 334, 345
Food Processor software program, 257
Foot problems, diabetes and, 129–30
Free radicals
    AGEs as cause of, 10
    antioxidants as fighting, 8–9, <u>8</u>, <u>14</u>
    avoidable sources of, 6
    calorie restriction for reducing, 9
    damage reduced by calorie
       restriction, 23
    defined, 5
    DNA damage from, 6, <u>7</u>
    hailstorm metaphor for, 7–8
    produced by immune cells, 12–13
    produced by mitochondria, 6, 7, 8, 23
    protein damaged by, 6
Fruits. *See also specific kinds*
    basket for, 107
    caloric density low in, 25
    in DASH diet, 46
    dried, ORAC content of (table), <u>341</u>
    lacking in American diet, 21
    ORAC content of (table), <u>44–45</u>
    phytochemicals in, 56–57
    primary guidelines for, 25
    for skin protection, <u>220</u>
    vitamin A content (table), <u>91</u>
    vitamin C content (table), <u>92</u>

G

Gallstones, 78–79
Garbanzo beans, 294
Garlic, 60, <u>162</u>
Gastroesophageal reflux disease
    (GERD), 73–75
Gastrointestinal system. *See* Digestive
    system
Genes, 3. *See also* DNA damage;
    Family history
Genistein, <u>59</u>
GERD (gastroesophageal reflux
    disease), 73–75
Gestational diabetes, 128
Ginger, <u>162</u>, 341
Gingerbread with Dried Cherries and
    Toasted Pecans, 340–41

Gingered Edamame with Fire-Roasted Tomatoes, 331
Glucocorticoids, 186
Glucose. See Blood sugar
Gluten intolerance, 76–78
Glycation, 10, 132. See also Advanced glycation end products (AGEs)
Glycemic index (GI) of foods, 137, 138–39
Glycemic load (GL) of foods, 138–39
Grains
    Barley Risotto with Wilted Greens, 305
    Cumin-Spiced Bulgur and Lentils, 308
    ORAC content of (table), 136
    Whole Grain Bread (or Buns), 306–7
    whole, health benefits of, 57, 170
    whole, lacking in American diet, 21
    Wild Rice with Radicchio and Dried Cherries, 309
Grapefruit juice, 278
Grapefruit Lassi, 278
Grapes, purple, 44
Green tea. See Tea
Green Tea Miso Soup, 297
Grilled Salmon with Almond Pomegranate Sauce, 320–21
Gum disease, 234–37

H

Hair changes, 231–33
Harris Benedict Equation, 30
HCAs (heterocyclic amines), 60
HDL cholesterol. See also Cholesterol
    about, 41
    heart disease risk and, 38–39
    increased by calorie restriction, 51
    ratio to total cholesterol, 48
    stroke prevention and, 159, 162
Heart
    about, 37, 40
    age-related problems, 40–41
Heart attacks, 40, 41, 342
Heartburn, 73–75
Heart disease. See also Atherosclerosis
    age-related problems, 40–41
    AGEs linked to, 10
    aging and risk of, 16, 38–39
    Alzheimer's and risk factors for, 166, 168
    biomarkers, 43, 46, 47–48, 52, 53
    diabetes and risk of, 137
    gender and risk of, 16
    gum disease and risk of, 20
    menopause and risk of, 145, 147

prevalence of, 16
reducing risk for, 147–48, 168
10-year risk estimate for, 38–39
Heart failure, 41, 42
Hemorrhagic stroke, 158–59. See also Stroke
Heparin, 186
Herbs, 274–75. See also specific herbs
Heterocyclic amines (HCAs), 60
High blood pressure. See Blood pressure, high
High-density lipoprotein. See HDL cholesterol
Homocysteine, 53, 163, 168
Honey, 15, 29
Hormones
    estrogen, 8, 61, 63
    linked to cancer, 55, 61, 63
    menopause and changes in, 142, 143, 145–46
    muscle strength and changes in, 198
    tests monitoring, 146
Hormone therapy, 145–46
Hot Chocolate, 277
Hot flashes, 144, 145–46, 149, 172
H. pylori bacteria, 74
Hydration. See Fluids or water
Hydrogenation, 49
Hydrostatic weighing, 199
Hypertension. See Blood pressure, high
Hyperthyroidism, 98
Hypotension (low blood pressure), 46
Hypothyroidism, 98

I

IBS (Irritable bowel syndrome), 81–82
Immune system
    age-related disorders and, 84, 85–86
    autoimmune diseases, 84, 85, 87–90
    biomarkers of impairment, 86–87
    free radicals produced by, 12–13
    important cells in, 85
    inflammation and, 84, 85–86, 87–90
    overview, 84–86
    strengthening, 90–96
Indian Olives with Citrus and Panch Puran, 292
Indoles, 59
Infections, 40, 130
Inflammation
    AGEs as cause of, 10
    Alzheimer's risk and, 166
    antioxidants for reducing, 13, 89–90
    chronic, 85–86

Inflammation *(cont.)*
C-reactive protein with, 52
damage caused by, 12–13
defined, 12
foods protecting you from, 13, 90
minimizing, 87–90
omega-3s for reducing, 13, 87–88
role in age-related conditions, 86
Insulin. *See also* Blood sugar; Diabetes
about, 42, 128
calorie restriction and, 23
chromium and metabolism of, 140
cinnamon and increased sensitivity,
274
high, problems from, 130
meal timing and, 27
white carbohydrates' effect on, 25
Insulin resistance, 42, 43, 153
Iron
fatigue reduced by, 101
sources of, 101–2, 284, 317, 327
Irritable bowel syndrome (IBS), 81–82
Ischemic stroke, 158. *See also* Stroke
Isoflavones, 59
Isothiocyanates, 59
Italian Vegetable Soup, 302

J

Joint aches during menopause, 144
Journaling, 113–14

K

Kidneys, diabetic damage to, 129
Kitchen
taking out the garbage, 107
tools for, 113

L

Labels, reading, 29
Lactase enzymes, 76
Lactobacillus acidophilus, 265. *See also*
Probiotics
Lactose intolerance, 75–76
Laughter, 155
LDL cholesterol. *See also* Cholesterol
about, 41
arterial damage from, 40
categories of levels, 48
reduced by calorie restriction, 51
soybeans for lowering, 331
stroke prevention and, 159, 162
Lebanese Kababs, 322–23
Legumes. *See* Vegetables and
legumes; *specific kinds*
Libido, loss with menopause, 144–45

Life expectancy. *See also* Longevity
greater for women, 3
reduced by heart disease, 16
Lignans, 59
Lima Beans with Parsley and Red
Cabbage, 335
Limonen, 59
Lipids. *See* Fat, body
Lipoproteins, 41–42. *See also* HDL
cholesterol; LDL cholesterol;
Triglycerides
Lips, 224, 243
Longevity
biomarkers, 23, 42
calorie restriction and increase in,
22–23
centenarians, 1, 3, 4, 20, 23
gender and chances for, 3
goal for, 2
growing numbers of centenarians, 1
heart disease as obstacle to, 16
life expectancy, 3, 16
as measure of health, 2
role of genes in, 3
Low-density lipoprotein. *See* LDL
cholesterol
Lung cancer, 16, 17
Lutein, 242, 312
Lycopene, 56, 311, 312
Lymphocytes, 85

M

Macular degeneration
age-related (AMD), 18, 238–39, 240
lutein for reducing risk of, 312
Magnesium, 261
Magnetic resonance imaging (MRI),
63
"Make One Change" strategies
about, 31
for bones and muscles, 204–5
for hormones and mind, 170–71
for outside parts, 241–43
for vital functions, 106–7, 110
Mammograms, 63, 114–15
Manganese, 294
Mango, 269, 286
Mango Butter, 286
Mango Mint Smoothie, 269
Mask recipes for skin, 228–29
Massage, 172
Meal timing, 27
Meats. *See also specific kinds*
AGE content of foods containing, 12
avoiding pickled, salted, or cured, 60

cancer risk and, 60, 62, 71
cholesterol in, 49
overcooking, avoiding, 60, 62
Medical advice, seeking for
   cholesterol, 51
   dental health, 235–36, 241–42
   diabetes testing, 131, 172
   fatigue, 98
   hair loss, 232, 245
   heartburn and GERD, 77
   high blood pressure, 51
   hormone therapy, 145–46
   menopause, 172–73
   skin health, 241
   vision problems, 239–40, 243–44
   Positively Ageless plans, 114, 204
Medical checkup, scheduling, 110, 114
Medications
   dental health and, 237
   osteoporosis dangers from, 186,
      188–89
Mediterranean diet, 167–68
Memory loss during menopause,
   144
Menopause
   biomarkers, 146
   defined, 143
   hair loss after, 232
   heart disease risk increase after, 16
   high blood pressure linked to, 42
   hormone therapy for, 145–46
   joys of, 142–43
   managing symptoms, 146–50
   menstrual diary for, 170–71
   not a disease, 142
   osteoporosis risk and, 145–46, 148,
      187
   perimenopause, 143, 146
   skin changes from, 222
   symptoms of, 142, 143–46
Menu plans
   adding 100 calories to, 116, 174, 208,
      246
   recipes in, 116, 174, 208, 246
   scheduling meals and snacks, 113
   scheduling snacks in, 116, 174, 208,
      246
   week 1, 116–23
   week 2, 174–81
   week 3, 208–15
   week 4, 246–53
Metabolic syndrome, 42–43
Metabolism
   of insulin, 140
   lowered by calorie restriction, 23–24

Methylhydroxy chalcone polymer
   (MHCP), 274
Mexican parsley, 319
Microdermabrasion, 223
Migraines during menopause, 144
Milk, 277, 333. *See also* Dairy foods
Mint, 271
Mirin (Japanese cooking wine), 287
Miso, 287, 297
Miso Marinade, 287
Mitochondria, 6, 7, 8, 23
Moroccan Fish Stew, 328
Motion sickness, easing, 341
MRI (magnetic resonance imaging),
   63
Muscles
   aging and loss of mass, 18, 195
   biomarkers for loss, 198–200
   importance of maintaining, 195–96
   maintaining, 201–3
   reasons for loss of strength, 197–98
Muskmelon, 272
Mustard, 281

N

Natural killer cells, 85
Nitrates and nitrites, 60
Nuts, 110, 111. *See also specific nuts*
Nutty Chocolate Shake, 270

O

Oatmeal, 347
Obesity or overweight. *See also*
      Weight loss
   cancer risk increased by, 61–62
   CRP increased by, 88
   health risks from
      BMI chart to assess, 134–35
      cancer, 57, 69
      GERD, 73
      high blood pressure, 47
      high cholesterol levels, 51
      inflammation, 88
      overview, 24
      type 2 diabetes, 42
   menopause and weight gain, 144
Okinawan diet, 20, 23
Old-Fashioned Breakfast Sausage, 259
Olive oil, 26, 150, 295
Olives, 292
Omega-3s. *See also specific kinds*
   about, 64
   conversion of, 64, 260, 283
   depression from deficiency of, 149
   fish rich in, 26

Omega-3s *(cont.)*
  for hair and skin health, 242
  health benefits of, 64
  as inflammation protection, 13, 87–88
  kinds of, 64
  in nutritional analyses, 257
  omega-6s vs., 64, 65
  organic milk as higher in, 277
  ratio of omega-6s to, 87
  recommended daily intake, 88
  sources of, 64, 90, 94, 112, 293, 325
  for stroke prevention, 159, 162
Omega-6s
  inflammation increased by, 88
  omega-3s vs., 64
  ratio of omega-3s to, 87
  reducing intake of, 65
Onion, 162
ORAC. *See* Oxygen radical absorbency
  capacity
Orange and Blueberry Compote in
  Green Tea-Ginger Syrup,
  344–45
Oranges, 278, 314, 345
Oregano, 274, 302
Organic foods, 110, 277
Osteoarthritis, 10
Osteoporosis
  avoiding injury, 193–94
  biomarkers, 189–90
  boron for preventing, 44
  consequences of, 186–87
  medications to beware of, 186, 188–89
  prevalence of, 185
  preventing after menopause,
    145–46, 148
  protection against, 190–94
  risk factors for, 17-18, 145–46, 148,
    187–89
  risk in women, 17-18
Overweight. *See* Obesity or
  overweight
Oxidation or oxidative stress, 6,
  165-66. *See also* Free radicals
Oxygen radical absorbency capacity
  (ORAC)
  amount needed daily, 14
  average daily consumption of, 14
  content of foods
    beans and legumes (table), 80
    cocoa and chocolate (table), 104
    dried fruits (table), 341
    fruits (table), 44–45
    herbs and spices (table), 274–75
    nuts (table), 111
    oils (table), 150
    sweeteners (table), 345
    tea (table), 69
    top foods in 15 categories (table),
      19
    vegetables (table), 312–13
    whole grains (table), 136
    wine (table), 325
  described, 14, 255

P

PAHs (polycyclic aromatic
  hydrocarbons), 60
Palpitations during menopause, 145
Panch puran, 292
Pans, nonstick, 107
Pap test, 115
Parkinson's disease, 13
Pecans, 291
Pelvic exam, 115
Peptic ulcers, 74
Perimenopause, 143, 146
Periodontal disease, 234–37
Periods, changes in, 143–44, 187–88.
  See also Menopause
Peristalsis, 72
Pets, stress reduced by, 155–56
Phagocytes, 85
Photoaging, 221–22
Phytochemicals, 56–57, 58–59, 323
Phytoestrogens, 66
Phytosterols, 316
Pickled foods, avoiding, 60
Pinolillo (Spanish Chocolate Shake),
  273
Plaques in neurons, 165
Plums, 44
Pollution, free radicals and, 6
Polycyclic aromatic hydrocarbons
  (PAHs), 60
Polyphenols, 90, 325
Pomegranate, 15, 282, 321, 343
Pomegranate Syrup, 282
Pork tenderloin, 259
Portions, measuring, 107
Positive thinking, 155
Positively Ageless Flax Cereal, 260
Post-traumatic stress disorder (PTSD),
  152
Potassium, 46, 317, 332, 345
Prediabetes, 10, 130–33
Probiotics, 95–96, 265, 297
Protein
  in black-eyed peas, 332
  as breakfast necessity, 259

cross-linked due to AGEs, 10
damaged by free radicals, 6, 23
in every meal, 243
figuring daily needs, 99–100
guidelines for, 25–26, 197–98
lack, contributing to fatigue, 99
during menopause, 147
needed for muscle strength, 197–98
in nutritional analyses, 257
RDA for, 197
for skin health, 230
in soybeans, 331
Provitamin A carotenoids, 91
PTSD (post-traumatic stress disorder), 152
Pumpkin, 339
Pyridoxine. See Vitamin B$_6$

Q

Quercetin, 59
"Quick Start" strategies
about, 32
for bones and muscles, 205–7
for hormones and mind, 171–72
for outside parts, 243–44
for vital functions, 110–12

R

Racial and ethnic background
cancer risk and, 69
diabetes risk and, 127
osteoporosis risk and, 187
Radicchio, 315
Rainbow Radicchio Slaw, 315
Reading labels, 29
Recipes. See also Menu plans; specific categories
beverages, 268–78
breakfast, 258–67
condiments, 279–89
desserts, 336–47
entrées, 318–29
grains, 304–9
listed in menu plans, 116, 174, 208, 246
nutritional analyses explained, 257
salads, 310–17
skin scrubs and masks, 226–29
snacks, 290–95
soups and stews, 296–303
vegetables and legumes, 330–35
Red beans. See Beans
Red Bean Mole Soup, 300–01
Red cabbage, 335
Red wine. See Wine

Reflux
defined, 73
dental health and, 236
GERD, 73–75
Resistance training, 201–3
Resveratrol, 59, 325
Rich Cocoa Sorbet, 342
Roast Pork Tenderloin with Citrus, Green Tea, and Spices, 329
Ruby Lemon Sorbet, 343
Rutin, 261

S

Salads
Arthur's Tomato Salad, 311
Baby Spinach Salad, 314
Broccoli Salad with Caramelized Onions and Toasted Almonds, 317
Rainbow Radicchio Slaw, 315
Sliced Avocados and Oranges with Tahini Yogurt Sauce, 316
Salmon, 293, 325
Salt, limiting intake of, 27
Salvestrols, 59
Savory Beef Stew, 298–99
Saturated fat
AGE content of foods containing, 12
cancer risk increased by, 57, 63
inflammation increased by, 88–89
limiting to prevent stroke, 159
maximum daily amount (table), 50
reducing intake of, 48–49
Scales, body fat, 200
Scalp, aging, 231–32
Scheduling meals and snacks, 113
Screening methods for cancer
breast, 62–63
colorectal, 70, 114
endometrial, 65
Scrub recipes for skin, 226–27
Seasonings, guidelines for, 27
Sedimentation rate (sed rate), 86–87
Selenium, 93, 93, 111, 162
Sesame seeds, 284
Sesame Turkey Stir-Fry with Cabbage and Green Beans, 326–27
Shopping list, 107, 108–9
Skin
AGEs in wrinkling process, 10
Avocado Banana Mask, 229
biomarkers for aging, 222–23
Carrot Coconut Scrub, 226
Cornmeal Yogurt Scrub, 227
damage increase with aging, 18

Skin (cont.)
  diet for healthy, <u>220</u>, 221, 225, 228–30
  factors in aging, 221–22
  free radicals and signs of aging in, 6
  guide to healthy, 223–25, 228–30
  lips, <u>224</u>, 243
  masks for, <u>228–29</u>
  menopause and changes in, 144
  microdermabrasion, <u>223</u>
  Oatmeal Exfoliating Scrub, <u>227</u>
  Omega-3 Egg Mask, <u>229</u>
  as an organ, 219–20
  scrubs for, <u>226–27</u>, 242
  Sesame Mint Scrub, <u>226–27</u>
Sleep
  antiaging benefits of, 243
  diabetes risk and, 141
  improving, 103–5, 171, 173
Sleep apnea, 105
Sliced Avocados and Oranges with
    Tahini Yogurt Sauce, 316
Smoking
  AGEs introduced by, 12
  free radicals introduced by, 6
  health risks from
    atherosclerosis, 40, 43
    cancer, 17, 55
    diabetes, 141
    GERD, 75
    gum disease, 236
    heart disease, <u>38–39</u>, 52
    high blood pressure, 47
    immune system problems, 96
    osteoporosis, 188, 193
    skin damage, 106, 222, 230
  quitting, 106–7
Snacks. See also Menu plans
  Asparagus Spears with Smoked
      Salmon and Tangy Mustard
      Sauce, 293
  Candied Pecans, 291
  dental health and, 236
  Indian Olives with Citrus and Panch
      Puran, 292
  in menu plans, scheduling, 116, 174,
      208, 246
  nuts for, 110
  for stress reduction, 154–55
  Whole Wheat Pita Chips, 295
  Zippy Hummus, 294
Sodium, 27, 46, 257
Sorghum flour, 307
Sorghum syrup, <u>29</u>
Soups and stews
  Green Tea Miso Soup, 297
  Italian Vegetable Soup, 302

Red Bean Mole Soup, 300–301
Savory Beet Stew, 298–99
Spanish Meatball Soup, 303
Southwest Salmon Burgers, 324–25
Soy foods
  cancer risk reduced by, 65–66
  edamame, 331
  LDL cholesterol lowered by, 331
  menopause symptoms reduced by,
      148–49
  milk, dairy milk vs., 333
  for osteoporosis prevention, 193
Spaghetti squash, 334
Spaghetti (Squash) with Basil-Cress
    Pesto, 334
Spanish Meatball Soup, 303
Sparkling Melon Agua Fresca, 272
Spices, <u>274–75</u>. See also specific spices
Spicy Chai, 276
Spicy Strawberry Frozen Yogurt, 337
Spinach, <u>14</u>
STDs, tests for, 115
Stews. See Soups and stews
Stomach cancer, 59–60
Strawberries, <u>14</u>, 337
Strength training, 201–3
Stress
  fight-or-flight syndrome, 151
  health risks from, 152–53
  IBS symptoms increased by, 82
  reducing, 154–56
Stroke
  aging and risk of, 17
  cocoa for reducing risk of, 342
  estimating risk of, <u>160–61</u>
  gender and risk of, 17
  hemorrhagic, 158–59
  ischemic, 158
  possible outcomes of, 157
  preventing, 159, 162–63
  signs of, <u>158</u>
Sugar, 147, 229, 257. See also
    Sweeteners
Sulfur compounds, 281
Sunglasses, 240, 244
Sun hats, 245
Sunlight
  protecting skin from, 223–25
  skin damage from, 221–22
Sunscreen, 224, 242
Superoxide dismutase, 294
Supplements
  antioxidants from food vs., 9
  calcium, <u>191</u>
  lactase enzymes, 76
  during menopause, 171

Sweeteners
  alternative, 28–29, 345
  artificial, avoiding, 28
  ORAC content of, 345
  primary guidelines for, 27–29
Sweet Potatoes with Onion Confit, 333
Sweet Pumpkin Polenta, 339

T

Tangles in neurons, 165
Tangy Mustard Dressing, 281
Tahini Yogurt Sauce, 284
T cell count, 87
Tea
  as antioxidant source, 15, 68–69
  blood pressure lowered by green, 47
  caffeine in, 103
  cancer risk reduced by green, 67
  experimenting with, 110
  green vs. black, 68–69
  health benefits of, 68–69
  nitrosamine formation reduced by, 60
  ORAC content of (table), 69
  steeping time and caffeine content, 276
Tests. See also Biomarkers
  breast exam, 62–63, 114
  cancer screening methods, 62–63, 65, 70
  diabetes, 114, 131–33
  hs-CRP, 52
  immune system impairment, 86–87
  mammograms, 63, 114–15
  monitoring hormones, 146, 171
  omega-3 deficiency, 89
  osteoporosis, 189–90
  pap test and pelvic exam, 115
  for STDs, 115
  thyroid, 115
Thyroid, 98, 115
Thyroxine, 186
Tissue sampling, breast, 63
Tofu, 270
Tomatoes, 56, 280, 311, 312
Tomato Ginger Vinaigrette, 283
Trans fat, 49
Triglycerides. See also Fat, body; Fat, dietary
  about, 41–42
  as biomarkers for heart disease, 47–48
  categories of levels, 48
  diabetes and elevation of, 130
  lowering, 48–49, 51–52
Turkey, 327

Turkey bacon, 60
Turmeric, 274, 328
Type 1 and 2 diabetes. See Diabetes

U

Ulcers, 74
Ultrasound
  bone densitometer, 189, 205
  cancer screening, 63
Ultraviolet light, breast cancer risk reduced by, 67
Unsaturated fats, choosing, 49
Urushiol toxin on mango skin, 286

V

Vegetables and legumes. See also specific kinds
  as antioxidant sources, 14
  Black-Eyed Peas with Garlic, 332
  caloric density low in, 25
  in DASH diet, 46
  Gingered Edamame with Fire-Roasted Tomatoes, 331
  lacking in American diet, 21
  Lima Beans with Parsley and Red Cabbage, 335
  ORAC content of beans and legumes, 80
  ORAC content of vegetables, 312–13
  phytochemicals in, 56–57
  primary guidelines for, 24–25
  for skin protection, 220
  Spaghetti (Squash) with Basil-Cress Pesto, 334
  Sweet Potatoes with Onion Confit, 333
  vitamin A content (table), 91
  vitamin C content (table), 92
Vision problems
  age-related macular degeneration (AMD), 18, 238–39, 240
  biomarkers, 239
  cataracts, 10, 18, 129, 239
  diabetic retinopathy, 239, 240
  preventing, 239–41
  risk factors for, 18, 129, 238–39, 240
Vitamin A. See also Beta-carotene
  immune system strengthened by, 90–91
  preformed, 91
  provitamin A carotenoids, 91
  for skin health, 230
  sources of, 13, 91, 263, 317
Vitamin B₆
  homocysteine lowered by, 53, 163
  immune system strengthened by, 95

Vitamin B₆ *(cont.)*
    RDAs, 95
    for skin health, 230
    sources of, 95, 263
Vitamin B₉. *See* Folic acid or folate
Vitamin B₁₂, 53, 163
Vitamin C
    eliminated during pasteurization, 282
    health benefits of, 312
    immune system strengthened by, 91–92
    for skin health, 225, 228–29
    sources of, 92, 263, 311, 314, 317, 337, 345
Vitamin D, 71, 148, 190–92
Vitamin E
    immune system strengthened by, 91
    sources of, 13, 93, 111, 284, 338

W

Water. *See* Fluids or water
Watercress, 288
Watercress Sauce, 289
Weight loss
    cancer risk reduced by, 57
    diabetes risk reduced by, 133
    high blood pressure lowered by, 47
    rules for, 133
White blood cell count, 87
Whole Grain Bread (or Buns), 306–07
Whole Wheat Pita Chips, 295

Wild Rice with Radicchio and Dried Cherries, 309
Wine. *See also* Alcohol
    as antioxidant source, 15, 112, 309
    drinking in moderation, 31, 112
    ORAC content of, 325
    polyphenols in, 325
    white vs. red, 112, 309, 325
Women
    cancer risk for, 16–17
    free radical protections in, 8
    heart disease risk for, 16
    high blood pressure risk factors for, 42
    life expectancy greater for, 3
    osteoporosis risk for, 17–18
    stroke risk for, 17
Wrinkles, 106, 222. *See also* Skin

Y

Yogurt, 220, 265
"Young for Life" strategies
    about, 32
    for bones and muscles, 207
    for hormones and mind, 172–73
    for outside parts, 244–45
    for vital functions, 113–15

Z

Zinc, 94, 94, 284
Zinger Green Tea, 271
Zippy Hummus, 294